THE SULTAN'S SEX POTIONS

ALSO BY DANIEL L. NEWMAN

The Exile's Cookbook: Medieval Gastronomic Treasures from al-Andalus and North Africa

The Sultan's Feast: A Fifteenth-Century Egyptian Cookbook

An Imam in Paris: Account of a Stay in France by an Egyptian Cleric (1826–1831)

Co-authored with R. Husni

A to Z of Arabic-English-Arabic Translation

Arabic-English-Arabic Translation: Issues and Strategies

Modern Arabic Short Stories: A Bilingual Reader

Muslim Women in Law and Society

The Sultan's Sex Potions

Arab Aphrodisiacs in the Middle Ages

Naṣīr al-Dīn al-Ṭūsī

A Critical Edition, Translated and Introduced by

Daniel L. Newman

SAQI

Saqi Books
Gable House, 18–24 Turnham Green Terrace, London W4 1QP
www.saqibooks.com

First published in hardback in 2014 by Saqi Books
This edition published 2025

ISBN 978-1-84925-075-7
eISBN 978-1-84925-076-4

A full CIP record for this book is available from the British Library.

The EU GPSR authorised representative is Logos Europe,
9 rue Nicolas Poussin, 17000 La Rochelle, France.
Email: contact@logoseurope.eu

Printed and bound by Clays Ltd, Elcograf S.p.A

Contents

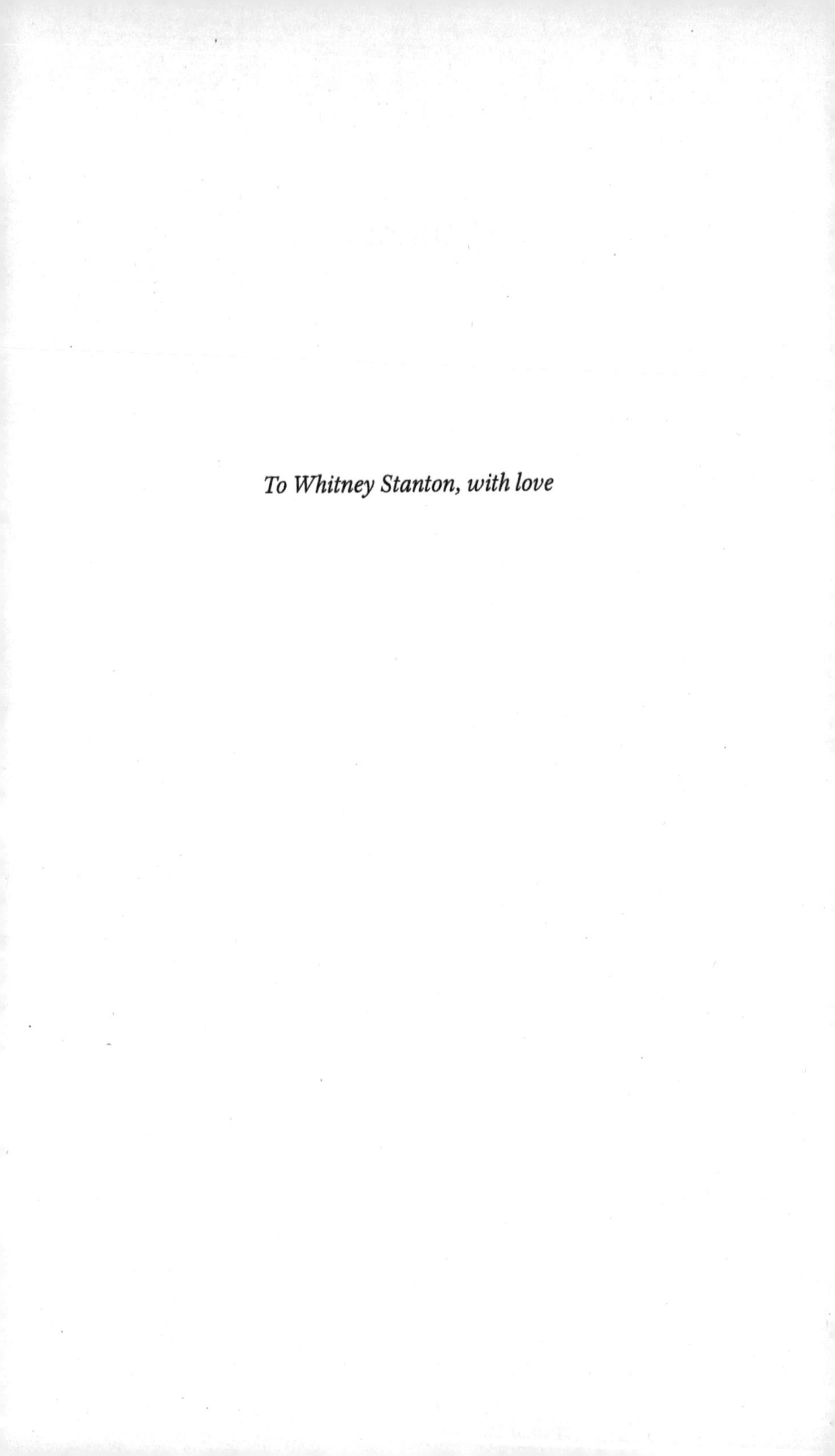

To Whitney Stanton, with love

Preface

When the Emirati-born family guidance counsellor Widād Lūtā published her book, *Sirrī li 'l-ghāya, muʿāshara al-zawjiyya: uṣūl wa ādāb* (usually translated as 'Top Secret: Sexual Guidance for Married Couples'), in 2009, it caused quite a furore in the traditional Gulf state. In the same period, there was a similar vehement reaction to the publication of other works deemed contrary to present-day mores, whether it be those offering an unorthodox interpretation of sexuality within Islam, such as *Ḥayra Muslima* ('A Muslim Woman's Confusion', 2009) by the Tunisian feminist Ulfa Yūsuf, or Muṣṭafā Fatḥī's novel *Balad al-Wilād* ('The Boys' Country', 2009), which chronicles homosexuality in contemporary Egyptian society.

In today's globally wired age, it is, of course, not just the printed word that must be considered, with satellite television and the Internet being much more pervasive, prominent and powerful media. In addition to the proliferation of private (usually foreign) sex channels, the past decades have also seen the appearance of programmes dealing with sexual health and relationships on mainstream Arab media, as well as on web forums and, of course, blogs. The response by Arab society in general to all of these has been one of severe censure, often including accusations of unreligiousness and transgression against local culture.

While, to the casual observer, this response may not be surprising within a modern context, it is less so when seen in its broader historical context. Arabic literature has a long and extremely rich tradition in sexology, with the first examples emerging as early as the ninth century. On the whole, contemporary Arabic-speaking readers are as unfamiliar with this aspect of their heritage as Western audiences are.

This book presents a critical edition, translation and study of one such text from the past – the thirteenth century, to be precise – which deals with a core subject within the genre, aphrodisiacs, and provides a unique insight into the role of sexuality in the Islamic world in the Middle Ages. Its author, a famous Persian scholar, wrote not in his native Persian, but in the scholarly lingua franca of his age, Arabic.

The Introduction will provide a brief overview of Arabic erotological literature and attempt to highlight some of its salient topics and authors, as well as the context of its creation.

It is something of a contradiction that a preface usually represents not the start of the book, but rather its end, as it is usually written when the creative work has been completed. As a revised second edition, this work has, in some ways, been completed not once but twice. Here, I use the opportunity to share three compelling reasons behind the decision to publish a second revised edition of *The Sultan's Sex Potions*: as a result of advances in the scholarship related to the field, there is a need to address certain shortcomings identified in the first edition. More importantly, this edition benefits from the addition of two manuscripts.

By far the most exciting development occurred when some years after the publication of the first edition I was at Oxford University's Bodleian and consulted an anonymous manuscript on sexual hygiene which was also said to contain recipes. There was no title and the copy clearly started in what was the middle of a text. However, almost immediately after I started reading the text, I realised that I was holding a previously unknown copy of al-Ṭūsī's book. The discovery of this new text, in combination with the British Library copy to which I had not had access when I first edited the text, revealed fresh perspectives and interesting insights. Together, these manuscripts not only enhance the primary material available for study but also provide a more comprehensive framework for understanding the subject matter. Incorporating their contents into the revised edition significantly strengthens the book's relevance.

Since the publication of the first edition, the academic landscape surrounding the book's subject matter has also evolved and new theories, methodologies, and interdisciplinary approaches have emerged, offering more nuanced interpretations and analyses. New publications and research have provided a more detailed understanding of some of the topics discussed and these have been included into the revised edition, enriching the book's arguments and providing readers with a more holistic view of the topic.

Another area of refinement involved the updating of bibliographic references and source material. Since the first edition's release, several key texts have become available, and the revised edition has incorporated these. Most notably, the list of known erotological works has been substantially expanded. All of these additions provide readers access to the most accurate and up-to-date resources when engaging with the book's arguments.

No scholarly work is immune to the possibility of errors, oversights, or areas in need of further clarification, and this book is no exception. Feedback from readers, reviewers, and scholars has identified areas where corrections are necessary, and the revised edition offers an opportunity to address these constructively.

This significantly augmented and revised new edition offers a richer, more accurate, and more comprehensive exploration of its subject and, hopefully, ensures its relevance for readers with an interest in this passionate subject.

This preface is also an opportunity to acknowledge assistance that has been provided by others that has facilitated the task – which always proves to be more arduous than was initially imagined, or indeed bargained for.

First and foremost, I should like to thank Ms Whitney Stanton for the unstinting support – both editorial and otherwise – that she has given me in the course of the making of the book.

Secondly, a particular word of thanks is due to the staff of the libraries in Paris (Bibliothèque nationale), Tunis (Dār al-Kutub al-Waṭaniyya), Berlin (Staatsbibliothek), Glasgow (University of Glasgow), Oxford (Bodleian Library), Cairo (Dār al-Kutub wa 'l-Wathā'iq al-Qawmiyya) and Alexandria (Bibliotheca Alexandrina). In Alexandria, my gratitude goes especially to Dr Ahmed Mansour, who generously provided me with some key resources.

The book constitutes part of a project that will result in the translation of a number of other medieval Arabic erotic works, and so the manuscripts that have been my companions for such a long time will remain so for the foreseeable future.

Note on Transliteration

The style of transcription of Arabic words in this book is that of the *Encyclopaedia of Islam* (2nd edn), with the following deviations: kh = kh; dj = j; sh = sh; ḳ = q. The kh, dj, sh transcription does not reflect the regressive assimilation (*idghām*) of the lateral in the definite article '*al*' with the so-called 'sun letters' (t, th, d, r, z, s, sh, ṭ, ẓ, ṣ, ḍ, n): for example *al-Shām* (and not *ash-Shām*). In line with common usage, *hamza* is not transcribed in word-initial positions, whereas the so-called 'nunation' (*tanwīn*) – regular indefinite inflectional noun endings – is dropped throughout (except in some cases for the accusative singular *-an*), as are the anaptyctic vowels of catenated speech. Place names appear in their common historical English forms – e.g. Cairo (instead of al-Qāhira) – or in transliteration, usually followed by an English equivalent in brackets, when it involves little-known towns or areas for which no established English form is available, such as 'Alamūt'. Arabic technical terms are transliterated and italicized, except for words that have gained currency in English, such as 'Islam', 'Muslim', 'hadith' or 'imam'. The plurals of isolated Arabic words appear in the singular with the English regular plural *-s* marker, as in, for instance, *dirhams* (instead of *darāhim)*.

As regards dates, only the Gregorian ones are given, with the dates of the Muslim (lunar) Hijra calendar (which starts in 622 CE, the year in which the Prophet Muhammad emigrated from Mekka to Medina) added in the event of overlaps or ambiguity, in which case the Hijra calendar year comes first, e.g. 1236/1820–21.

Symbols and Abbreviations

[A]	Berlin manuscript
[B]	Glasgow manuscript
BN	Bibliothèque nationale de France (Paris)
[C]	Cairo manuscript
[D]	British Library manuscript
[E]	Bodleian (Oxford) manuscript
CA	Classical Arabic
EI^2	*Encyclopaedia of Islam*
fol.	folio
GAL	C. Brockelmann 1937–46
GALS	C. Brockelmann 1937–46, Supplement
GAS	F. Sezgin 1967–84
Gr.	Greek
pl.	plural
sg.	singular

(أ)	Bodleian (Oxford) manuscript
(غ)	Glasgow manuscript
(ب)	British Library manuscript
(ق)	Cairo manuscript
{ }	text in margin of manuscript
+	addition in manuscript
-	omission from manuscript
?	doubtful reading

INTRODUCTION

CHAPTER ONE

Arabic Erotic Literature

In spite of the recently increased attention for gender and sexuality in modern Islamic societies, the history of the discourse of sexuality and eroticism in the Arab-Muslim tradition remains to be written. This is all the more surprising in view of the unparalleled richness of erotological and erotic literature.

Until the 1960s, interest in the subject was driven by the prurient appetites of a segment of the Victorian readership for whom the reputedly sexually permissive East exerted an irresistible attraction. The leading exponent in this movement was, of course, Sir Richard Burton (1821–1890), who was only too willing not only to pander to, but also to invigorate this myth, particularly through his translations. A typical example is *The Perfumed Garden* (1886), a rather free rendition of a fifteenth-century erotic manual written by the Tunisian scholar al-Nafzāwī, entitled *al-Rawḍ al-ʿāṭir fī nuzhat al-khāṭir* ('The Perfumed Garden of Sensual Delight').

Burton's translation is weighed down by Oriental(ist) views – or, rather, prejudices – about Arab-Muslim sexuality, couched in a pseudo-scholarly purple prose, complete with mock critical apparatus offering the author's salacious comments on the arcana and idiosyncrasies of 'Muhammedan' sexual practices (particularly homosexuality), often invoking divine endorsement by proxy.

This resulted in a translation that inflates the thin source text to several hundred pages. For instance, Chapter 5 ('On Intercourse') is one of the shortest – a mere seven lines in the Arabic printed edition – but takes up to three pages in Burton's text. The following is a brief example of the translation strategy. The chapter ends as follows in Arabic:

> *fa idhā qaḍayta ḥājataka fa-lā taqūmu ʿanhā qiyāman tatarāmā fīhi al-ʿajala wa la-yakun dhālika ʿalā yamīnika yarfaq*[1]

This is rendered by the most recent translator as: 'when you have satisfied your desire, do not be in a hurry to rise from her but do so gently, on your right hand side.'[2]

Burton's rendition is, to put it mildly, somewhat 'expansive':

> And after the enjoyment is over, and your

> amorous struggle has come to an end, be careful not to get up at once, but withdraw your member cautiously. Remain close to the woman, and lie down on the right side of the bed that witnessed your enjoyment. You will find this pleasant, and you will not be like a fellow who mounts the woman after the fashion of a mule, without any regard to refinement, and who, after the emission, hastens to get his member out and to rise. Avoid such manners, for they rob the woman of all her lasting delight. In short, the true lover of coition will not fail to observe all that I have recommended; for, from the observance of my recommendations will result the pleasure of the woman, and these rules comprise everything essential in that respect.
>
> God has made everything for the best![3]

Burton's translation was based on the earliest French published version (1886), authored by the mysterious 'Baron R***', rather than on the Arabic text.[4] It was, however, entirely in keeping with Burton's own *modus operandi* in his rendition (1885–88) of *The Thousand and One Nights* (revealingly titled *The Arabian Nights' Entertainments*) – this time from the Arabic original – in which the translator is highly 'visible', to use a popular term in contemporary Translation Studies,[5] on almost every page, whether through textual embellishment or notes replete with foreign phrases, especially for the more 'delicate' passages. Though clearly aimed at conveying the scholarly credentials of the author, the commentary only increased the already considerable exoticness – or 'foreignization', if you will – of the convoluted Victorian prose, which often collapses under the weight of its own pretentiousness. Secondly, and more importantly, it also conveyed much of Burton's views on sexuality, in general, and that of the 'Orientals', in particular.

The kaleidoscope of Orientalist tropes on display would have a lasting effect on perceptions of the East, and Bernard Lewis rightly pointed out that 'the cause of cultural communication has suffered ... damage from a sort of Anglo-Arabese favored by many, particularly Victorian, translators — a pseudo-biblical, neogothic, mock-Elizabethan, bogus Oriental style which finds its ultimate form in Burton's translation of the *Thousand and One Nights*.'[6]

One might say that the *text* clearly chose its mediator, who became an *actor*, rather than a 'trans-actor', as the translation became a rewriting of 'the Other' within a preconceived framework, which is dealt with in great detail in the 'Terminal Essay'[7] to his translation of the *Arabian Nights*. The fourth part of the essay deals with the 'Social Condition' and it is here that Burton expounds on the '*turpiloquium*' in Eastern societies. It includes sections on 'Woman', 'Pornography' and, most controversially, 'Pederasty', which he proceeds 'to discuss (...) sérieusement, honnêtement, historiquement; to show it in decent nudity not in suggestive fig-leaf or feuille de vigne'![8]

One of the more famous sections is that on the so-called 'Sotadic Zone', which in the Burtonian *Weltanschauung* encompasses areas whose populations are inclined towards pederasty. It includes parts of Europe (Southern France, Spain, Italy and Greece), Northern Africa and most of Asia, but its epicentre is 'Asia Minor and Mesopotamia now occupied by the "unspeakable Turk," a race of born pederasts.'[9]

In the world of Victorian pornography, Burton's *Perfumed Garden* was an instant hit, and inspired others to produce their own 'translations' of Eastern sexual culture. In the first half of the twentieth century the 'genre' subsided, but it is clear from A. Edwardes's *Jewel in the Lotus* (1963) that the Burtonian view and attitude towards Oriental(ist) sexuality perdured for much longer.

Arabic erotic literature is a wide-ranging subject, cutting across many centuries and genres. Whilst the output is primarily associated with *belles-lettres* (*adab*), particularly the *mujūn* (dissolute) poetry by the likes of Abū Nuwās (756–814) and Bashshār Ibn Burd (714–784), the present discussion will centre on works that fall under the heading of erotological literature written in Arabic, irrespective of author origins.

A comprehensive study of medieval Arabic medieval erotological and sexual literature has yet to be written, not least because of the large number of primary sources that are still in manuscript form, whereas others have scarcely been studied. That is not to say that the field is still a blank canvas, as a number of scholars have produced ground-breaking work dealing with Islamicate[10] sexuality in history.[11] Recent decades have also seen a growing interest in specific themes, such as homosexuality, both in history[12] and the present,[13] transvestism,[14] hermaphroditism,[15] transsexualism,[16] Islamic jurisprudence (especially with regard to homosexuality)[17] and the role of sexuality in contacts between Muslim and Western cultures.[18]

The spectre of Orientalism is never far away, albeit cloaked in a more modern, and far more surreptitious, guise; for instance, in a number of cases the discourse regarding homosexuality in the Muslim (Arab) world has borrowed – and re-gendered – tropes from historical Orientalism concerning Eastern women. Within this discourse, the submissive Eastern temptress is replaced by her masculine counterpart, the lascivious virile Eastern catamite.[19]

The first observation is that the overwhelming majority of scholarship on sexual and erotological literature has been conducted by Western scholars. Secondly, the interest in the subject as an academic field has hitherto resulted in only a handful of scholarly editions of the primary sources. Many re-editions of books are emendated, with the editors' barely veiled distaste causing them to omit references that run counter to prevailing morals. In the most extreme cases, this involves the removal of entire chapters that are deemed inconsistent with the shariah.[20]

This distinctly modern, Victorian-inspired morality extends to high literature as well, with modern editions of Abū Nuwās's work excluding his *mujūn* verse, to the extent that the poems in question were the object of a separate edition, enticingly titled *al-Nuṣūṣ al-muḥarrama* ('The Forbidden Texts').[21]

Translations of the primary texts are few and far between, and those that exist are problematic, as many are based on non-authoritative sources (often unidentified by the translator), in the above-mentioned Victorian style, or are 'secondary' renditions, i.e. relayed through a third language.[22]

The Genre: History and Typology

Chief among the erotological and sexological literature we find sex manuals and guides, (semi-)fictional works, and medical treatises – and often a combination of all three – which generally contain details on sexual health, hygiene, regimens and disorders, as well as various treatments, remedies and medicines.

The genre first emerged at the turn of the ninth century, with a large number of works being produced especially in the period up until the thirteenth century. The overlap between the sexual and erotic, on the one hand, and the technical–medical and 'spiritual', on the other, is a salient aspect of this type of literature, as religious injunctions are often juxtaposed with medical prescription and erotic titillation.

Several are known only by their titles, while a large number remain in manuscript form. In principle, this category excludes works that deal with profane, chaste love, such as *Kitāb al-Zahra* ('The Book of the Flower') by Muḥammad Ibn Dāwūd al-Ẓāhirī (d. 910) and *Rawḍat al-qulūb wa nuzhat al-muḥibb wa 'l-maḥbūb* ('The Garden of Hearts and the Delight of the Lover and the Beloved') by al-Shayzarī (twelfth century).[23] But things are never straightforward, and even these contain some stories and anecdotes associated with the erotic/erotological genre.

The majority of the erotological texts include aphrodisiacs, with some authors devoting an entire treatise to them – for example *Adwiyat al-Bāh* ('Medicines for Coitus') by al-Qusṭanṭīnī (d. 1568), the anonymous *Risāla fī dhikr adwiyat al-bāh* ('Treatise on Medicines for Coitus') and al-Ṭūsī's *Kitāb albāb al-bāhiyya wa 'l-tarākīb al-sulṭāniyya*, which forms the object of this study.[24]

Sexual health and erotology were often discussed in the medical literature, which may conveniently be subdivided into a number of categories.[25]

The first includes the medical encyclopedias, the most famous of which are *al-Kitāb al-Manṣūrī fi 'l-ṭibb* ('Manṣūr's Book on Medicine') and *Kitāb al-Ḥāwī fi 'l-ṭibb* ('The Medical Compendium') by Abū Bakr al-Rāzī (d. 925; Lat. *Rhazes*);[26] *Kitāb Kāmil al-ṣinā'a al-ṭibbiyya* ('Complete

Book of the Medical Art') – also known as *al-Kitāb al-malakī* ('The Royal Book') – by ʿAlī Ibn al-ʿAbbās al-Majūsī (d. late tenth century; Lat. *Haly Abbas*); *al-Qānūn fī 'l-ṭibb* ('Canon of Medicine') by Abū ʿAlī al-Ḥusayn Ibn Sīnā (d. 1037; Lat. *Avicenna*); *Tadkhirat ulī ʿla-albāb wa 'l-jāmiʿ li 'l-ʿajab al-ʿujāb* ('Memorandum for The Wise and a Collection of Marvelous Wonders') by Dā'ūd Ibn ʿUmar al-Anṭākī (d. 1599); *ʿUmdat al-iṣlāḥ fī ʿamal ṣināʿat al-jarrāḥ* (The Principal Guide to Pratising the Surgeon's Art) and *al-Shāfī fī 'l-ṭibb* ('The Healer in Medicine') by Abū 'l-Faraj Ibn al-Quff (1233–86).[27]

Hygiene literature devoted attention to sexual hygiene practices, including their possible therapeutic functions: e.g. Ibn al-Khaṭīb's *Kitāb al-wuṣūl li ḥifẓ al-ṣiḥḥa fī 'l-fuṣūl* ('Book on Preserving Health') and the *Taqwīm al-ṣiḥḥa* ('Almanac of Health') by Ibn Buṭlān (eleventh century).[28]

Sexual hygiene was also dealt with in dedicated treatises, including Qusṭā Ibn Lūqā's (820–912) *Kitāb fī 'l-Bāh wa mā yuḥtāju ilayhi min tadbīr al-badan fī istiʿmālihi* ('Book on Coitus and The Regimen that Is Necessary to Practise It') and *Kitāb fī 'l-Bāh*; al-Rāzī's *Kitāb al-Bāh wa manāfiʿuhu wa maḍārruhu wa mudawātuhu* ('Book on Coitus, Its Benefits, Harmful Effects and Remedies').

Sexuality, particularly sexual health, appears frequently in religious literature, in hadith literature (the sayings of the Prophet) and, especially, as part of the so-called 'Prophetic medicine', which refers to a voluminous body of literature that provides therapy based on a combination of herbal medicine and tradition.[29] The most celebrated works in this category include *al-Ṭibb al-nabawī* ('Prophetic Medicine') by Ibn Qayyim al-Jawziyya (d. 1350) and Shams al-Dīn al-Dhahabī (d. 1348); *al-Manhaj al sāwī wa 'l-manhal al rāwī fi 'l-ṭibb al nabawī* ('The Correct Method and Refreshing Source for Prophetic Medicine'), *Mukhtaṣar al-ṭibb al nabawī* ('Abridgement of Prophetic Medicine') and *al-Raḥma fi 'l-ṭibb wa 'l-ḥikma* ('Compassion in Medicine and Wisdom'),[30] by Jalāl al-Dīn al-Suyūṭī (d. 1505); and *Kitāb shifā' al-ālām fī ṭibb ahl al-Islām* ('Book on The Treatment of Pain in the Medicine of the Believers in Islam'), by al-Surramarrī (d. 1374).

Treatises devoted to sexual diseases may also be considered a subgenre, and concentrated on sexually transmitted ailments and their treatment, especially syphilis. Their authors included the Moroccan ʿAbd al-Wahhāb Muḥammad Adarrāq (d. 1746) and the Tunisians al-Bājī al-Masʿūdī (d. 1879) and Aḥmad al-Dihmānī (eighteenth century). It was, in fact, through this 'imported' sexual disease – which became known as *ḥabb al-Ifranj* ('the Frankish chancre') and was first referred to in Arabic medical literature as early as the fifteenth century – that Muslims developed a perfunctory interest in European medicine.[31] This was a major development since, until the nineteenth century, it was deemed devoid of merit. Generally speaking, the Arab-Muslim world showed little interest in European sciences, due to an unwavering conviction of the completeness, self-sufficiency and, indeed, superiority of Muslim achievements in this field. This was particularly true for medicine as medieval Muslim scholars were far ahead of their Christian European counterparts.

Another category is comprised of literature that deals with sexual ethics, of which the most famous exponents are Abū Ṭālib al-Makkī (d. 996), *Qūt al-qulūb* ('Nourishment of the Hearts'); Abū 'l-Faraj Ibn al-Jawzī (d. 1200), *Dhamm al-Hawā* ('The Condemnation of Love'); al-Ghazzālī (1058–1111), *Iḥyā' 'ulūm al-dīn* ('The Revival of the Religious Sciences');[32] Ibn Qayyim al-Jawziyya, *Rawḍat al-muḥibbīn wa nuzhat al-mushtaqīn* ('The Garden of Lovers and Excursion of the Longing'); al-Aqfahsī (d. 1406) *Raf' al-janāḥ 'ammā huwa min al-mar'a al-mubāḥ* ('The Raising of the Wing On What Is the Lawful Woman'); al-Ḥakamī's *Aḥkām al-Nikāḥ* ('Rules of Lawful Intercourse'); and 'Abd Allāh al-Mawṣulī's (tenth century) *al-Ikhtiyār li-ta'līl al-mukhtār* ('The Selection in the Explanation of the Chosen [legal opinions]').

Travel has always played a large part in Islam, not only as a means of seeking knowledge – as witnessed by the famous hadith *uṭlub al-'ilm wa law bi 'l-Ṣīn* ('Seek knowledge even in China!') – but also because of the injunction on all believers to perform the pilgrimage (*ḥajj*) to the Muslim holy site of Mekka. This gave rise to a distinct subgenre of travellers' medical manuals addressing specific health issues facing travellers, especially pilgrims, and contained specific advice on matters relating to sexual hygiene. Examples include

Ibn al-Jazzār's (d. 1004) *Zād al-musāfir wa qūt al-ḥāḍir* ('Provisions for the Traveller and Nourishment of the Sedentary')[33] and Qusṭā Ibn Lūqā's *Risāla fī tadbīr safar al-ḥajj* ('Treatise on the Regimen of the Pilgrimage Journey').[34]

The rich Arabic pharmacological literature dealt with all aspects of human well-being, including sexual health, how to enhance and treat it. Examples of these works are compendia like *al-Jāmiʿ li mufradāt al-adwiya wa 'l-aghdhiyya* ('The Comprehensive Book on Simple Drugs and Foods') by Ibn al Bayṭār (d. 1248), or formularies, like the *Aqrābādhīn* (Medical Formulary) by Sābūr Ibn Sahl (d. 869),[35] and *Minhaj al-dukkān* ('The Running of an Apothecary's Shop') by al-Kūhin al-ʿAṭṭār (thirteenth century).

Finally, as love is sometimes said to go through the stomach, the extensive medieval culinary literature commonly included information on the medicinal properties of certain foods, with a number of recipes for dishes, condiments, beverages and sauces with alleged aphrodisiac qualities.[36]

Questions arising from this overview include why and how sexuality, eroticism and erotology became such a significant element in Arabic literature, whether scientific or *belles-lettres*. Although there is no single ready-made answer to this question, it is true to say that initially various elements combined that formed the basis of Arabic sexual literature.

Firstly, sexual enjoyment, as opposed to procreative

intercourse, has been recognized in Islam since the beginning. For instance, while in Christianity *coitus interruptus* is condemned as 'the sin of Onan', in Islam it is viewed as an acceptable sexual outlet without the goal of procreation.[37] It is also against this background that one should interpret the lawfulness (for some time at least) of the so-called *nikāḥ al-mutʿa*, the 'marriage of enjoyment' – a temporary union (especially for soldiers and pilgrims), in which the believer could lawfully practise his sexuality in a short-term relationship that was religiously endorsed. Also, the famous Qur'ānic verse, 'your wives are a tilth for you, so go to your tilth as you will' (II: 231) is often interpreted as meaning that the man may exercise his conjugal right whenever and *however* he pleases, which for some – but by no means all – legal authorities includes anally (*fī duburihā*).

The distinction is also evidenced in the use of terminology, with *nikāḥ* being the term reserved for sexual intercourse during marriage and, by extension, also denotes marriage itself. The act of coitus is more commonly referred to as *bāh* (which also means potency) – a cognate of the Hebrew verb *bô' 'el* ('to enter into'), which connoted sexual intercourse for purposes of procreation – and *jimāʿ*, with *waṭ'* being employed in Islamic law (*fiqh*).[38] When not practised within a lawful context of marriage (or a bond of ownership, such as that between master-slave/concubine), coitus is considered unlawful (*ḥarām*) and falls within the remit of fornication (*zinā'*).

The second key element, to some degree an extension

of the first, was the attention given to the subject of sexuality in medicine, where it was an integral component of the holistic approach to physical well-being – a concept that ultimately went back to the Greek medical tradition. The influence and significance of medicine may be summarised as follows:

'medicine ... and the sexual script it produced provided the scientific basis for most sex-oriented discourses in Muslim Middle Eastern societies. Its injunctions and prohibitions, believed to originate in scientific knowledge, were subsumed by other discursive arenas, from literature to sacred law, almost intuitively, as part of their basic assumptions about the world.'[39]

Although the erotic was present as far back as pre-Islamic poetry,[40] it was the sophistication and hedonism of the first centuries of the Abbasid caliphate (750–1258) that would provide the breeding ground for the creation of both erotic and erotological literature.[41] Possibly the oldest known (but unfortunately lost) work is that by the Persian-born scholar Jibrīl Ibn Bukhtīshū' (late eighth to early ninth century), who served as private physician to the caliphs Hārūn al-Rashīd and al-Ma'mūn. The ninth century witnessed a boom in the number of works. To some extent, this may be explained by the fact that they responded to a trend that was also visible in *belles-lettres*; alternatively, it may point to a development in the genre, rather than its starting point. Some indications are provided by Ibn al-Nadīm's bio-bibliographical encyclopedia *Fihrist* (*Index*), which dates from the tenth century. It contains the names of a number of erotological and erotic works, revealing the substantial output in the field. In addition to details of individual authors (al-Ṣaymarī and al-Ṭahirī),[42] the text contains extensive lists of anonymous works, arranged in various categories: 'passionate lovers during the pre-Islamic period';[43] 'loving and fickle girls';[44] 'passionate lovers from the rest of the people, about whose traditions books were written';[45] 'passionate lovers whose traditions enter into the evening stories'.[46] As none of the titles mentioned is found anywhere else, it is impossible to trace the growth of the genre prior to the ninth century, when it suddenly appears.

Sources

Erotology in all of its aspects – views on male and female sexuality, coital practices, illnesses and treatments – was entirely subsumed in the framework of medieval Islamic medicine, which owed much to the ancient Greek tradition, represented in particular by Rufus of Ephesus (Rūfūs al-Afsīsī, late first and early second centuries),[47] Pedanius Dioscorides (Diyusquridīs, ca. 40–ca. 90),[48] Galen of Pergamon (Jālīnūs, 131–200)[49] and Hippocrates (Buqrāṭ, ca. 460–ca. 375 BCE).[50]

It was Abbasid rulers such as Hārūn al-Rashīd (766–809) and his son al-Ma'mūn (813–33), the founder of the famous 'House of Wisdom' (Bayt al-Ḥikma), who provided the impetus for the first translation movement in Muslim history, when many Greek scientific works were translated into Arabic, often through Syriac.[51] Key actors in this movement included Nestorian Christian physicians, such as Ḥunayn Ibn Isḥāq[52] and Ibn Māsawayh (d. 857, known in Latin as Mesue).[53] Nestorians were renowned for their medical knowledge, and many served as physicians to the Abbasid rulers; in some cases, this resulted in veritable dynasties, such as the Ibn Bukhtīshūʿ family, several generations (eight in total) of which acted in this capacity.[54]

When they were in turn translated into Latin from the eleventh century onwards, these texts, and the medical scholarship that was influenced by them, would have an impact that went beyond the Muslim empire. In many cases, it is thanks to the Arabic versions that Greek originals have survived. This is of particular relevance to authors like Rufus and – especially – Galen, nearly all of whose works were translated into Arabic and whose theories would be extremely influential in medieval and Renaissance Europe. From the point of view of historical scholarship, the translations provide invaluable clues for the reconstruction of the original Greek texts that survived only in later versions, as well as an insight into the history of medical terminology.[55]

In the field of erotology and sexology, the Greek influence was often direct. Firstly, all of the above-named scholars make an appearance in many erotological works, either through quotation or reference. The thirteenth-century author Ibn Māssa even devoted a chapter of his book to a paraphrase of the pseudo-Aristotelian *Problemata Physica.*[56] Secondly, views on women's sexuality and medicine in the Arabic tradition can also be traced back to Greek texts.[57]

As Greek erotic handbooks were a prolific genre in Greek literature, it is tempting to speculate a link and/or influence in this field, too. Any discussion of this question is complicated by the fact that only fragments of the Greek works have been preserved. One isolated piece of evidence is a reference by the tenth-century author al-Kātib to a Greek erotica book that included 'almost all the subjects to be found in Indian books'.[58] But the author does not specifically mention actually using – or even having seen – this work. Upon closer examination, a Greek influence here would seem unlikely in light of the significant differences in both format and content. Firstly, the Greek works were all attributed to (fictional) women (usually *hetairai* – 'courtesans'), on whose professional experience they were putatively based; 'restricted primarily to a tabulation of schemata for intercourse',[59] the manuals were intended as a guide to an art or skill (*technê*).

What the Arabic and Greek works also have in common is the fact that the female protagonist is of a lower social status; equally, there is a 'close connection [with] other genres, principally medical writings, and other encyclopedic, scientific and culinary works'.[60]

The translation movement provides us with a second

reason for the emergence of erotological literature, which also played a role in the development of Greek sex manuals. The Greek medical and philosophical works, with their emphasis on taxonomy and analysis, held a powerful attraction for Muslim scholars, whose propensity for classification covered all fields and lay at the heart of the hadith literature, with the Prophet's sayings being methodically and meticulously arranged and ordered. In this sense, the genre may be seen as a 'continuance of the Aristotelian ... tradition of analysis and classification, wherein the continua of the world are broken into discrete, nameable and hence controllable quanta'.[61]

One of the core elements of medieval Islamic medicine was the theory of humorism, whose origins lay in the Hippocratic corpus but was expanded by Galen. It was the latter's version of it that was imported.[62] Within this framework, human beings were seen as the microcosm of nature, subject to the interaction of the four elements (*arkān*) that make up all things: air, water, fire and earth.[63] Each of these was associated with two of the 'primary qualities' (hot, *ḥārr*/cold, *bārid*; moist, *raṭb*/dry, *yābis*): fire was hot and dry; air, hot and moist; water, cold and moist; earth, cold and dry. The basic elements were thought to be concentrated in one of the four so-called 'humours' (< Gr. *khumos*; Ar. *khilṭ*, pl. *akhlāṭ*, 'mixture'), essentially the bodily fluids: air in blood (*dam*); water in phlegm (*balgham*, < Gr. *phlegma*); fire in yellow bile (*mirra ṣufrā'*); and earth in black bile

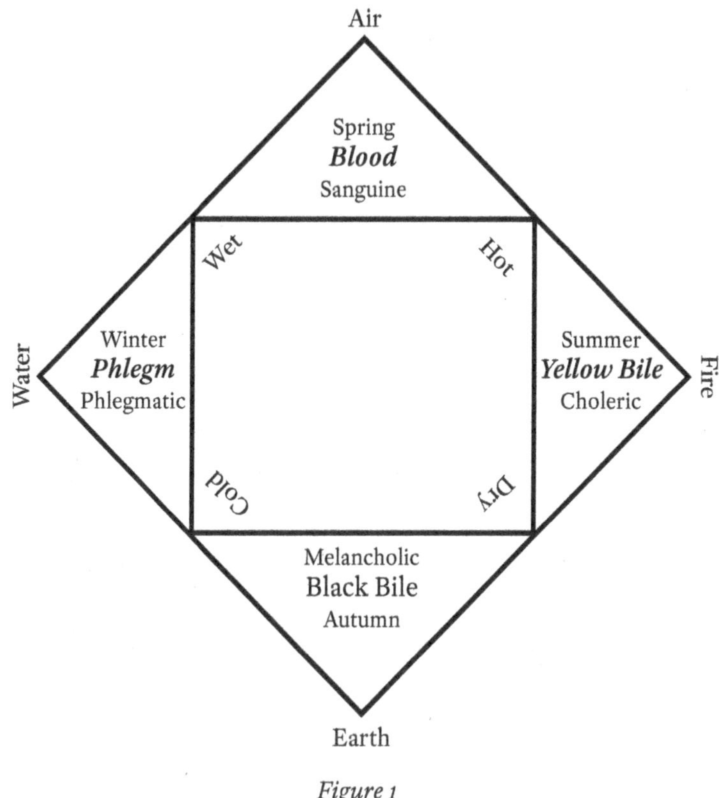

Figure 1

(*mirra sawdā'*). As a result, each of the humours was endowed with the primary qualities associated with the element: blood was hot and moist; phlegm was cold and moist; yellow bile was hot and dry; and black bile was cold and dry. The humours were also associated with a season: blood with spring, yellow bile with summer, black bile with autumn and phlegm with winter. This may be illustrated as in Figure 1.[64]

According to Galenic theory, a human being's physical health relied on the balance in the mixture (Gr. *krasis*;

Ar. *mizāj*) of the humours, i.e. the temperament (or 'complexion') and the equilibrium (Ar. *i'tidāl*) of the qualities, a state which was known in Greek as *eukrasia* or *symmetria*. For instance, if black bile was predominant, this resulted in a cold and dry (or melancholic) temperament, making the individual prone to sadness (melancholy). Similarly, sanguine temperaments were characterized by a predominance of blood, choleric ones by yellow bile and phlegmatic ones by phlegm, each of which was associated with differences in character.[65] Another crucial component within the Galenic system was the view (originally Aristotelian) that men and women shared a common reproductive system, with that of women being essentially a mirror-image of men's.[66]

The treatment of ill health was aimed at making the temperament balanced (*mu'tadal*) through therapies, medication or diet to counterbalance the humours or qualities that caused the disequilibrium (Gr. *dyskrasia*; *sū' al-mizāj*).

Spices and other foods were also associated with humours and with (varying degrees of) the above-mentioned qualities, and prescribed accordingly. For instance, cardamom was hot and dry, whereas cucumbers were said to be cold and moist. Whether a fruit or plant was dried or fresh could also affect its qualities: for instance, fresh figs were hot and moist in the second degree, while dried ones were hot in the first degree, but moderately moist and dry.

A related concept was that of living beings' 'innate

(or 'vital') heat' (Gr. *emphuton thermon*, Lat. *calidum innatum*; Ar. *ḥarāra gharīziyya*), which was said to be created by the heart and circulated through the body by blood, with its amount determining the place of a species within the biological hierarchy. As human beings were thought to have the greatest innate heat, they were at the top of the pyramid. Similarly, men were considered 'hotter' (and 'drier') than women – and thus superior to them – which explained, for instance, the fact that the former's genital organs were on the outside.[67]

It has been claimed that the medieval Arabic medical scholars did not aim 'to discover new knowledge, or to reinterpret the processes which go on in the human body, or to develop new and more adequate therapies', and that 'the literature of the ancients is both example and authority'.[68] The implicit argument is that they made few original contributions. However, the Greek theories were not only borrowed, digested and assimilated, but also expanded and developed. The erotological literature includes a number of examples not only of innovation but also of empirical research. For instance, Ibn al-Jazzār refers to recipes invented (and tested) by both his predecessors[69] and himself – and when discussing the effectiveness of a pill for the retention of menstrual blood, he adds that he has 'tried it and approved of it'.[70]

The next question is whether authors drew on an existing pool of traditions and conventions. Although it is difficult to address this issue in the absence of a complete picture, there are a number of clues. The first are the references by some authors to predecessors in the genre (for example, al-Tīfāshī and al-Kātib).

The first mention of non-Arabic sources can be found in the famous *Kitāb al-ḥayawān* ('The Book of Animals') by the belle-lettrist al-Jāḥiẓ (d. 868), where a number of Arab poets are mentioned, as well as an unnamed Indian (*Hindī*) author of *Kitāb al-Bāh* ('Book on Coitus') – which one may speculate is a reference to the *Kama Sutra* – who is quoted as the source for the claim that the elephant has the biggest penis of all animals and the gazelle the smallest.[71] However, the Indians' reputation in sexual matters was not based on this solitary author, as:

'the Indians are like the Arabs in all respects, except for the circumcision (*khitān*) of women and men, but they were driven to it by their pursuit of sexual prowess, for which they took medicines; they wrote books on the art of sex (*ṣināʿat al-bāh*) and instructed their sons.'[72]

Further references to an Indian connection are given by other authors, such as the poet Abū Tammām (788–845),[73] the legal scholar Ibn al-Jawzī (508–97),[74] the encyclopedists Ibn al-Nadīm[75] and Ibn Abī Uṣaybiʿa (1200–79),[76] as well as, of course, in erotological works, such as al-Kātib's erotological compendium, *Jawāmiʿ al-ladhdha* ('The Encyclopaedia of Pleasure').[77]

Among the Indians there was, it seems, a woman who was known as *al-alfiyya* ('The Thousander'), in reference to the number of men she had had intercourse with. Her expertise turned her into an oracle on matters sexual – a

Dr Ruth *avant la lettre*. Her legend was transmitted by al-Jāḥiẓ and others, including al-Tīfāshī, who relates that

> Groups of women gathered to visit her. They would say to her: 'Sister, tell us what is required and we will do it. What is it that makes women settle in men's hearts, what gives them pleasure and what morals do they abhor? What should we do in order to arouse their love and affection?'
>
> She replied: 'the first thing is that the look of a man should be on a body that is healthy, not smelly but fragrant, in which case [the woman's] beauty will be enhanced.'
>
> 'What does a man have to do in order to capture a woman's heart?'
>
> 'He should be playful prior to coitus and shudder before ejaculation.'
>
> 'What is the reason for mutual love and concord [between a man and a woman]?'
>
> 'Their simultaneous orgasm.'[78]

While no translation of the *Kama Sutra* into Arabic has ever been found, or is even known to have existed, a number of Indian medical texts were translated into Persian and/or Syriac (and then into Arabic) very early on by scholars in the city of Gondēshāpūr (a former city in southwestern Iran), which was known for its physicians, and Indian medical knowledge thereby filtered through into Arabic-Islamic medical thought.[79] One may cite the famous *Ladhdhat al-Nisā* ('The Pleasure of Women'), which was a Persian translation of a Hindi text called *Kok-shastar* (or *Kokasara*), attributed to a certain Koka (Koka pandit) and based on a Sanskrit text entitled *Ratirahasya* ('On the Art of Love').[80] In Arabic medical literature, there are a number of Indian references. For instance, the last chapter of the famous *Firdaws al-Ḥikma* ('The Paradise of Wisdom'), by the Persian ʿAlī Ibn Rabban al-Ṭabarī (ninth century), is devoted to Indian medicine, with quotations from a number of works. Although it is possible that al-Ṭabarī was able to access the original Sanskrit, it is more likely that he based himself on Syriac or Persian translations. The encyclopedias by Ibn Qutayba (d. 885),[81] Ibn al-Nadīm[82] and Ibn Abī Uṣaybiʿa[83] also include references to Indian physicians (such as Cāṇakya/Shānāq[84] and Maṅka) and works, whereas al-Rāzī quotes a number of (unnamed) Indian sources.[85] Indian medical knowledge was highly respected and it is said that Hārūn al-Rashīd called for Maṅka when he was ill and, together with a compatriot by the name of Ibn Dham, the latter translated a medical text on poisons.[86]

The second clue regarding the construction of the erotological genre involves similarities in approach and/or content in the various works. Examples include the 'comparatist' approach in some of al-Jāḥiẓ's and al-Suyūṭī's works, discussions of sexual positions[87] and sexual frequency related to sexual age,[88] and the lists of substances that invigorate coitus which many of the authors have in common and whose creator is sometimes identified.[89]

Indirectly, the above question regarding the existence of an established tradition and corpus is inextricably linked to the extent to which the works spread across the Muslim world. When talking about a time when manuscripts were the currency, this is a particularly thorny issue and can only be addressed tangentially.

There are indications that, at least in some cases, the spread took place not only across genres, but also across languages. An example combining the two movements involves stories on homosexual prowling (*dabb*), which can be found in al-Tīfāshī, Abū Nuwās and, more surprisingly perhaps, the work by the sixteenth-century Turkish author Deli Birader, whose discussion of the various positions of anal intercourse is redolent of those found in al-Tifāshī's work.[90] And at least one author (al-Kātib) acknowledges a Persian source.[91]

This leads us to another indication regarding the spread of the works, namely the translations into other languages, which also attest to the popularity – perceived or imagined – of the source text. In the case of al-Ṭūsī's work, there were translations into both Turkish[92] and his native Persian.[93]

Features

The list of 141 titles in the appendix to this volume is the most extensive bibliography to date of literature devoted wholly, or for the most part, to erotology. It is worth pointing out that it is by no means exhaustive since it is more than likely that other works are held in collections that cannot be readily explored. As has been noted, the list does not include erotic poetry, which continued to be produced (and/or collected) in the post-classical age by, for instance, Khalīl Ibn Aybak al-Ṣafadī (1297–1363),[94] Ṣafī al-Dīn al-Ḥillī (1279–1348)[95] and Shams al-Dīn al-Nawājī (1386–1455).[96]

A number of elements merit discussion, including the authors, themes, formats, sources, and so on. A. Jarkas classified what he called 'erotic books' into the following categories, according to the topics they deal with:

- 'books dealing with the ethics, art, kinds, time and condition of coition;
- books dealing with the sexual capacity of men and women; kinds of invigorating food and drugs that keep sexual capacity normal; different kinds of medicinal prescriptions, consisting of tablets, powders, suppositories, ointments, and so on;
- books that deal with the subjects of former categories so that benefits may be more general;

- books dealing with one specific subject, such as prostitution, sodomy, lesbianism, masturbation, and the like.'[97]

The multitude of overlapping genres, intersecting fields of application and levels of discourse means that any classification of this type will be at once too narrow and too broad, as far too many exponents of the genre defy simplistic categorization.

It makes more sense to view the works along a continuum in relation to the approach taken by the authors and the extent to which certain elements are present. On one end of the spectrum, for instance, one may put *belles-lettres* (*adab*) works in which the erotic fictional component predominates, as in the works of al-Jāḥiẓ or al-Suyūṭī. On the other end, we find treatises that deal with erotology from a scientific (medical) perspective, such as those by Ibn Sīnā, Ibn al-Jazzār, Qusṭā Ibn Lūqā, Maimonides, or the author of the work that is presented here, al-Ṭūsī.

Neither of these subgenres exists in a 'pure' form, and varying elements associated with the other are present in both. For instance, even the 'fictional' type often deals with medical issues attendant upon sexuality – enhancing libido and performance, recommended practices, sexual positions, aphrodisiacs, and so on. In the case of al-Tīfāshī's *Rujūʿ al-shaykh ilā ṣibāh fi 'l-quwwa wa 'l-bāh* ('Returning the Old Man to his Youth and Coital

Vigour'), this results in a neatly compartmentalized construction, with the 'medical' prefacing the fictional.

As for the 'scientific' type, it does not eschew the more frivolous and/or literary features associated with its counterparts' output. It might also include, for instance, some lines of relevant poetry – but generally no erotic stories.

In the middle of this continuum are texts distinguished by their form rather than their content. This category includes erotological works with high literary aspirations, expressed either in their use of poetic quotations or by the composition of the treatise itself in verse (for example, Ibn Kannān, Ibn Sīnā), or those with a lexicographical and taxonomical focus, such as al-Suyūṭī's *al-Wishāḥ fī fawā'id al-nikāḥ* ('The Sash in the Advantages of Sexual Intercourse'), which contains a veritable thesaurus of terms denoting the sexual organs, intercourse, and so on. This may be presented diagrammatically as in Figure 2.

What all of these works have in common, to a lesser or greater degree, is their didactic intent: irrespective of the genre or medium (poetry versus prose), the aim and tone are avowedly pedagogic, practical and scientific. In this sense, the books serve as teaching manuals or handbooks; even the ribald stories and obscene poetry (some of which would put Catullus to shame) regarding past *roués* contain lessons – often a 'moral' of sorts – deemed useful to the reader. The target readership also merits some attention. It has been claimed that the

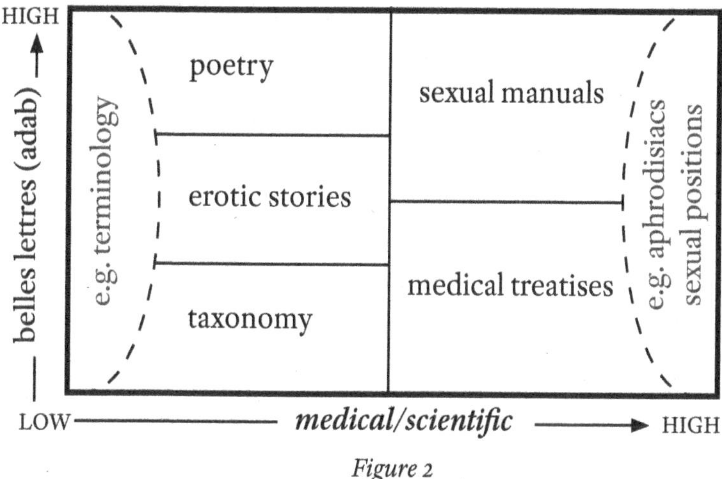

Figure 2

authors' motive was to 'write sexual instructions that mothers gave their daughters on their wedding day'.[98] However, this is highly unlikely, not least because the books were written *for* men, *by* men.

In fact, the typical reader would be a fellow medical scholar or, as some authors inform us, a member of a courtly audience (often the ruler himself), whereas the medical treatises might also be used as self-medication manuals, as is the case for al-Ṭūsī's work. It is likely that a number of the works – or appropriate parts of them (such as stories, poems) – would be read at social gatherings of the elite, which would be exclusively male and, as such, 'tend<ed> to spread information – one might say in certain cases a kind of initiation – by placing their science in the service of an art of living'.[99] This also underlies the link between sexuality and food as another constant in erotological literature, while references to the aphrodisiacal properties of food were, as we have seen, an integral part of culinary manuals. A similar connection can be found in classical Greek erotic works, albeit as part of a spirit of overindulgence and immoderation not present in the Arabic tradition, the 'association between the ethics of sex and ethics of food [being] a constant factor in ancient culture'.[100]

Another dimension of variation is the number of topics covered, ranging from the encyclopedic to texts that focus on only one area (such as aphrodisiacs). The erotological corpus runs the full gamut of sexuality and erotology, generally combining *ars amatoria* and *scientia sexualis*: types and positions of intercourse, penis size, homosexuality, lesbianism, pederasty, hermaphroditism, impotence, nocturnal emissions, priapism, anilingus, cunnilungus, voyeurism, bestiality, sadomasochism, hymen restoration, contraception, prostitution, fetishism, and so on. Interestingly enough, the extant works do not contain any discussions of fellatio,[101] which was prominent in the Greek and Roman traditions (which also included *irrumation* – forced fellatio), both in literature (Catullus) and pictorial art, where it is often represented both between men and between men and women. Many of these themes also formed the object of the (pure) medical literature – though devoid of the fictional narrative content – which further consolidates the link between the medical and the erotological/erotic.[102]

It is difficult to overstate the importance and relevance

of erotological literature for what it teaches us about various aspects not only of Islamic medicine but also, and more importantly, of Muslim society, gender relations and sex-power relations. Most of all, it provides a unique vantage point on the experience of sexuality – that is, 'the correlation between fields of knowledge, types of normativity, and forms of subjectivity in a particular culture', to use Michel Foucault's words.[103] Though Foucault was discussing sexual discourse in the West from the seventeenth century onwards, this comment is equally applicable to medieval Arabic sexual discourse. One of the questions that lies at the heart of his framework is deceptively simple: 'what were the effects of power generated by what was said?'[104]

Like Greek erotic literature, Arabic erotology is decidedly phallocentric in that the emphasis is on (active) male penetration. The role of women is subordinate to the penis, with remedies including the tightening and narrowing of the vagina 'like that of a virgin'; women are often unnamed, invisible as secondary characters. As one author put it, coitus is 'the greatest pleasure given to *men*'.[105] The terminology, too, is inscribed into this discourse, as the words for coitus (see above) tend to identify the male rather than the female as the 'primary' actor.

And yet, perhaps surprisingly in light of this, both the Arabic erotological and medical works paid attention to female pleasure and Ibn Sīnā, for instance, clearly placed the onus of pleasuring a woman on the man: 'if a man can't make her orgasm, some of them (*sc.* women) turn to lesbianism (*musāḥaqa*)'. Furthermore, female coital pleasure does not result from male ejaculation, but from her own ejaculation and the movement of her womb.[106] This was a notion originating in the Greek tradition, with Galen referring to women deriving sexual pleasure from the release of female semen.[107] The more active role of women – albeit with concomitants of predatoriness and deviousness – is also evidenced by the many stories about the wiles of women in seeking out and securing the amorous affections of invariably well-endowed men.[108] The same notion emerges from *belles-lettres*, whether it be in poetry or prose, with a number of examples in the *Thousand and One Nights*. It has been argued that this view of female sexual aggressiveness, combined with artfulness, runs throughout Muslim culture and contributed to the spread of the veil.[109]

The erotological works have a number of things in common, the most important of which is the varying degree of pedagogic and/or literary intent when discussing sexual behaviour outside the 'norm', whether it be homosexuality or bestiality, which tend either to be presented without judgement[110] or treated as *medical* 'deviations', and worthy of study.

Use of the word 'norm' in this context does not in any way imply a moral judgement, and the same was broadly true in the Greek and Roman traditions, whose 'moral reflection concerning the pleasures was not directed towards a codification of acts, nor towards a hermeneutics of the subject, but towards a stylization of attitudes and an aesthetics of existence. A stylization, because the rarefaction of sexual activity presented itself as a sort of open-ended requirement.'[111]

However, as Holt Parker has pointed out, this statement does not apply to all Greek erotic texts, and sex manuals were considered to be 'shameless'[112] – a perception absent from Arabic erotological literature, which, it seems, bears out the saying that *'lā ḥayā' fī 'l-'ilm* ('there is never any shame in science'). That is not to say that the concept of (il)licitness did not exist in Arabic erotological literature. In order to discuss this, it is useful to introduce the Foucaultian contrast between 'moral code' and 'moral behaviour'. The former denotes 'a set of values and rules of action that are recommended to individuals through the intermediary of various prescriptive agencies',[113] whereas the latter, which is equated with 'morality', involves the actual behaviour of individuals 'in relation to the rules and values that are recommended to them', and 'thus designates the manner in which they comply more or less fully with a standard of conduct, the manner in which they obey or resist an interdiction or a prescription; the manner in which they respect or disregard a set of values'.[114] The 'moral code' is sometimes implicit, and sometimes – as in al-Tīfāshī's statement regarding the aims of his work – explicit:

> In the writing of this book I did not aim to increase corruption, to encourage sin, or assist those seeking pleasure and sinfulness

> by trying to make lawful what Allah the Almighty has made unlawful; rather, my aim is to help those whose passion is reduced to achieve pleasure in a lawful context (*fi 'l-ḥalāl*), which is the basis of civilized society and procreation.[115]

This passage provides us with a great deal of food for thought. Seemingly, it sets out the contours of the subject: the individual's relation towards sexuality, particularly the part that is divinely endorsed, and the aims of the sexual experience. Most saliently, it pre-emptively guards against accusations of irreligiousness due to the inclusion of topics that may arouse censure. This applies to sex that is considered illicit by religious precept – outside the confines of marriage or an ownership bond – and to homosexuality (and pederasty), the treatment of which provides a particularly good case in point.

Several verses of the Qur'ān[116] mention sexual actions between men in relation to the People of Lot (*qawm Lūṭ*), which gave rise to the word *liwāṭ*, with the active male homosexual being known in Classical Arabic as *lūṭī*, *lā'iṭ*, or *mulāwiṭ*.[117] Lesbianism (*musāḥaqa, siḥāq*) is not mentioned in the holy text.

The Qur'ān refers to homosexual intercourse as a depravity (*fāḥisha*), and it is equally condemned in various hadiths, the most famous one stating, 'anyone finding those committing the act of Lot, kill both the active and passive party' (*man wajadtumūhu ya'mal 'amal qawm lūṭ fa-uqtulū al-fāʿil wa ʾl-mafʿūl bihi*). Though *liwāṭ* is often equated with 'homosexuality' in its contemporary (Western) acceptation, it is important to state that the modern concept had no equivalent in Islamic society, law or language.[118] Similarly, there was (and still is) no word in Arabic for 'heterosexual(ity)'. For the purposes of punishment, homosexuality tended to be equated with *zinā'* in law (*fiqh*), with varying penalties, depending on the school of Muslim of jurisprudence.[119] The association with *zinā'* is based on the fact that, like heterosexuality, homosexuality was viewed as a binary construct involving an active/penetrating and passive/penetrated partner.[120] The same notion underlay views of the lesbian sexual experience, which, in addition to entailing friction, as the terms for it indicate (*siḥāq, musāḥaqa* < *saḥaqa*, 'to grind'), was thought to be penetrative, by means of dildos.

Homosexual intercourse took place within a hierarchical relation, with the 'passive' partner (or 'bottom', to use the modern jargon) being invariably subordinate in age (with a preference for the *amrad*, the 'beardless youth') and/or status (as in the case of a servant or slave). It is because of this inequality that the passive partner, known as *ma'būn* (compare the *cinaedus* of Roman times), comes in for greater criticism, whereas a predilection for it (*ubna*) was commonly classified as a disease.[121]

Despite the censure embedded in the 'moral (religious) code', the erotological (and erotic) literature demonstrates that male sexual intercourse, within the above constraints, was part of 'moral behaviour' inasmuch as it derived from the established sexual script. In other words, compliance with the established code was endorsed by socially accepted practice. As a result, the immanent contradiction of al-Tīfāshī's prefatory claims and the ostensible breaches of religion in the course of the book are superseded by what was considered 'moral behaviour'. Al-Kātib is one of the few erotological authors to discuss anal intercourse from a religious point of view – but only as a preamble to extolling the virtues of the rectum over the vagina.[122]

In other texts, particularly medical treatises, the legal aspect was clearly divorced from the pursuit of science. Ibn Sīnā, for instance, simply stated that intercourse with youths (*ghulmān*) 'is reprehensible to the masses (*al-jumhūr*) and prohibited under the shariah',[123] before discussing it from a purely physical point of view. No author links homosexuality with a lack of 'morals' (*akhlāq*), or immoral behaviour.

The treatment of homosexuality and pederasty in erotic poetry and erotology reinforced the Victorian view that the practice had been historically condoned, and even encouraged, in Arab-Muslim society, as it was said to have been in ancient Greece.[124] Despite being thickly tarred with an Orientalist brush, it is a view that has some merit, albeit with the provisos mentioned above. In recent times, this perception has been rejected in its entirety on the grounds that, for instance, the severe legal constraints on evidence for homosexuality (a confession, or four witnesses to the act) explain the absence of legal action against individuals in the pre-Modern period.[125]

Just as there is no single type of erotological work, there is no 'typical' author. Irrespective of the often raunchy contents of the works, the authors should by no means be considered seedy pornographers driven by scurrilous licentiousness. For a start, nearly all of the known authors were scholars (mainly physicians), many of whom became part of the canon of Islamic science for their activities in other fields – for example, Qusṭā Ibn Lūqā, Ibn Sīnā, al-Rāzī, Ibn al-Jazzār and Maimonides in medicine; al-Tīfāshī in mineralogy; al-Suyūṭī in jurisprudence; and al-Ṭūsī in astronomy. Secondly, the importance of the subject as a scientific field of study to these (and other) scholars is further demonstrated by the fact that they also addressed it in their specialized medical works – this was true of Ibn Sīnā,[126] Maimonides[127] and al-Rāzī,[128] for example.

A second factor that often emerges is the authors' association with the rich and powerful of the day, often their patrons. They not only dedicated their works to such figures, but also received commissions from them to produce a treatise on the subject.[129] This relationship of patronage served a twofold purpose. On the one hand, it confirmed the writer's status within the establishment and, on the other, neutralized any accusations of immorality, shamelessness or frivolousness. It is also within this context that one should interpret the references to past scholars, especially Greeks, in order to corroborate statements, while anecdotes and erotic stories are sometimes 'defictionalized' by reference to past historic characters or unnamed dignitaries, such as judges, princes and the like.

Finally, it is striking that, except in some of the medical works, the authors do not appear as *actors*, but variously as *narrators* and/or diagnosticians. When they do appear as actors (as in the case of Ibn al-Jazzār), it is to endorse this or that remedy of their own making and attest to its efficaciousness.

The list allows us to draw up some interesting statistics. Firstly, of the 141 titles identified, 32 have been lost and 66 remain in manuscript form to this day. The remaining 43 texts are available in either editions (often incomplete) or translations. Finally, 32 of the entries are anonymous.

A number of the authors wrote several works: Ibn Sīnā, al-Kātib, al-Rāzī, Ibn Lūqā, al-Namlī, and al-Nafzāwī each wrote two; al-Tīfāshī and al-Ẓāhirī produced three; and al-Saymarī wrote six. But by far the most prolific in the field was the Egyptian polymath al-Suyūṭī, who wrote no fewer than 23 treatises on various aspects of erotology.[130] If known dates of these texts are correlated with the origins of the authors, the picture is also revealing (see Table 1).

The data demonstrate that the heyday of erotological literature fell between the ninth and fourteenth centuries, after which it tapered off considerably, with a few isolated works in the seventeenth, eighteenth and nineteenth centuries. The nineteenth century also marks the end of Arabic erotological literature. While, as we have seen,

Table 1

Century	al-Andalus (Muslim Spain)	Bilād al-Shām[131]	Egypt	Iraq	Morocco	Persia	Sudan	Tunis	Turkey	Yemen
9th		1		6		2				
10th				2		1				
11th				2		2		1		
12th	1		2		1			1		
13th						2		2		
14th		2	3							1
15th			3		1					
16th								3		
17th		1			2					
18th							1			
19th			1							

the dawn of the genre is cloaked in mystery, its demise is less enigmatic, as it coincides with increasing Western influence on Muslim societies and, through missionary movements, the importation of a Western-style morality – Victorian or otherwise.

The authors' origins are also of interest, with seven of Persian origin, both geographically and linguistically, while one is Turkish. Secondly, although I have been referring to the 'Islamicness' of the works, this should be taken to refer to a broad cultural tradition that the authors were a part of, rather than to their religious affiliation, as five of them were Christians and three Jews. Finally, certain regions – Tunis and Iraq – were clearly dominant in terms of output, which may be explained by the importance of these two places as cultural centres during certain periods.

When East Meets West

We have seen that at least some of the works spread throughout the Arabic-speaking world, and sometimes even as far as Turkey. Thanks to the Latin translations of Arabic works in the eleventh and twelfth centuries, the Arabic medical tradition (both original and borrowed from the Greeks) would go on to influence not only medicine in Christian Europe, but also its views on sexuality.[132]

Greek medicine arrived in medieval Europe either

via translations into Latin from the Greek source texts, or through Arabic as the relay language. The earliest results of the former activity took place in the fourth and fifth centuries in North Africa,[133] where some of the works (including one on gynaecology) of Soranus of Ephesus (*fl.* 100)[134] were translated. Over the next few centuries, the centre of activity moved north across the Mediterranean, to Ravenna in northern Italy.[135]

But it was in the south of the country, in Salerno, which became a centre of medical training in the tenth century, that the first translations of Arabic medical works into Latin were carried out.[136] The protagonist was a Muslim convert from Carthage by the name of Constantine the African, who arrived in Salerno in 1077, but became associated with the monastery of Monte Cassino through the offices of Alphanus (d. 1085), the archbishop of Salerno and abbot of the monastery, who was also a physician.[137] Constantine had brought a number of manuscripts from his native land, and during his translation career he rendered some twenty Arabic works into Latin, often with the help of his assistant (and fellow Muslim convert), Johannes Afflacius. The first was the *Isagoge*, a translation of Ḥunayn (known in Latin as Johannitius) Ibn Isḥāq's *Masā'il fi 'l-Ṭibb* ('Medical Questions'), an abridgement of an introduction to Galen's *Techne iatrike* ('The Art of Medicine'), known in Latin as *Tegni* (also *Ars parva* and *Ars medica*). The *Isagoge Ioannitii ad Tegni Galieni* ('Johannitius' Introduction to the Art of Galen'), to give it its full title, is the earliest known Latin translation of an Arabic medical text, and subsequently became the core of the *Articella,* a collection of medical writings on the basics of Hippocratic and Galenic medicine that would become a core textbook at medical schools across Europe for many centuries.[138] Constantine's translation of Ibn al-Jazzār's *Zād al-Musāfir* (*Viaticum peregrinantis*) and, especially, of al-Majūsī's *Kāmil* (*Liber Pantegni*)[139] gained equal authority and currency among students of medicine.

An additional avenue opened up in the twelfth century, at Toledo, where a circle of translators applied themselves to the rendering of Arabic scientific works – including many on medicine – into Latin.[140] The leading light in the Toledan group was the Italian-born Gerard of Cremona (d. 1187),[141] to whom over seventy translations in various fields were ascribed, among them Ibn Sīnā's *Qānūn* (*Canon Medicinae*)[142] and al-Rāzī's *Kitāb al-Manṣūrī,* the ninth book of which became particularly popular in the paraphrase by the founder of modern anatomy, Andreas Vesalius (1514–64), which was published in 1537.[143] The dissemination of the new scientific output was further ensured through the foundation during the same period of medical faculties in a number of cities – including Montpellier, Paris, Bologna, Naples and Padua.[144]

Through the translations of the Arabic medical texts, European scholars were introduced to the Islamicate views (and knowledge) of sexuality – which, it is worth remembering, was coupled with erotology. This influence, which manifested itself in a number of guises, developed at an interesting time, when perceptions of sexuality could not have been more different between the Christian European West and the Muslim East. In the West, Christian dogma condemned all sexual activity that was extramarital and non-procreational. What is more, even if conception was the aim, taking pleasure in the act was considered sinful.[145] As we have seen, this attitude was completely absent from – and indeed alien to – the Islamic tradition and its treatment of sexuality. Equally significant was the gap in gynaecological knowledge between the two medical traditions.

The translations of Arabic medical works would profoundly alter the perceptions and study of sexuality and women's medicine. First, Constantine's translation of al-Jazzār's *Zād al-Musāfir* included a lengthy section on sexual matters, including aphrodisiacs and contraceptives.[146] Another treatise ascribed to Constantine was *De Coitu* ('On Coitus'), which would inspire a number of homonymous works.[147] Another *De Coitu* was a thirteenth-century translation of Maimonides' *Fi 'l-Jimā'* by John of Capua, an Italian Jewish convert, who also translated Maimonides' work on hygiene (*De regimine santitatis*)[148] and *Kitāb al-Taysīr fi 'l-Mudāwāt wa 'l-Tadbīr* ('The Book of Facilitation in Remedies and Regimen') by the Andalusian physician Ibn Zuhr (Lat. *Avenzoar*, 1094–1162).[149]

In addition to translations, original work was soon

produced dealing with matters sexual in ways that would have been unthinkable prior to the introduction of the Arabic tradition. Two examples may be cited. The first was the *Thesaurus Pauperum* by Peter of Spain (d. 1277), the future Pope XXI, who included a large number of fertility and contraception prescriptions, as well as emmenagogues and abortifacients, and aphrodisiacs.[150] The second is a Catalan work, entitled *Speculum al foderi* ('A Mirror for Fuckers'), which bears a strong resemblance to some of the Arabic erotological works.[151] Of particular interest is the fact that, from the outset, the author acknowledges a debt to an Arabic original – which, however, would seem to be a fictional device intended either to absolve the author or to add authority to the content. Whatever the case may be, it highlights the reputation of Muslims in the field.

Another direct Arabic influence, in terms of both content and format, can be observed in the so-called 'Secrets' literature (*Secretum Secretorum*, Ar. *Sirr al-asrār*), which can be traced back to Aristotle's advice to princes, and is of course part of the 'Mirrors for Princes' tradition. Taking the form of a dialogue (usually between two clerics or a cleric and a layman), it discussed how men should behave with women, but also contained medical information, for instance on physiognomy and regimen. An offshoot of this genre was the 'Secrets of Women' literature, which provided some semblance of sexual education.[152]

By the end of the thirteenth century a profound change, driven by the 'new' Arabic tradition (especially Ibn Sīnā, whose *Canon* had become the standard reference), had taken place in female medicine, the understanding of the female body and, concurrently, the medical ideas of maleness and femaleness, as shown by the works of European doctors between the twelfth and fourteenth centuries.[153] Among them was a female doctor from Salerno called Trotula (eleventh–twelfth century), the first female professor of medicine, to whom a number of treatises have (spuriously) been ascribed that show a clear influence from Arabic medicine.[154] Though it would take a few more centuries before the anatomy of the female sexual organs would be described and its functions understood, this could not have happened without the impetus provided by the Arabic texts.

A related development was the upheaval in the perceptions of sexuality and eroticism. Here, too, there was an undeniable influence from Ibn Sīnā, in particular – not least in making 'Arabic erotic lore ... a component of the didactic message'.[155] Ibn Sīnā, in effect, paved the way for the emergence of an erotic art with a medical preoccupation – a science offering a way out of the religious constraints that had hampered any clear perception, let alone discussion, of sexual matters.

This resulted in a split between theology, with its focus on reproduction within a marital context, and medicine, within which the sexual act and experience became a physiological necessity that was both beneficial and pleasurable. As we have seen, the latter was a key component in Arabic sexology and erotology.

The new ideas on sexual positions and, more importantly, of pleasure during sex – most of them mediated by Ibn Sīnā's *Canon* – filtered through very early on into European writings, including literary texts, in troubadour poetics and Capellanus' *De Amore*.[156] The focus on the importance of female pleasure during coitus and the benefits of kissing was at the heart of another innovation attributable to the Arabic tradition: foreplay.[157]

In the area of medical terminology, too, the Arabic works made substantial contributions; the Latin translators were forced to grapple with new concepts for which new terms had to be coined, necessitating a quest for precision. In the field of sexuality, a particularly apt example is the translation of the word 'clitoris' (Ar. *baẓr*), which had eluded even some of the Arabic physicians, and was translated by Constantine the African as *badedera* and by Gerard of Cremona as *batharum*.[158] Though neither of these withstood the test of time, others did, with research into terminology resulting in new insights into the human body.

Is there any evidence of Arabic erotological works (other than Maimonides' *De Coitu*) having travelled to the West? The simple answer would appear to be 'no'. However, the chronology provides some interesting clues. First, the period of the Latin translations coincides with considerable erotological output being produced in the Muslim world. Second, we know that a number of the works were widely disseminated. Third, it is hardly far-fetched to speculate that 'bestsellers' such as those by an al-Tīfāshī – who was active in Tunisia, which had significant trading links with Italian territories – would have found their way across the Mediterranean, together with other Arabic science manuscripts.

The influence of Arabic sexology and erotology would endure beyond the Middle Ages; as a way of presenting a 'carnal technique',[159] it is difficult to ignore its influence on the erotica of the Italian Renaissance, with authors like Pietro Aretino (1492–1556), whose name lives on in one of the favourite topics in Arabic erotology – sexual positions (*modi*) – even though he merely wrote the sonnets accompanying the engravings by Marcantonio Raimondi (d. 1534).

Aphrodisiacs

In the *Oxford Companion to Food*, Alan Davidson concludes his entry on aphrodisiacs by stating that 'the concept of a truly aphrodisiac food is on a par with that of finding a crock of gold at the end of a rainbow.'[160] Its opening is of the same tenor: 'Aphrodisiacs in the usual sense of foods or drinks which stimulate the sexual appetite and improve performance, are prominent on the list of human 'wannahaves', but virtually non-existent.' He argued that they simply reflected human psychology, as 'sexual appetite ... [may be] increased for some people if they eat something which they know has an aphrodisiac reputation (oysters); or which is thought to bear some resemblance to sexual organs (carrots, figs); or which is so rare and expensive that it creates an atmosphere of luxury or thoughts of wealth and power (such thoughts being sometimes linked to sex).'

The multitude of purportedly aphrodisiac products and concoctions in many cultures would appear to gainsay Davidson's comments, even if, for the most part, Western medicine has not been able to provide supporting evidence.

In medieval Islamic medicine, sexual health was considered an important feature of good health. For instance, in the pharmacological encyclopedia *Minhāj al-bayān fīmā yasta'miluhu al-insān* ('The Pathway of Explanation Regarding That Which Human Beings Use') by the Baghdadi physician Abū 'Alī Yaḥyā Ibn 'Īsā, known as Ibn Jazla (d. 1100), ten per cent of the entries reference sexual potency – only slightly behind the top three of the most frequently encountered conditions, which affected, in ascending order, tumours, the liver, and ulcers. This also explains aphrodisiac properties of the medicines discussed in general medical works. It is, however, important to add that in nearly all cases, sexual potency is mentioned alongside other health benefits provided by the *materia medica*.

Aphrodisiacs in Arabic medical literature are variously referred to as 'increasing' (*zāda*), 'stimulating' (*hayyaja*) or 'strengthening' (*qawwiya*) sexual vigour (*al-bāh*) or intercourse (*al-jimāʿ*), and stirring coital lust (*hayyaja/ḥarraka al-shahwa/shahwat al-jimāʿ*), while individual ingredients are sometimes known as sexual 'strengtheners' (*muqawwiyāt* [*li 'l-jimāʿ/'l-bāh*]).

What makes something an aphrodisiac is linked to a number of factors. At the most general level, they are, to use Maimonides' words, 'foods that produce good, wholesome blood and all those that heat and moisten and that contain flatulence necessary for the erection that is released from the food with the third digestion.'[161]

There was always a link with the individual's temperament as well, and so extremely hot substances, such as pepper, would not be suitable for young people, who already have hot temperaments.

Al-Ṭūsī's book reveals that the substances cut across a number of categories and could be spices, herbs, nuts, tree bark, flowers, cereals, fruits, animals or animal parts and flowers. In all cases, they have other beneficial properties; there are no dedicated aphrodisiacs. Besides the temperament, shape (phallic) or function could be determining factors. Examples of the former include carrots, whereas the latter was particularly related to procreation, as in the case of musk or animal testicles and penises (especially of bulls and wolves), which were thought to be effective as a sexual stimulant because they also increased semen. Some features could clearly trump others; despite being cold and moist, cucumbers were still considered aphrodisiacs by some authors.[162]

The book also prescribes wine on a number of occasions, which is not as surprising as it may seem at first blush since, despite being unlawful in religion, it was considered to be highly potent. The prevailing view is best summed up by Maimonides, who stated that:

> More beneficial than any food or remedy in this regard is wine. There is nothing that can replace it in this respect, because the blood that is produced therefrom is abundant, hot, and moist, and it rejoices the soul and strongly incites to sexual intercourse – because of a specific property it has in addition to its nature, it fills the vessels with beneficial vapor and therefore stimulates an erection – if it is ingested with moderation and after a meal and after leaving the bath. Its effect in this regard is greater than that of anything else.[163]

Rather surprising is the fact that a number of substances that were generally considered very powerful aphrodisiacs in the literature are omitted by al-Ṭūsī. Examples include asparagus[164] or skink (*siqanqūr*), which was considered 'so potent that it continues to stimulate desire unless countered with a broth of lettuce or lentils'.[165]

CHAPTER TWO

The Author

The thirteenth century marks a dramatic turning point in Arab-Islamic history. It witnessed the end of the great ʿAbbāsid caliphate, which had been founded by descendants of ʿAbbās Ibn ʿAbd al-Muṭṭalib, the Prophet's paternal uncle, in 750, following the defeat of the Umayyad dynasty that had succeeded the four 'Rightly Guided Caliphs' (*al-khulafāʾ al-rāshidūn*), who were at the head of the Muslim community (*al-umma*) after the Prophet Muḥammad's demise in 632 CE. The period of the ʿAbbāsid caliphate, which soon after its establishment moved the centre of power from Damascus to Baghdad, built by al-Manṣūr (754–75), is commonly considered the Golden Age of Islam, during which culture, literature, philosophy and the sciences flourished.

That is not to say that the ʿAbbāsid caliphate constituted a monolithic empire between 750 and 1258, or that its cultural and scientific advances continued with unabated vigour throughout its reign. Relatively early on, 'Abbāsid dominion was successfully challenged across its expansive empire, with the emergence of several powerful dynasties, such as the Fatimids (in Northern Africa, including Egypt) and the Seljuqs (in Persia and Central Asia).[166] For a while, the 'Abbāsid caliphs had been reduced to mere vassals of the Būyids, a Persian Shī'ī dynasty, which ruled over Iran and Iraq (10th–11th centuries).[167]

It was in the Seljuq-controlled Tus (Ṭūs)[168] – close to Mashhad in Khorasan province (northeastern Iran), high in the valley of the Kashaf River – that Abū Ja'far Naṣīr (also sometimes Nāṣir) al-Dīn Muḥammad Ibn Muḥammad Ibn al-Ḥasan al-Ṭūsī (al-Shī'ī), usually known as Naṣīr al-Dīn al-Ṭūsī,[169] was born on 11 Jumādā I 597 AH/17 February 1201 CE.[170]

The name of Tus was famous in Arab history as the place where Hārūn al-Rashīd died, though it was eclipsed in importance by the much more famous Nishapur, which had been the capital of the Seljuq dynasty. In the year of al-Ṭūsī's birth, the city was going through a particularly difficult time. Less than a year before it had been a victim in the struggle between the Khwarezmid dynasty (the rulers of Tus) and the Ghūrid empire, which conquered Khorasan. In the process, Tus was besieged and, after surrendering, sacked.

Al-Ṭūsī received his early education under his father's guidance in his native area, and at first focused on the Arabic language and religion, as was common for all scholars of the age. He concentrated in particular on Imāmism, the largest branch of Shī'a Islam, followers of which are also known as 'Twelvers', in reference to their belief in twelve divinely decreed leaders (imams). In his early teens, he left for Nishapur, which was a centre for medicine, and was instructed in mathematics, philosophy, natural science and medicine by former pupils of two famous scholars – the Ash'arite theologian Fakhr al-Dīn al-Rāzī (d. 606/ 1209) and Ibn Sīnā.

It was during al-Ṭūsī's stay in Nishapur that he acquired first-hand experience with those who would eventually destroy Baghdad and establish an empire that stretched across the whole of Asia, the Mongols, when their forces, headed by Genghis Khan's generals Jebe and Sübetey, arrived in the city. As we shall see, this was not the last time that al-Ṭūsī would have direct contact with the Mongols.

After Nishapur, al-Ṭūsī travelled to Iraq, where he completed his training in Islamic (Shī'ī) jurisprudence, followed by mathematics and astronomy in Mosul. In 1233, he went to Sartakht, in Persia's southwest Khuzistan province, and joined the court of the Ismaili governor Muḥtasham Nāṣir al-Dīn 'Abd al-Raḥīm Ibn Abī Manṣūr. It was here that he would start composing his first major works, including two treatises on ethics, both of them dedicated to his patron – *Akhlāq-i Nāṣirī* ('Nāṣirī Ethics') and *Akhlāq-i Muḥtashamī* – as well as an autobiography, *Sayr wa sulūk* ('The Path and Behaviour'), which outlines his spiritual journey towards Ismaili esoteric philosophy.

In the mid-1240s, al-Ṭūsī appeared in Alamūt – the stronghold of the Ismaili community of the Assassins (*ḥashshāshīn*) in the Alburz mountains of northern Iran that had been founded by Ḥasan al-Ṣabāḥ (d. 1124). The reasons behind his journey remain open to debate, but al-Ṭūsī ended up staying there for two decades, and in 1255 was sent to Hülegü, the Mongol Khan, who was about to attack Persia. The Assassin fortress fell to the Mongols a year later, as they swept through the region and headed west towards Baghdad. Al-Ṭūsī joined Hülegü's entourage on his campaigns, and was present at the capture of the capital of the Sunni caliphate in February 1258, which also resulted in the murder of the last caliph, al-Mustaʿṣim bi-llāh. Al-Ṭūsī enjoyed the favour of the Mongol ruler and it was thanks to the scholar that many of the Shīʿī sanctuaries were spared destruction. However, even before the sacking of Baghdad, al-Ṭūsī had been given a number of official duties, including court astrologer, and was put in charge of the religious endowments (*awqāf*) and finances – duties he continued to discharge under Hülegü's son and successor, Ābāqā (1265–82).

In 1259, al-Ṭūsī oversaw the construction of an observatory (*raṣadkhāneh*) in Marāgha (currently in Iran's East Azerbaijan Province), which Hülegü had made his capital. The observatory, which also comprised a large library and school, became a hugely important scientific institution and centre of learning that attracted many leading scholars of the day, including Chinese astronomers. In addition to heading the observatory, al-Ṭūsī compiled astronomical tables (*al-Zīj al-Īlkhānī*, 'Ilkhanate Tables') for calculating the positions of the planets.[171] Astronomy earned him great fame for many centuries to come, as did his work on planetary theory, which would later inform the work of Copernicus and others. Extracts of the tables were translated into Latin by John Greaves (1602–52), who was then the Savilian Professor of Astronomy at Oxford, as well as an accomplished Arabist and Persianist. The text was published in 1648, together with the astronomical and chronological tables of the Timurid scholar-sultan Ulugh Beg (1394–1449).[172] Although the observatory was short-lived (it remained in operation for about fifty years), it would have a large impact on astronomy in both China and Europe in subsequent centuries.

Shortly before his death, al-Ṭūsī left Marāgha for Baghdad, where he died a few months later, on 18 Dhū 'l-Ḥijja 672 AH (25 June 1274 CE), at the age of seventy-two. His body was laid to rest near the tomb of Mūsā al-Kāẓim (744–99), the seventh of the Twelve Imams (and son of the sixth, Jaʿfar al-Ṣādiq).

A prolific polymath, al-Ṭūsī, who has been called the most important Shīʿī scholar of his age, built up a huge oeuvre (in excess of 150 works in both Arabic and Persian) across a wide range of fields, including mathematics, physics, geometry, mineralogy, astronomy, medicine, philosophy, ethics, mysticism and Islamic law (*fiqh*). In addition to composing original works, he prepared editions and wrote commentaries on Greek and Arabic mathematical works (including those of Euclid, Archimedes and Thābit Ibn Qurra), which became crucial resources in the spread of the Greek sciences in the Muslim world.

In the field of medicine, al-Ṭūsī wrote three other works besides the one treated here: *Qawānīn al-ṭibb* ('The Principles of Medicine');[173] *al-Risāla al-dhahabiyya fī tadbīr ḥifẓ al-ṣiḥḥa* ('Golden Treatise on the Regimen of Health');[174] and *Sharḥ qawl al-shaykh al-ra'īs anna 'l-ḥarāra taf'alu fi 'l-raṭab sawādan wa fī ḍiddihi bayāḍan* ('Commentary on the Statement by the Great Master [Ibn Sīnā] that Heat Causes Blackness in Moistness and Whiteness in the Opposite').[175]

Al-Ṭūsī's reputation spread very quickly throughout Islamic territories, and his commentary on Ibn Sīnā's *Kitāb al-ishārāt wa 'l-tanbīhāt* ('Book of Hints and Pointers'), entitled *Ḥall mushkilāt al-ishārāt* ('The Solution to the Problems in the *Ishārāt*'), was singled out for praise by none other than the Tunisian historian Ibn Khaldūn (1332–1406), who applied the Qur'ānic verse (XII, 76) *wa fawqa kulli dhī 'ilmin 'alīmun* ('and over every lord of knowledge there is one more knowing') when comparing al-Ṭūsī's work to that of others.[176]

Later on, others bestowed equally grand epithets on the Persian scholar, such as *ustādh al-bashar* ('the teacher of mankind'), *al-mu'allim al-thālith* 'the third teacher' – the other two being Aristotle and the philosopher al-Fārābī (d. 950) – or, most commonly, *al-Khwāja* ('Master').[177]

CHAPTER THREE

The Sultan's Potions

Contents and Structure

The text translated here was the only book written on the subject by al-Ṭūsī, and is modest in its aims inasmuch as it treats only aphrodisiacs. The title, *Kitāb albāb al-Bāhiyya wa 'l-tarākīb al-sulṭāniyya,* literally translates as 'The Book of Choice Sexual Stimulants and the Sultan's Mixtures.'[178] Dedicated to 'the Sultan of Qāzān' (the Ilkhanid Ābāqā Khan, r. 1265-1282), al-Ṭūsī mentions that the book was written at the ruler's request, since he had a child suffering from paraplegia. The motive behind the request is predicated in the belief that the quality and strength of sexual intercourse impact on the offspring that results from it, with the disability of the child being linked to the father's coital deficiency.

As for the intended readership, the author

recommends his treatise as a self-study manual: 'Anyone reading this treatise will no longer need a physician for medical treatment as it contains all the reader requires to treat ailments and diseases.' In the introduction the author states that the book is a compendium of existing knowledge, which raises the question of sources. In addition to Greek authors (Galen, Hippocrates, Aristotle), the only Arabic physician named is al-Rāzī, whereas the author's Shīʿa affiliations are revealed by a quote from ʿAlī Ibn Abī Ṭālib. Other sources are referred to, simply, as 'past scholars'. In none of these cases, however, is there a mention of the works from which the information was allegedly culled.

Despite its declared focus on aphrodisiacs, the treatise touches upon many of the topics addressed in erotological literature, and may therefore be put at the 'scientific/medical' end of the continuum discussed in Chapter 1. Like other works in this category, it combines the fields of medicine, dietetics, hygiene and erotology, but is devoid of anecdotes, poetry and stories intended for titillation. The author's approach appears by then to have become firmly established, as it is shared by many other authors.

The text comprises an introduction and eighteen chapters of uneven length, with some very brief ones alternating with more extensive ones. As is customary for many manuals of the period, the introduction outlines the reason for writing the treatise and the author's expert credentials in the field. It also provides a table of contents, which includes not only the titles of the chapters (or variants thereof) but also a brief description of their contents. This is followed by general information on key medical concepts, such as semen and the need, lawfulness and advantages of coitus, as well as the best seasons to engage in it. While there is 'no greater human pleasure than that of sexual intercourse', the author warns against excess, as this reduces innate heat. This was in line with the prevailing (Galenic) orthodoxy that frequent ejaculation resulted in a loss of *pneuma* (Ar. *rūḥ*) and its vitalizing power.

Chapter 1 addresses the link between sexual potency and lust for coitus, on the one hand, and physiognomy and the individual's temperament, on the other. At the top end of the scale, it appears, are those with coloured skins as well as some with white skins, though another section of the latter are incapable of having sex. This leads to a discussion of the reasons for the weakness of organs (including, of course, the penis), the symptoms and how each of them can be treated through syrups, electuaries and broths. The author identifies four *loci* which, when afflicted with weakness, cause limpness in the body's organs: the brain, heart, liver, penis and testicles. As for the weakness in the (male) genitals, this can be due to one of three factors: innateness, excess intercourse from an early age, or being over the age of forty. Despite the author's claim that the book is a compendium, the information is sometimes tantalizingly compressed; the author refers, for instance, to a multitude of benefits for this or that concoction (for example, musk and spikenard electuaries) but these are omitted for reasons of conciseness.

Chapters 2 and 3 list simple foodstuffs that are used to increase libido and potency, whereas Chapter 4 concentrates on compounds that serve the same purpose, in addition to restoring temperament imbalances and increasing innate heat. The various concoctions, ingredients and cooking methods are given in detail, including when to consume them. When it comes to the effects, hyperbole is never far away; the reader is advised that eating a particular dish will enhance his stamina to the extent that he is able to pleasure ten women every night!

The following three chapters plough the same general furrow, outlining syrups, electuaries and stomachics, which, in addition to acting as aphrodisiacs, restore the temperament and purify the blood (Chapter 5); strengthen various organs, remove excess humours, open up blockages (Chapter 6); and eliminate various qualities and humours (Chapter 7). Enemas intended to increase potency, as well as remedying colic and back weakness, constitute the object of Chapter 8. The next chapter discusses the types of clothing fabric that should be worn in each of the seasons, and how they assist in preventing illness.

Chapter 10 devotes attention to the sexual positions that are to be preferred, which ones to avoid, and the possible harmful effects they may cause. The next four chapters are squarely phallocentric, enumerating ointments to be rubbed on the penis to stiffen and lengthen it (Chapters 11 and 12); or in between the fingers and toes in order to maintain an erection, even after having intercourse with ten women (Chapter 13).

Moving on from penile prowess, Chapter 14 contains recipes for pleasure- and potency-enhancing pills. In Chapter 15, the woman is brought into the equation, with suggestions for various concoctions to ensure ecstasy during coitus for both partners. Chapter 16 continues the focus on the woman, albeit from the man's point of view, offering recipes aimed at narrowing the vagina and 'restoring' it to that of a virgin, which was in keeping with the prevailing – and religiously endorsed – gender orthodoxy. Besides potions for the same purpose, the final chapters provide concoctions for the purposes of contraception (Chapter 17) and conception (Chapter 18). Interestingly enough, recipes in the former have gall as their main ingredient which also appears in a number of aphrodisiacs.

The potions, drugs and therapies are gendered in that they are mainly aimed at improving the man's coital performance and experience, with a focus on frequency of intercourse and penile strength. Coitus within marriage is conspicuous by its absence, as the sexual partners referred to are generally hierarchically inferior (servants) – which, as we have seen, is a prominent feature of both erotological and erotic literature.

How innovative was al-Ṭūsī and what was his

influence, if any, on the genre and subsequent works? While some elements are similar to those of other treatises, others are unique to al-Ṭūsī. We have seen that the work was translated into Persian and Turkish, which would suggest that it was held in high esteem, if only because of the reputation of its author – which he himself expounds upon at length at the beginning of his book, referring to himself as the 'erudite *shaykh*', the 'king of scholars' and the 'teacher of scholars of all time'. It is, therefore, surprising to note that the extant erotological works do not contain any mention of the treatise or seem to have availed themselves of al-Ṭūsī's contribution. However, the Bodleian manuscript, which will be discussed in the next section, shows that substantial parts of al-Ṭūsī's text circulated and became part of other collections. A more detailed study of the erotological corpus will undoubtedly uncover new insights into al-Ṭūsī's influence on the field.

The Manuscripts

No autograph copy of the text is known to have survived. This critical edition is based on five manuscript copies, which are considered below. There is a sixth known manuscript of the text (Istanbul, Shahid Ali No 1/2068),[179] which, however, was excluded because it proved impossible to consult it.

1. Berlin, Staatsbibliothek, Wetzstein II 1189 – Ahlwardt 6383; dated 1208 AH/1793 CE, 35 folios (68pp), with fifteen lines per page, and catchwords. This is the oldest dated copy of al-Ṭūsī's treatise. Although the copyist is not mentioned, the name of Muṣṭtafā al-Kaftānī is included at the end of the second medical manuscript (an untitled translation of an anonymous Turkish treatise)[180] with which it is bound, and which bears the same date. The oriental *naskh* script of both texts is clearly identical and thus it is highly likely that the same copyist also produced this version of al-Ṭūsī's text. The Berlin manuscript contains a number of errors and marginal additions and corrections (indicated in the Arabic and English texts by braces). Many of the errors involve interference from the vernacular. In addition, there are also numerous orthographic and grammatical inconsistencies and mistakes (for instance, subject-verb agreement, declensions and conjugation patterns). As it is the oldest and most complete of the three manuscripts, it has been chosen for the critical edition, where it is referred to as [A].[181] The page numbers in the English translation also refer to it.

2. Glasgow University, MS Hunter 144.4 (T.7.3), eleven folios (22pp), twenty-seven lines per page. The manuscript is the fourth in a bound collection including three other treatises on medicine.

The first is a commentary by Muḥammad al-ʿAskarī, entitled *Ḥall al-Mūjiz* ('Solution of the Abridgement'), on the abridgement of Ibn Sīnā's *Qānūn* (*Mūjiz al-Qānūn*), composed by the Syrian physician Ibn al-Nafīs (d. 1288). The second is an Arabic translation of the famous epitome of the *Qānūn*, entitled *al-Qānūnja*, by the fourteenth-century Persian physician Maḥmūd Ibn Muḥammad Ibn ʿUmar al-Jaghmīnī.[182] The third is an Arabic translation of an (anonymous) Turkish work on colds (*Risālat al-Nāzila*). The Glasgow manuscript, whose date, copyist and origin are unknown, was copied in a tighter Farsi *nastaʿlīq* hand. It is almost identical with [A], save for a few minor variations and omissions. One may conjecture that it was copied after [A], which may have served as the original. It has far fewer language errors than [A]. This manuscript is referred to as [B] in the present edition.

3. Cairo, Dār al-Kutub, *Ṭibb* 582; dated 18 Rabīʿ I 1334/03.05.1809; eleven folios (20pp), nineteen lines per page, with catchwords and some marginalia. This manuscript is incomplete and also the most recently dated. It is unclear whether it was copied from any of the others, and thus significantly emendated and/or poorly copied, or whether it should be traced back to another, hitherto unknown copy. In addition to

substantive omissions, which include an entire chapter (4), there are a number of colloquialisms and orthographic and grammatical errors. This manuscript is referred to as [C] in the present edition.

4. London, British Library, Or 11213, thirty-one folios, 208 x 135mm (153 x 100mm written area); thirteen lines per page; black ink with red rubricated headings, and black double frames around text areas on each page; some marginalia (folios 15v., 19r., 20r. 21v., 22r., 25r.). The text is written in a clear *naskh* script, with catchwords. The name of the scribe is given as Muḥammad ʿAlī Ibn Ḥusayn bn Ḥasan al-Jazāʾirī (fol. 31v, lines 6–7). This copy was purchased in 1930 from the German Orientalist – and avid manuscript collector – Oskar Rescher (1883–1972), who had acquired it during his residence in Istanbul. According to the catalogue, the copy dates from the nineteenth century. This manuscript is referred to as [D] in the present edition.

5. Oxford University, Bodleian, MS. Marsh 530 (item 3), forty-three folios (108r–151v.), fifteen lines per page, medium-large casual *naskh* script with headings in red (sometimes gold-sprinkled, as on folio 131b) and yellow/orange, while folio 149 is dyed yellow. There are catchwords, some

marginal headings and a few marginalia. The manuscript is part of the collection bequeathed to the Bodleian by Narcissus Marsh (1638–1713), who was successively Archbishop of Cashel, Archbishop of Dublin and Archbishop of Armagh. The manuscript is undated but according to the most recent catalogue 'the paper, ink and script suggests a dating of the eleventh/seventeenth to twelfth/eighteenth century'. Until now, this text was not identified as a copy of al-Ṭūsī's work, and is listed in the catalogue as an anonymous 'essay on sexual hygiene, with recipes'.[183] In another catalogue, it was said to be part of a copy of Ibn al-Bayṭār's *Kitāb al-Mughnī*.[184] The text is the third item in Marsh 530, and is preceded by a work entitled *al-Īdāhiyya fi 'l-umūr al-nikāhiyya* (fols. 1r.–59r.), described as a 'collection of pieces with sexual hygiene transcribed from various unidentified writers',[185] and an anonymous 'collection of medical and magical extracts and recipes [which] includes sections on the treatment of haemorhoids and diseases of the head and eyes, as well as magcial names useful against poisons' (fols. 59v–107r.).[186] It is followed by a short treatise on the properties and benefits of the radish (fols. 152v.–153v.)[187] This copy of al-Ṭūsī's work is the least reliable, as it is incomplete and jumbled up. Chapter 4 is on folio 116r., the fifth on 118r. and the eleventh on 120r., which is followed by the thirteenth on folio 120v. and the eighteenth on folio 124v. It jumps from Chapter 7 to Chapter 11, while it lacks a section from Chapter 11 and the entirety of Chapter 12. As a result, it does not contain the eighteen chapters referred to in the Bodleian catalogue. In addition, there are two recipes missing from Chapter 6. Conversely, it adds recipes not included in any of the other copies. There are some indications that, at least in part, it was based on [D]. The text starts (fol. 108r.) with a recipe on penis lengthening, which is part of Chapter 12 in the other manuscripts, and is followed by the discussion of principal organs, which is usually in the Introduction. The volume has a nineteenth-century European library binding, but it is possible, and even likely, that the manuscript acquired by Marsh was already jumbled up. On the whole, it it is a very corrupted copy with a large number of lapsus calami, which often hampers comprehension, as in, for instance, *'āqir qarḥā* ('pellitory') being rendered by the nonsensical *qīrāṭ 'araq al-qirāṭ*. Finally, the Bodleian catalogue also fails to specify that al-Ṭūsī's text only goes to folio 126r., after which there are a series of other recipes clearly drawn from a variety of sources. Confusingly, the musk electuary and the recipes following it in chapter 1 are repeated on folio 146r., after a recipe for coughs, with other recipes relating to a variety of subjects, including itch, sleep, and so on. The text reveals a not uncommon practice of cherry-picking sections on a particular topic from multiple sources to produce an eclectic manual or digest of sorts. These types of works were often anonymous and enjoyed not inconsiderable circulation. This manuscript is referred to as [E] in the present edition.

Notes

1. al-Nafzāwī n.d.: 28.
2. al-Nafzāwī (J. Colville trans.) 1999: 33.
3. al-Nafzāwī (R. Burton trans.) 1886: 34.
4. The passage is as follows in the original:
Et, lorsque la cessation de la jouissance aura mis un terme à vos ébats amoureux, gardez-vous de vous lever brusquement, mais restez près de la femme, couchez-vous sur le côté droit dans le lit témoin de vos plaisirs et retirez votre membre avec précaution; car c'est en agissant ainsi que vous trouverez le bien, et vous ne serez pas comme celui qui monte sur la femme ainsi qu'un mulet, sans avoir égard aux vrais principes de l'art, et qui, dès qu'il a éjaculé, s'empresse de se relever en retirant son membre. Une telle manière d'agir doit être écartée, car elle ne peut qu'éloigner tout bien des femmes. En résumé, il appartient au véritable amateur du coït de n'omettreaucune de mes recommandations; car, c'est de leur observation que résulte le bonheur de la femme, et ces règles comprennent tout ce qui convient en pareille matière. Dieu a tout fait pour le bien!
Mohamed Lasly, ed., Le jardin parfumé, Paris: Philippe Picquier, 2002, pp. 155–6. The earliest preserved French translation dates from 1848 (mss Paris BN SG MS8-60 [1336]).
5. For background and a discussion of this term, which is often used in conjunction with 'foreignization' and 'domestication' of the source text, see L. Venuti, *The Translator's Invisibility: A History of Translation*, London: Routledge, 1995.
6. B. Lewis 1993: 71.
7. R. Burton 1885–89: X, 173ff.
8. *ibid.*, 205.
9. *ibid.*, 206ff.
10. This term is used in preference to others, such as 'Arab' or 'Islamic', as the former would imply that the authors involved were ethnically Arabs, which was not the case. The term 'Islamicate' was coined by Michael Hodgson (1977: 59), who reserved 'Islamic' for 'pertaining to Islam *in the proper, the religious, sense*' (emphasis in the original), with 'Islamicate' referring 'not directly to the religion, Islam, itself, but to the social and cultural complex historically associated with Islam and the Muslims, both among Muslims themselves and even when found

among non-Muslims'.

11. Ṣ. al-Munajjid 1957, 1969, 1975; M. ᶜAbd al-Wāḥīd 1961; Y. El-Masri 1962; G. H. Bousquet 1966; R. Devereux 1966; L. Giffen 1971; A. Bouhdiba 1975; A. L. Al-Sayyid-Marsot 1979; B. Musallam 1983; D. Ze'evi 2006. To these, one may also add the 'popularizing' works on the subject by Malek Chebel (1984, 1986, 1988, 1995, 2004, 2006).
12. F. Rosenthal 1978; S. Murray and W. Roscoe 1979; A. Abu Khalil 1993; B. Nathan 1994; J. Wright and E. Rowson 1997; J. Dakhlia 2007; K. El-Rouayheb 2005; E. Rowson 1991b, 1997, 2003, 2004, 2006, 2008; P. Steckler 2007–8. Most of these centre on male homosexuality, with lesbianism being the focus in H. Samar 2007 and S. Amar 2009. An Iranian perspective on the issue is offered by A. Najmabadi 2005.
13. M. Cervulle 2008, 2009; M. Ghoussoub and E. Sinclair-Webb 2000; F. Lagrange 2000; O. Lahoucine 2006; A. Schmitt and J. Sofer 1992; M. Schildt 1988.
14. S. Amar, 'Cross-Dressing and Female Same-Sex Marriage in Medieval French and Arabic Literatures', in K. Babayan and A. Najmabadi 2008; E. Rowson 1991a.
15. P. Saunders 1991.
16. U. Wikan 1977 (in present-day Oman).
17. K. Ali 2006; N. J. Coulson, 'Regulation of Sexual Behavior under Traditional Islamic Law', in A. L. Al-Sayyid-Marsot 1979: 63–8. In this area, too, homosexuality has received a great deal of attention: H. El Menyawi; A. Shalakany 2008; S. Yep 2012; A. Schmitt 2001–2.
18. D. Hopwood 1999.
19. For a discussion, see J. Massad 2002.
20. This is the case, for instance, for a chapter on homosexuality and the reasons why some men prefer sexual intercourse with teenage boys to women in al-Isrā'ilī's *Nuzhat al-aṣḥāb fī muʿāshirat al-aḥbāb* ('A Jaunt amidst Lovers' Copulation'): 2007: 49. A few pages down, the word *nayk* ('fucking') is emendated, while a footnote states: 'A word meaning "sexual intercourse", which we have preferred not to mention' (52).
21. Ed. J. Jumʿa, Beirut: Riad El-Rayyes, 1994.
22. For instance, al-Tīfāshī's *Tuḥfat al-albāb fīmā lā jūjad fī kitāb*, whose (abridged) English translation (Edward A. Lacey, *The Delight of Hearts: Or, What You Will Not Find in Any Book,* Los Angeles: Gay Sunshine Press, 1988) is based on the French text (R. Khawam, *Les délices des coeurs,* Paris: Jérôme Martineau, 1971; rev. eds, Paris: Phébus, 1981, 1988), rather than on the original Arabic.
23. David Semah and George J. Kanazi, Wiesbaden: Otto Harrassowitz, 2003. See also D. Semakh, '*Rawḍat al-Qulūb* by al-Shayzarī: A Twelfth-Century Book on Love', Arabica 24 (1997): 187–206.
24. See also *EI*[2], s.v. 'muḳawwiyāt' (F. Sanagustin).
25. For an overview of Islamic medicine, see P. Pormann and E. Savage-Smith 2007.

26. The 'Compendium' was first translated into Latin as *Liber Continens* by the Jewish physician and translator Faraj Ibn Sālim (Lat. *Farraguth*) for King Charles of Anjou (1226–85) in the last quarter of the thirteenth century. It was printed for the first time in 1515, in Lyon.
27. *EI*², s.v. 'Ibn al-Ḳuff' (S. H. Hamarneh). For the part dealing with simple drugs, see H. G. Kircher 1967.
28. It was first translated into Latin in the thirteenth century, by the already-mentioned Farraguth, and published in 1531 as *Tacuinum Sanitatis* (Strassburg: J. Schott). It was a key medical text in Europe for many centuries.
29. cf. I. Perho 1995; F. Rahman 1989; W. Rasslan 1934; 'A. al-Sharīf 1990. On sexuality in this literature, see U. Weisser 1983; J. Bummel 1999.
30. al-Suyūṭī n.d.: 24–6, 159–67 (recipes of various aphrodisiacal electuaries).
31. See R. Serjeant 1965; O. Spies 1969.
32. See Madelain Farah (trans.), *Marriage and Sexuality in Islam: A Translation of Al-Ghazali's Book on the Etiquette of Marriage from the Ihya 'ulūm al-dīn*, Salt Lake City, UT: University of Utah Press, 1986. Extracts from the erotological sections were also published separately, in *al-Jins 'inda 'l-'Arab*, vol. 3, 127–47.
33. The whole of Book 6 is devoted to the subject (see G. Bos 1997).
34. G. Bos [al-Jazzār] 1992: 23–7.
35. O. Kahle 2003.
36. See, for instance, cookery books from Egypt dating to the fourteenth (Anonymous 1993: Nos. 75–6, 185, 187–8, 376, 478, 518; Appendix No. 68) and fifteenth (D. Newman 2020: No. 111) centuries, from ninth-century Baghdad (al-Warrāq 1987: 54, 110–1, 312, 318–9) and thirteenth-century al-Andalus (D. Newman 2023: No. 19).
37. For a discussion, see B. Musallam 1983; A. Bouhdiba 1975 (esp. 143ff); *EI*², s.v. ''azl' (G. H. Bousquet).
38. See Franke 2012; *EI*², s.vv. 'bāh' (G. H. Bousquet), 'djins' (Ch. Pellat), 'nikāḥ' (J. Schacht et al.); 'zinā'' (R. Peters); Davidson 2011: 10; E. Lane: I, 315; IV, 451; VIII, 102; al-Suyūṭī 2001: 119ff.
39. D. Ze'ev 2006: 16.
40. See for example J. C. Bürgel, 'Love, Lust and Longing: Eroticism in Early Islam as Reflected in Literary Sources', in A. al-Sayyid-Marsot 1977: 81–117.
41. See *EI*², s.v. 'djins' (C. Pellat).
42. See list at the end of the Introduction.
43. Ibn al-Nadim 1871–72: II, 306 (trans. II, 719–23) – 51 entries.
44. *ibid.*, 307 (trans. II, 721) – 12 entries.
45. *ibid.*, 306–7 (trans. II, 720–1) – 28 entries.
46. *ibid.*, 307–8 (trans. II, 722–3) – 38 entries.
47. For the introduction of Rufus's works in Islamic medicine, see *GAS*, III: 64–8; M. Ullmann 1970: 71–6; *EI*², s.v. 'Rūfūs al-Afsīsī' (M.

Ullmann). Ibn Lūqā 1974: 26 (trans. 34); 1973: 43 (trans. 29), 47 (trans. 31). For one of Ibn Lūqā's translations of Rufus, see Hakim Syed Zillur Rahman, ed., *Risalah al Nabidh' of Rufus by Qusta bin Luqa* (on wine) and *Risalah fi Auja al Niqris by Qusta Ibn Luqa* (on gout ache) both published by Ibn Sina Academy of Medieval Medicine and Sciences, Aligarh, 2007.

48. *EI*², s.v. 'Diyuskuridīs' (C. E. Dubler); *EI*³, s.v. "Dioscorides" (Leigh Chipman); M. Ullmann 1970: 257–63; John M. Riddle, *Dioscorides on Pharmacy and Medicine*, Austin: University of Texas Press, 1986. For the Arabic transmission his work, see Manfred Ullmann, *Untersuchungen zur arabischen Überlieferung der Materia medica des Dioskurides*, Wiesbaden: O. Harrassowitz, 2009.

49. For the introduction of Galenic works in Islamic medicine, see M. Ullmann 1970: 35ff; *GAS*, III, 274ff; *EI*², s.v. 'Djālīnūs (R. Walzer).

50. For Hipocrates in the Arabic tradition, see M. Ullmann 1970: 25–35; *GAS*, III, 23–47; *EI*², s.v. 'Bukrāṭ' (A. Dietrich); P. E. Pormann (ed.), *Epidemics in Context: Greek Commentaries on Hippocrates in the Arabic Tradition*, Berlin: de Gruyter, 2012.

51. See D. Newman 2015; D. Gutas 1998; R. Walzer 1962; D. Jacquart and F. Michaud 1990: 32–33. For the developments in literature, see J. Ashtiany *et al.* (eds) 1990.

52. *EI*², s.vv. 'Ḥunayn b. Isḥāḳ al-'Ibādī' and 'Isḥāḳ b. Ḥunayn' (G. Strohmaier). For Ḥunayn's biography, see G. Bergstrasser, 'Hunain ibn Ishaq, Über die syrischen und arabischen Galen-Übersetzungen', *Abhandlungen für die Kunde des Morgenlandes* XVII: 2 (1925), XIX: 2 (1932).

53. *EI*², s.v. 'Ibn Māsawayh' (J.-C. Vadet).

54. On Ibn Bukhtīshū[c] and his family, see *EI*², s.v. 'Bukhtīshū[c]' (D. Sourdel); *Encyclopaedia Iranica*, s.v. "Boktīšū'" (Lutz Richter-Bernburg); A. Contadini, . *A World of Beasts: A Thirteenth-Century Illustrated Arabic Book on Animals (the Kitāb Na't al-Ḥayawān) in the Ibn Bakhtīshū' Tradition*, Leiden: Brill, 2012.

55. D. Jacquart and F. Micheau 1990; H. H. Biesterfeldt, 'Zur medizinischen Terminologie des arabisch-islamischen Mittelalters', in D. Jacquart 1994: 66-90; *EI*², s.v. "Djālīnūs (R. Walzer).

56. This work consists of thirty-eight chapters each dealing with a particular medical subject in the form of questions and answers. Chapter X had previously inspired an earlier translation/adaptation by the physician Thābit Ibn Qurra (Chapter X), whereas Ibn Māssa (1971: 33–4) used Chapter IV (No. 31). For a discussion, see R. Kruk 1976.

57. P. Pormann and E. Savage-Smith 2007: 105–8.

58. al-Kātib 1977: 334ff.

59. See H. N. Parker 1992: 92.

60. *ibid.*

61. *ibid.*, 100.

62. For more details, see, for example: M. Dols 1984: 3–24; P. Pormann and E. Savage-Smith 2007: 41ff; M. Ullmann 1970: 97–100, 108–84; M. Green 1985: 323–7; Ibn Sīnā 1999: I, 28–35.
63. The theory was also an integral part of prophetic medicine; see, for example, al-Suyūṭī n.d.: 2–5.
64. Adapted from www.calvin.edu/academic/medieval/medicine/overview/overview.htm.
65. See Ibn Sīnā 1999: I, 19–23; R. M. Stelmack and A. Stalikas, 'Galen and the Humour Theory of Temperament', *Personality and Individual Differences* 12: 3 (1991), pp. 255–63.
66. D. Jacquart and C. Thomasset 1988: 36ff.
67. For a discussion of the Galenic view on sexual differences between men and women, see for example Gadelrab 2010, and M. Levey and S. Souryal, 'Galen's On the Secrets of Women and on the Secrets of Men: A Contribution to the History of Arabic Pharmacology,' *Janus* 55 (1968), pp. 208–19.
68. M. Ullmann 1978: 23–4.
69. G. Bos 1997: 135 (trans. 266) – Ibn Māsawayh; 136 (trans. 267) – Isḥāq Ibn 'Imrān.
70. *ibid.*, 138 (trans. 267).
71. al-Jāḥiẓ 1938: VII, 226. See also, in the same work: II, 216 (wolves and dogs), V, 218–19 (on birds); and al-Kātib 1977: 365ff.
72. *ibid.*: VII, 29.
73. Abū Tammām, *Diwan*, 172, 11.
74. Ibn al-Jawzī 1902: 142.
75. Ibn al-Nadīm 1871–72: II, 303.
76. Ibn Abī Uṣaybiʿa 1882: I, 34, 69.
77. al-Kātib 1977: 216, 229, 251, 332ff., 370; 2002: 23, 29.
78. al-Tīfāshī 1892: 64; S. al-Munajjid 1975: 154–5; al-Kātib 1977: 75.
79. See P. Pormann and E. Savage-Smith 2007: 21–3; M. Meyerhof, 'On the Transmission of Greek and Indian Science to the Arabs', *Islamic Culture*, 1937, 11, pp. 17–29; *GAS*, III, 191ff. The traditional view regarding the importance of Gondēshāpūr as a centre for medical care (including a hospital), training and scholarship has recently been called into question on the grounds that the earliest report on the hospital dates from the thirteenth century, in the work of the Egyptian historian al-Qifṭī. Even if this is true, the reputation of the town as a medical centre is less uncertain, as it is already referred to in the ninth century, by al-Jāḥiẓ. See *EI*[2], s.v. 'Gondēshāpūr' (Cl. Huart-Aydin Sayili); P. Pormann and E. Savage-Smith 2007: 20–1; M. Dols 1984: 5–6; R. Serjeant 1997: 86.
80. C. Storey 1972: 321–322.
81. Ibn Qutayba 1925–30: I, 24–5, 27–8, 30.
82. Ibn al-Nadīm 1871–72: II, 303.
83. The whole of Chapter XII is devoted to Indian physicians.
84. Ibn al-Nadīm (trans. B. Dodge) 1970: II, 738; *GAS*: III, 193–6.

85. al-Rāzī 1955–68: III, 210; V, 179; VI, 30, 47, 214; VIII, 205, X, 18, 133, 331; XII, 219.
86. Ibn al- Nadīm 1871–72: II, 245, 303.
87. *vide post.*
88. al-Tīfāshī 1970: 13ff. (trans. 27ff.) vs Ibn Sīnā (Cairo 519, f. 6).
89. For instance, Ibn al-Jazzār mentions a decoction of roots created by Ibn Māsawayh (G. Bos 1997: 135 – trans.: 266) and a powder composed by Isḥāq Ibn ʿImrān (*ibid.*, 136 – trans.: 267).
90. al-Tīfāshī 1892: 76ff/Deli Birader [S. Kuru 2000]: 208ff./al-Kātib 2002: 105ff.; trans. 299ff. (anal intercourse positions); Abū Nuwās 1994: 71 (trans. P. Kenney 2005: 40–2)/Deli Birader [S. Kuru 2000]: 193; al-Tīfāshī 1992: 207ff./Deli Birader [S. Kuru 2000]: 202ff./al-Kātib 1977: 323ff. (homosexual prowler).
91. al-Kātib 1977: 57, 330, 331.
92. Gotha 105; Gotha 124; Dresden 172.
93. For example, Bodleian 1622.
94. The most famous of his works is *Lawʿat al-shākī wa damʿat al-bākī* ('The Anxiety of the Complaining Lover and the Tears of the Weeper'). ʻU. al-Kaḥḥāla n.d.: IV, 113; XIII, 385; 'al-Ṣafadī' *EI*[1], (F. Krenkow); *EI*[2], (F. Rosenthal); *GAL* II: 39–41, *GALS* II: 27–9.
95. *EI*[2], s.v. 'al-Ḥillī' (W. P. Heinrichs). His works include *Risālat al-ashwāq fīmā yataʿalliqu bi 'l-ʿushshāq* ('Treatise on Longings Connected with Lovers') for instance, BN 3074.
96. *EI*[2], s.v. 'al-Nawādjī' (I. Kratschkowsky). He is most famous for his anthologies of erotic poetry, especially related to the love of boys, for example, *Khalʿat al-ʿidhār fī waṣf al-ʿidhār* ('Throwing Off All Restraint in the Description of the First Growth of Beard') (BN3041), and *Kitāb ṣaḥā'if al-ḥasanāt* (BN 3041).
97. Al-Kātib 1977: 35.
98. *ibid.*: 36.
99. D. Jacquart and C. Thomasset 1988: 126.
100. M. Foucault 1978–90: II, 50; H. N. Parker 1992: 98.
101. Even references to fellatio are quite rare in the literature: al-Tīfāshī 1892: part II, 65; *idem* 1992: 285.
102. For example, Ibn Sīnā 1999: II, 746–7 (penis size), 746 (hermaphroditism), 730–1 (impotence), 728–9 (benefits of coitus), 744–5 (priapism), 745–6 (*ubna*), 745 (*ʿudhaywiṭ*, involving orgasm-induced defecation).
103. M. Foucault 1978–90: II, 4.
104. *ibid.*: I, 11.
105. al-Ghazlāwī (BN 3069): 1.
106. Ibn Sīnā 1999: II, 746.
107. For Galen, see Siegel 1976: 185; de Lacy 1992: 150–1. This was also discussed by Ibn al-Quff (d. 1286) in his commentary on the Hippocratic Aphorisms (see Selove and Batten 2014; Batten 2018: 113), and Maimonides' aphorisms (G. Bos 2022: 327). Also see: P.

Myrne 2020: 13-14, 22-4, 32-4.

108. See, for instance, the stories in al-Tīfāshī 1892: 70–9; al-Nafzāwī n.d.: 55–6, 45–50. Also see S. S. Gadelrab 2010.

109. For example, Fatima Mernissi, 'The Muslim Concept of Active Female Sexuality,' *Women and Sexuality in Medieval Societies* (Istanbul: Women for Women's Rights/Kadinin Insan Haklan Projesi, 2000), pp. 19–35.

110. al-Jāḥiẓ 1938: I, 370–2; II, 203–4; IV, 117–18; al-Tīfāshī 1892: 90 (story of a woman having sex with a donkey), 92 (about a woman and a bear).

111. M. Foucault 1978–90: II, 92.

112. H, N. Parker 1992: 91, 98.

113. M. Foucault 1978–90: II, 25.

114. *ibid.*, II, 25–6.

115. al-Tīfāshī 1892: 2.

116. Qur'ān, VII, 80, 81; XXVI, 165–8; XXVII, 54–6; XXIX, 28–9.

117. The usual contemporary term, *mithlī*, is a late-twentieth-century neologism.

118. For a full discussion, see K. El Rouayheb 2005.

119. See *EI*[2], s.v. 'liwāṭ' (ed.). For discussion of the views on male homosexuality in Islamic jurisprudence, see A. Schmidt 2001–2; Shalakany 2008.

120. K. El-Rouayheb 2005; 15. The same has been observed for ancient Greece and Rome: see K. Dover 1984: 143–57; C. Williams 1999: 200.

121. See F. Rosenthal 1978 (on a treatise by al-Rāzī devoted to *ubna*).

122. Al-Kātib 1977: 237ff.

123. Ibn Sīnā 1999: II, 729.

124. See for example A. Abu Khalil 1993; K. El Rouayheb 2005.

125. A. Shalakany 2008: 51–2.

126. The *Qānūn* devotes a whole chapter to reproductive organs and the sexual instinct: Ibn Sīnā 1999: II, 725–47. See also E. H. Hoops, 'Die sexologischen Kapitel im '*Canon Medicinae*' des Avicenna, vergleichen mit der Schrift De coitu des Maimonides', *Aesthetische Medizin*, 1967, 16, pp. 305–8.

127. Maimonides, *Fī tadbīr al-ṣiḥḥa* ('Regimen of Health'), Chapter 4 (Ariel Bar-Sela, Hebbel E. Hoff, Elias Faris, 'Moses Maimonides' Two Treatises on the Regimen of Health: *Fī Tadbīr al-Sihhah* and *Maqālah fī Bayān Ba'ḍ al-A'rāḍ wa-al-Jawāb 'anhā*'', *Transactions of the American Philosophical Society*, New Series, 54:4 [1964], pp. 3–50); *Fuṣūl Mūsā fi 'l-ṭibb* ('Medical Aphorisms of Moses'), Treatise 17 (English trans. F. Rosner and S. Muntner, *The Medical Aphorisms of Moses Maimonides*, New York: Yeshiva University Press, 1973; G. Bos, *Medical Aphorisms. Treatises 16–21*, Chicago: Chicago University Press, 2013) (= *idem* 2022: 142–459).

128. See the chapter on coitus in al-Rāzī, *Kitāb al-Murshid aw al-fuṣūl.*

129. For example, Maimonides dedicated his work to Sultan al-Muẓaffar 'Umar Ibn Nūr al-Dīn of Hama; al-Isrā'ilī to Nūr al-Dīn Muḥammad Ibn Qārā Arslān of the Artuqid dynasty; al-Nafzāwī to Muḥammad al-Zawāwī, grand vizier of the Ḥafṣid ruler of Tunisia, 'Abd al-'Azīz al-Hafṣī; Ibn Raqīqa to the Ayyubid ruler al-Ashraf; and al-Ṭūsī to Ābāqā Khan.
130. For a discussion of al-Ṣuyūṭī's erotological and erotic works, see H. Jughām 2001.
131. This term is used for the area covered by the historical Greater Syria, which includes present-day Jordan, Syria, Lebanon.
132. For general overviews, see H. Schipperges 1964 *idem* 1976; D. Jacquart 1996.
133. M. Green 1985: 134–40.
134. On this physician's work, see *ibid.*, 91–101.
135. *ibid.*, 140ff.
136. See *ibid.*, 195–413; Green 2002: 3–7; V. Nutton, in L. I Conrad et al. 1995: 139–46; D. Jacquart and F. Michaud 1990: 87–130.
137. M. Green 1985: 218ff; 2002: 10–11; D. Jacquart and F. Michaud 1990: 96–107; V. Nutton, in L. I. Conrad et al. 1995: 140–1.
138. See, for instance, Jon Arrizabalaga, *The 'Articella' in the Early Press, c. 1476–1534,* Cambridge: Cambridge Wellcome Unit for the History of Medicine, 1998. For an extensive and erudite analysis of the *Isagoge*, which confirms Constantine as the translator, see Francis Newton, 'Constantine the African and Montecassino: New Elements and the Text of the Isagoge', in C. S. F. Burnett and D. Jacquart 1994: 16–40.
139. For background, see the various contributions in C. F. S. Burnett and D. Jacquart 1994. Constantine's translation was, in fact, incomplete, and a few decades later the Pantegni was retranslated in its entirety by Stephen of Antioch (*Liber regalis dispositionis*), who had studied in Salerno.
140. For an overview, see C. Burnett 2001.
141. D. Jacquart and F. Michaud 1990: 147–52.
142. The first three books of the Latin *Canon* were printed in 1472 in Milan, with the complete edition appearing one year later. The book would remain the authoritative medical text until the seventeenth century.
143. Gerard's translation, *Liber Medicinalis ad al Mansorem*, was published for the first time in Milan in 1481; other printings followed in Venice (1497) and Lyon (1510). Vesalius' redaction was entitled *Paraphrasis in nonum librum Rhazae medici arabis clariss: ad regem Almansorem, de singularum corporis partium affectuum curatione* (Basel: Robert Winter) and remained a core textbook in European medical schools for many centuries. For the influence of al-Rāzī on Vesalius's thought and oeuvre, see A. Compier 2012.
144. See D. Jacquart and F. Michaud 1990: 167ff.; D. Jacquart 1996; C. O'Boyle 1998; P. Pormann and E. Savage-Smith 2007: 164–7.

145. D. Jacquart and C. Thomasset 1988: 89, 90, 93.

146. See G. Bos 1997. For discussion of the impact of the *Viaticum*, see H. Schipperges 1964: 40–3; *idem* 1976: 106–8; Mary E. Wack, *Lovesickness in the Middle Ages: The Viaticum and its Commentaries*, Philadelphia: University of Pennsylvania Press, 1990.

147. It is now accepted that *De Coitu* was in fact an adaptation of the work of Ibn al-Jazzār. See D. Jacquart and C. Thomasset 1988: 116–20, 221; E. Montero Cartelle, ed., *Constantini Liber de Coitu. El tratado de andrologia de Constantino el Africano*, Santiago de Compostella: Universidad de Santiago de Compostella, 1983.

148. Dedicated to Pope Bonifacius VIII, it was first printed in 1480. For Maimonides in Latin, see G. Hasselhoff 2002; *idem*, 'Mediaeval Translations of the Maimonidean (Medical) Oeuvre', in G. Tamer, ed., *Die Trias des Maimonides. Jüdische, arabische und antike Wissenskultur/The Trias of Maimonides. Jewish, Arabic and Ancient Culture of Knowledge*, Berlin/New York: Walter De Gruyter, 2005, pp. 395–410.

149. D. Jacquart and C. Thomasset 1988: 120–1; C. F. S. Burnett, 'The Latin Versions of Maimonides' *On Sexual Intercourse (De Coitu)*', in F. E. Glaze and B. K. Nance, eds, *Between Text and Patient: The Medical Enterprise in Medieval and Modern Europe*, Florence: SISMEL/Edizioni del Galluzzo, 2011, pp. 467–80.

150. D. Jacquart and C. Thomasset 1988: 91–2.

151. *ibid.*, 135ff.

152. *ibid.*, 126–8. The first *Secrets Secretorum* was translated by John of Seville (who also translated one of Qusṭā Ibn Lūqā's works on the soul and the spirit, *De differentia spiritus et animae*) around 1120, and dedicated it to the first ruler of the kingdom of Portugal, Queen Teresa – daughter of the Spanish king Alfonso VI. See Steven J. Williams, *The Secret of Secrets: The Scholarly Career of a Pseudo-Aristotelian Text in the Latin Middle Ages*, unpublished PhD dissertation, Northwestern University, 1991.

153. For detailed discussions of this, see for instance D. Jacquart and C. Thomasset 1988: 7–8, 12–14, 22–40; J. Cadden 1993; A. Lindgren 2005; Helen Rodnite Lema, *Women's Secrets: A Translation of Pseudo-Albertus Magnus' De Secretis Mulierum with Commentaries*, Albany, NY: State University of New York Press, 1992; Sarah Alison Miller, *Virgins, Mothers, Monsters: Late-Medieval Readings of the Female Body Out of Bounds*, unpublished PhD dissertation, University of North Carolina at Chapel Hill, 2008.

154. The 'Trotula texts' comprise three treatises: the 'Trotula major', known also as *De passionibus mulierum curandarum* ('Diseases of Women') or by the *incipit* 'cum auctor', which is devoted to gynaecological medicine; the 'Trotula minor' ('*ut de curis*'), on medical matters and cosmetics; and *De ornatu mulierum*, on cosmetics. See R. Benton 1985; M. Green 2002: 51–115. The texts have been translated by M.

Green (2002). On the Arabic medical influence, see D. Jacquart and C. Thomasset 1988: 121–2, 132.

155. D. Jacquart and C. Thomasset 1988: 133.
156. *ibid.*, 96–110.
157. *ibid.*, 130–5.
158. Arab physicians like Ibn Sīnā and al-Rāzī were unclear about the clitoris, whereas al-Majūsī confused it with the labia. It would take until the mid-sixteenth century for its function to be 'discovered' – at least by men! The same confusion existed about the female genitals in general, with the vulva, for instance, signifying the vagina, the womb, or both, until the late Middle Ages. See D. Jacquart and C. Thomasset 1988: 44ff; A. Lindgren 2005: 95; T. Laqueur 1992: 64ff.
159. D. Jacquart and C. Thomasset 1988: 137.
160. A. Davidson 2014: 25–6. Taking an opposing angle, J. Turner (2004: 186) holds that 'If there is a single, solid conclusion to be drawn from the deeply bizarre study of aphrodisiacs, it is that practically everything remotely edible has at some time or another been credited with sexually enhancing powers—and many inedible substances besides.'
161. G. Bos 2019: 32–3 (= 2022: 462).
162. Al-Tīfāshī 1892: 48. However, for many scholars, temperament superseded shape in this case. Maimonides, for instance, said the cucumber was extremely harmful for coitus (as were melons and other 'sour substances'); Maimonides ([F. Rosner 1984]: *idem* [F. Rosner 1995]: 307–8; 170; *idem* [M. Meyerhof 1940]: Nos. 343 (*qiththā'*), 388 (*khiyār*).
163. G. Bos 2022: 462.
164. G. Bos 2019: 50–1 (= 2022: 466).
165. Al-Tīfāshī 1892: 60.
166. See P. M. Holt 1992.
167. J. Kraemer 1986.
168. See *EI*[2], s.v. 'Ṭūs' (C. E. Bosworth).
169. The author's name is also sometimes given as Naṣīr al-Dīn Abū Jaʿfar Muḥammad Ibn Muḥammad Ibn al-Ḥasan al-Ṭūsī (M. Sharif 1963–66, I: 564) or Naṣīr al-Dīn Muḥammad Ibn Muḥammad al-Ṭūsī (C. Storey 1972, II: 2, 216).
170. For biographical details, see the following, from which the information in this section has been drawn: *EI*[2], s.v. 'al-Ṭūsī' (al-H. Daiber/F. J. Ragep) (with extensive bibliography); Jon Mcginnis, in El-Rouayheb and.S. Schmidtke 2017: 326–47; H. Dabashi 1996; *GAL* I: 670–6; *GALS* I: 924–33; *GALS* III, 1245–7, 1314–5; C.A. Storey 1972, II: 1, xl, xlii–xliv, 6–7, 52–60, II: 2, 216–17; ʿU. Kaḥḥāla n.d.: XI.
171. See J. Boyle 1963.
172. Ulugh Beg, *Binae tabulae geographicae una Nassir Eddini Persae, altera Ulug Beigi Tatari*, London: J. Flesher, 1652.
173. *GALS* I: 932.

174. *ibid.*
175. *ibid.*
176. F. Rosenthal 1986, III: 148 (where al-Ṭūsī is also called 'an Iraqi', i.e. one hailing from non-Arab Iraq).
177. Originally derived from the Turkish and Persian words for teacher (*khōja*), it was a title used for a variety of people, including scholars, teachers, merchants and ministers. It also became a term of reference for non-Muslims, especially Europeans, in which sense it is still used in modern Egypt (*khawāga*). *EI*², s.v. 'Khwādja' (ed.).
178. *GAL* I: 676 refers to *albāb al-bāhiyya fi 'l-tarākīb al-sultāniyya* as a health manual (*Gesundheitsbuch*), 'the last part of which deals with coitus and aphrodisiacs'.
179. A. Ihsanoglu 1984: 378.
180. This manuscript is much longer (104 folios) and includes sixty-one chapters (besides an introduction and conclusion) on a wide variety of medical conditions.
181. This was also the manuscript used by Ghassan Ammari for his edition (unpublished PhD dissertation, Universität Erlangen-Nürnberg, 1974).
182. *EI*², s.v. 'al-Djaghmīnī' (H. Suter-[J. Vernet]); *GAL* I: 473; II: 213; C. Storey 1958, II: 1, 50, 219. The Glasgow catalogue misspells the author's name as 'al-Yaghmini'.
183. Savage-Smith 2011: 433–4 (No. 110).
184. Uri 1787: 144 (entry No. DCXXIV).
185. Savage-Smith 2011: 433–4, 431– (No. 109).
186. Savage-Smith 2011: 785–6 (No. 238).
187. Savage-Smith 2011: 780–1 (No. 234).

بسم الله الرحمن الرحيم

الحمد لله رب العالمين وصلى الله على سيدنا محمد
خاتم النبيين وعلى اله وصحبه اجمعين
وبعد فان الله تعالى قد اكمل النفوس الناطقة
الانسانيه بمواهب انعامه وحلاه باد
خواطر الحكما باعلامه لهم جواهر حكمته
كما قال الله تعالى ولقد اتينا لقمان الحكمة
الايه فالفضل بيده كما قال الله تعالى ان
الفضل بيد الله يوتيه من يشاء والله
ذو الفضل العظيم ونشرع الان في بيان
سبب تاليف هذا الكتاب وكشف اسرار
الحكما واظهار رموزاتهم في هذا الكتاب
هو ان خليفة الزمان سلطان قاران كان
له ولد ذات جمال وبها تحصل في بدنه الريح
الفالج وابطل شقته فسال الشيخ العالم ملك
علما

Illustration 1: Facsimile of first page of Berlin Mss 6383

٥٨٢ طب عمومية ٤٤٨٦٧

هذا الكتاب الباهيه في التراكيب السلطانيه
تاليف الشيخ العلامه والبحر الفهامه ابي البركات
ناصر الدين الطوخي رحمه الله
تعالي وجميع المسلمين
امين امين
امين

بسم الله الرحمن الرحيم وبه نستعين الحمد لله الذي
شهدت بوجوده جميع الكائنات والصلاة والسلام
علي افضل الانام سيدنا محمد المبعوث بالآيات الواضحات
وعلي اله وصحبه والتابعين لهم في المكرمات وبعد
فان الله تعالي قد اكمل النفوس الناطقه الانسانيه
بمواهب انعامه وملا معادن خواطر الحكماء باعلامه
لهم جواهر حكمته كما قال سبحانه ولقد اتينا لقمن الحكمه
فالاحسان منه والفضل بيده كما قال سبحانه وان الفضل
بيد الله يؤتيه من يشاء والله ذو الفضل العظيم ونشرع
الآن في بيان تاليف هذا الكتاب وكشف اسرار العلماء
واظهار رموزاتهم وذلك ان خليفة الزمان سلطان
فازان كان له ولد ذو جمال وبهاء فحصل له في بدنه ريح

Illustration 2: Facsimile of first page of Cairo Mss No. 582

بسم الله الرحمن الرحيم

الحمد لله رب العالمين وصلى الله على سيدنا محمد خاتم النبيين وعلى
آله وصحبه اجمعين. وبعد فان الله تعالى قد اكمل النفوس الناطقة
الانسانية بمواهب انعامه و ملأ معادن خواطر الحكماء باعلامه لهم
جواهر حكمته كما قال الله تعالى سبحانه ولقد آتينا لقمان الحكمة الآية فالفضل
بيده كما قال الله تعالى وان الفضل بيد الله يؤتيه من يشاء والله
ذو الفضل العظيم. و نشرع الآن في بيان سبب تأليف هذا الكتاب
وكشف اسرار الحكماء واظهار رموزاتهم في هذا الكتاب هو ان
خليفة ارباب سلطنة تاتارخان كان له ولد ذات جمال وبهاء فحصل له
في مرضه الريح الفالج والجلال (?) شفقة فسأل الشيخ العالم ملك علماء العصر
واستاد فضلاء الدهر قطب الاسلام والمسلمين وعرنين (?) الملوك والسلاطين
ابو البركات الخواجه ناصر الدين الطوسي ان يؤلف كتابا في الطب
مشتملا (?) بجميع كثير الفوائد لينتفع به المسلمين فاجابه الى سؤاله وألف
على ارشاده وجمع فوائد تامة من كتب المتقدمين والمتأخرين
وجعلها حاوية لفوائد نافعة وكافية لحفظ صحة بدن الانسان
وسبب وقوع العلة وعلاجها لا يحتاج احد بسبب مطالعتها الى معالجة
طبيب ويكتفي بها عن مداواة ما يحدث من العلل والامراض وغير ذلك
من الفوائد المجربة والمنافع والخواص المنتخبة ورتبها على ثمانية عشر بابا
وسماها كتاب الباهية والتراكيب السلطانية وهذه فهرسة
1 الكتاب. الباب الاول في بيان تدبير بدن الانسان وبيان امزجته
2 وغير ذلك. الباب الثاني في بيان اغذية المفردات وبيان منافعها
3 وخواصها وغير ذلك. الباب الثالث في بيان الادوية المفردة التي
هي خلاصة الادوية خصوصا لتقوية الافعال وزيادة الباه والشهوة
4 والمني وغير ذلك. الباب الرابع في بيان الادوية المركبة لدفع الامراض
وتقوية افعال الجماع ووقع موانعه وزيادة المني والشهوة وبيان

Illustration 3: Facsimile of first page of Glasgow University Mss Hunter 144 (T.7.3)

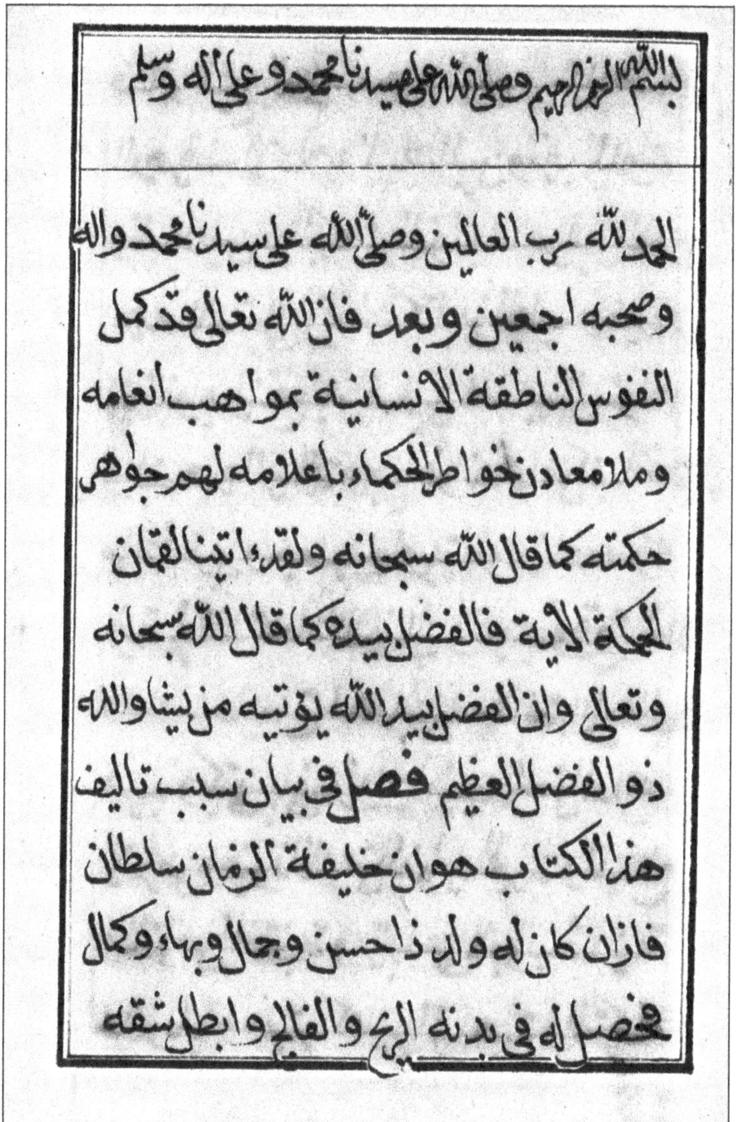

بسم الله الرحمن الرحيم وصلى الله على سيدنا محمد وعلى آله وسلم

الحمد لله رب العالمين وصلى الله على سيدنا محمد واله
وصحبه اجمعين وبعد فان الله تعالى قد كمل
النفوس الناطقة الانسانية بمواهب انعامه
وملا معادن خواطر الحكماء باعلامه لهم جواهر
حكمته كما قال الله سبحانه ولقد اتينا لقمان
الحكمة الاية فالفضل بيده كما قال الله سبحانه
وتعالى وان الفضل بيد الله يؤتيه من يشا والله
ذو الفضل العظيم **فصل** في بيان سبب تاليف
هذا الكتاب هو ان خليفة الزمان سلطان
فاران كان له ولد ذا حسن وجمال وبهاء وكمال
فحصل له في بدنه الريح والفالج وابطل شقه

Illustration 4: Facsimile of first page of British Library Mss Or 11213

صفة بتطويل الذكر قال محمد الدامغاني والامام
الرازي رحمهما الله عن افلاطون هذا العمل لتطويل
قال يوخذ الحسك الذي نبت اكثر من سنة
ويغسل نظيفا ويجففه غاية ويسحقه ناعما وينخله
ناعما ويدخل الحمام ويدلك ذكره بالماء دلكا قويا
حتى يحمى ويذر عليه من اصل الحسك المسحوق بعد
ذلك تمريخه بدهن السعد المسحوق معه وزن نصف
درهم جوز الهند وتكون سحقتهما واحضرتهما عندك
في الحمام تطلي به ذكرك ثلاثة مرات الى ان تخرج من
الحمام فانه غاية ونهاية لكن حكمه الى عشرة ايام فقط
نوع اخر تركيب غريب من اسرار الحكما بطول الذكر
ويجعله قد ضعفه مرتين وذلك ان ياخذ بعر الغنم
الطري المرق والبعر اليابس مقدار ما تطلي به ذكرك
وتاخذ قيراط مسك وتسحقه وتاخذ جوز الهند
اربع دراهم وتدقه في غاية النعومة وتخلط الجميع

Illustration 5: Facsimile of first page of Bodleian Mss Marsh 530, fol. 108

TRANSLATION

The Book of Sexual Stimulants and the Sultan's Potions[1]

[1v.][2] In the name of Allah, the Compassionate, the Merciful.

Praise be to Allah, Master of the Two Worlds. May He bless our lord Muḥammad, the seal of the Prophets, his family and companions.[3] Allah the Almighty has perfected human beings with the gifts of His grace, and He has filled the mines of the sages' thoughts by revealing the gems of His wisdom, as He said: 'And verily We gave Luqmān[4] wisdom'[5] and the bounty is in His hand. The Almighty also said 'that the bounty is in Allah's hand to give to whom He will. And Allah is of Infinite Bounty.'[6]

We begin by explaining the motive behind the writing of this book, the discovery of scholars' secrets and the revelation of their lucubrations. The caliph of Qāzān[7] had a beautiful son, whose body was struck by paralysis which incapacitated one side of his body. The caliph asked the erudite *shaykh*, the king [2r.] of scholars of the age, the teacher of scholars of all time, the pillar of Islam and all Muslims, preceptor of kings and sultans, one who is full of blessings, Master (*Khwāja*)[8] Nāṣir[9] al-Dīn al-Ṭūsī – may the Almighty have mercy on him! – to compile a book on medicine that is small in size but has many benefits that will be useful to Muslims. He acceded to the request and compiled the present book, in which he has gathered the wisdom culled from the works of past scholars and made it a compendium including that which is most useful and beneficial for the preservation of a healthy body, and the causes for the appearance of illnesses and their treatment. Anyone reading this treatise will no longer need a physician for medical treatment as it contains all the reader requires to treat ailments and diseases that are described in terms of tried and tested benefits and selected specialist remedies.

I have divided the book into eighteen chapters and named it *The Book of Choice Sexual Stimulants and the Sultan's Potions*. Here is the index [3r.] of the book for reference purposes:

Chapter 1: explanation of the organization of human beings, their temperaments, etc.;

Chapter 2: description of simple remedies, their benefits, properties, etc.;

Chapter 3: description of simple drugs,[10] which are the main medicines, especially for the strengthening of bodily functions, sexual potency, lust, sperm, etc.;

Chapter 4: description of compound drugs[11] that ward off illnesses, strengthen performance during coitus, protect against obstructions, increase sperm and lust;

description of compound remedies and sweets that are beneficial for the human temperament and restore it, remove paralysis in the body and limpness of the limbs, and increase sexual potency;[12]

Chapter 5: description of wines that restore spoiled temperaments, purify the blood and body, invigorate coitus and are of great benefit; [3r]

Chapter 6: description of stomachics[13] that raise the spirits and ward off boredom, are highly beneficial for the stomach and strengthen it; remove jaundice and phlegm; cut short melancholy; are beneficial for the brain; open up blockages in organs; reduce foul wind; strengthen the lungs; protect against headache and catarrh; and strengthen innate heat and all bodily actions;[14]

Chapter 7: description of the remedies[15] that extract and expel wind and coldness arising from the hip, back and organs; that remove moistness, yellow and black bile[16] from the stomach, intestines and other parts of the body;

Chapter 8: description of enemas which remove joint ache; protect against foul wind and expel it from the body and lungs; cure sciatica; remove back pain, colic; strengthen the back [3v.] and hip, and all functions;[17]

Chapter 9: description of the bandages that are tied around the hip during the four seasons and of everything that is appropriate for each season in order not to upset human nature and cause illness;[18]

Chapter 10: description of the conditions and manner [of coitus] so as to avoid harm and impotence;[19]

Chapter 11: description of medicines to rub on the penis so that it becomes strong, long, and erect;

Chapter 12: description of medicines to rub on the penis so that it becomes erect and long, as is desirable;[20]

Chapter 13: description of medicines that are rubbed in between the fingers and toes so that they are useful during coitus, strengthen it, and prevent impotence resulting from frequent intercourse;[21]

Chapter 14: description of pills that are placed in the mouth during coitus to increase the individual's pleasure; [4r.]

Chapter 15: description of the positions during coitus that provide pleasure to both the man and the woman, as reported by physicians;[22]

Chapter 16: description of medicines which, if used by women, colour their faces and cheeks pink, with intercourse becoming highly pleasurable, to the extent that no one can have sex with them anymore due to their hotness and tightness [of their vaginas'];[23]

Chapter 17: description of medicines that prevent pregnancy in a woman so that she remains like a virgin forever;[24]

Chapter 18: description of the medicines that make a woman become pregnant, if Allah the Almighty wills it.[25]

This concludes the list of chapters,[26] which we have provided to make it easier for the user who is looking for something to find it without effort or difficulty. I seek help from Allah. 'Allah is Sufficient for us! Most Excellent is He in Whom we trust!'[27]

[4v.] Know, student,[28] that Allah grants us success in achieving obedience to Him and that Allah, praise be to Him, the Sublime, has created animals and brought them into being out of nothing. He has created them in pairs and given them a soul so that they need and yearn for each other in pairs.[29] He has given preference to human beings over all others and favoured them with intellect, adorned them and bestowed His honour upon them, as Allah the Almighty has said – and He is the most truthful of utterers:[30] 'Verily, We have honoured the children of Adam. We carry them on the land and the sea.'[31] He made their food the finest of all animals. We have extended the discussion in this chapter because there is no more awful cause[32] for the destruction of the soul than sexual intercourse. Every disease can be treated, except those that are caused by frequent intercourse, which douses the innate heat, for which there is no treatment or therapy that can offer solace. May Allah save us from that!

Sperm, when it flows, comes from the principal organs and from all [5r.] extremities;[33] as ʿAlī[34] (may Allah be pleased with him!) said:[35] 'Your sperm is your soul, the light of your eyes, the brain in your head and legs. If you want to, conserve it.' When you have learned about intercourse and practise it as it should be, you will acquire twenty-four benefits;[36] for instance, it cures melancholy, protects against bilious and phlegmatic diseases, and causes happiness and high spirits, as described by past scholars, sages and physicians, who based themselves on their experiments and experience.[37]

As for the view held by a number of scholars that sexual intercourse is bad and harmful, and that it is not necessary for anyone to practise it, but rather that it should be abandoned, this is devoid of foundation, and erroneous because [a person's] dignity and beauty is rooted in five things – namely, the five faculties: hearing, sight, smell, taste and touch.[38] Taste mostly refers to taste in sexual intercourse and lust. [5v.]

The result of pleasure during sexual intercourse is the creation of living beings and, thus, the reproduction and propagation of the human species. Hence, any talk about the inadmissibility of sexual intercourse is a falsehood.

It is clear that this statement is nonsensical and only applies to those who engage in coitus whilst being ignorant of the time and circumstance when it should or should not take place, and of the conditions and regimen it requires. When coitus takes place in these cases, it results in the above-mentioned ailments and the individual's destruction, in contrast with those who know how to manage coitus and its conditions. In the latter case, sexual intercourse does not cause any harm; rather, it is hugely beneficial,[39] as we have mentioned, whereas there is no greater human pleasure than that of sexual intercourse. It is part of the natural disposition and it is mixed into the make-up of human beings and all other animals. It is rooted in their very being, which is why there is no animal in whose soul and brain such lust is not present, except if it has [6r.] a defect in its temperament, limpness in the limbs, or its libido has died.

Know that a man grows weak and becomes afflicted by illness and pain, only if the principal organs are aching. As long as the principal organs remain strong[40] because of medicines and treatments, and by avoiding wrong conduct and guarding against harm, the limbs will remain sound and free from defects and illness, and will not be afflicted by pain until the moment of death, if Allah the Almighty wills it. Death cannot prevent anything; its verdict cannot be changed and its judgement cannot be opposed.[41]

The principal organs are the brain, heart, liver and testicles, together with their organs [*sic*]. Some scholars also count the lungs among the principal organs; others include the kidneys.[42] Human beings should strengthen these organs and the stomach with medicines, electuaries, syrups [collyria][43] and unguents, [6v.] whose properties and preparation will be explained later, Allah the Almighty willing, in line with what was said about this in the books by ancient philosophers and physicians, who relied on their experiments and experience. They include Plato, Aristotle, Hippocrates, Palladius,[44] Aristo[45] and scholars like them.[46]

Description of the benefits and harmful effects of sexual

intercourse during the four seasons, which are spring, summer, autumn and winter. [47]

Note that spring is the best and most beneficial season for sexual intercourse, as it is the most temperate[48] and its air the most agreeable.[49] It purifies the blood, restores balance and increases the pneuma in the veins, which strengthens the innate heat, enhances vitality and taste, eliminates weakness in the penis and makes it powerful. If this is the case,[50] sexual intercourse in this season is not harmful, does not make the body sluggish or cause illness and pain, regardless of whether sexual intercourse occurs after taking medicines, electuaries, [7r.] etc.[51] Sexual intercourse in any other season is harmful, except with the use of medicines since, in truth, passion is derived from the potency of the latter as it does not come from within the individual. So, sexual intercourse during summer, autumn and winter requires treatment through medication and electuaries for it to be beneficial and not harmful.[52]

CHAPTER 1

The regimen required for each person and a description of the signs referring to the temperament of each individual.

Know that those with brown or wheat-coloured skin, with either strong or limp flesh,[53] wide veins and black hair, who are temperate and clean, with bluish-black eyes, thick eyebrows and powerful testicles, are endowed with a hot and dry temperament. Those who fall into this category are eager [7v.] for sexual intercourse[54] and are not spoilt by it. Those who have a yellow colour, red face, white skin and big belly, have a cold and moist temperament. Those with a moist temperament desire to engage in coitus but are not sufficiently strong to do so. If such a person increases the frequency of intercourse, it weakens him.[55] Those with a black colour, a clean skin and body, of lean and slight build,[56] with small eyes and very red gums have a hot temperament and a strong desire for sexual intercourse. As for those who are white-skinned, they come in two categories; either they have a clear colour, beautiful eyes, or the whiteness of the skin tends towards yellow, with blond hair.[57] The second group have a high libido. Those who have a white colour and a phlegmatic temperament have flaccid limbs and are not strong enough to have sexual intercourse.[58] If they practise it to excess [8r.] they will die and thus have to take great care when engaging in coitus.[59]

The weakness in limbs and the limpness of organs derives from a weakness in the brain, which is called 'brain weakness'. Its signs are as follows: vertigo, sunken eyes, poor eyesight,[60] weak physical strength, variable colour, increased shame at having a limp penis and feeble coital activity, without experiencing ecstasy.[61] If such a person has intercourse, he has no strength to repeat it a second time due to the weakness of his limbs. Someone like this should remedy these ailments by strengthening the brain, the treatment for which is sugar syrup because the defects arise from increases in moistness;[62] it dissolves superfluities, strengthens the sperm and invigorates coitus. Sugar syrup has many other benefits, whose explanation would take too long.[63]

Recipe for sugar syrup: take ginger[64] and cinnamon[65] [8v.], two-fifths of a *dirham* of each,[66] two *dirhams* of cardamom[67] and two *dirhams* of cloves.[68] Pound all of these separately and then mix everything together. Place the mixture in a pot, add seven times the amount of fresh water and bring to a boil over a low heat until the strength of the medicines has been extracted and the required substances have been cooked thoroughly. Then, strain the water and throw away the sediment. Take four times the weight of the mixture in sugar, which amounts to thirty-two *dirhams*, and boil all the ingredients so that everything becomes mixed, without thickening. If you want to reduce it, add half a *dirham* of saffron.[69] Remove from the fire and take a spoonful each day on an empty stomach. Wait until dawn before eating it. It is beneficial and curative, Allah the Almighty willing.[70]

The second cause for the weakening of limbs and limpness of organs, which leads to [9r.] sexual impotence, is weakness of the heart. The sign of a weak heart is that during forceful movements or walking, as when crossing a threshold; when being angry with someone; when good news is received; when gazing upon the object of one's desire, or by being in a large group, the individual will experience the following symptoms:[71] heart palpitations, trembling hands and knees, sadness, shortness of breath and a change in colour. Anyone suffering from this will experience weakness during coitus, after which there will be palpitations.

{People like this should guard against these ailments by strengthening the limbs and the limpness of organs with apple syrup so as to remove the symptoms,}[72] increase stomach secretions, and heat up and proliferate the sperm. This syrup has many other benefits, but a description of this would take too long, and this is sufficient.

The apple syrup is made as follows: take an apple,[73] peel and core it. Pound it and strain its juice through a thin piece of cloth or a fine sieve. [9v.] Add the same measure of rosewater[74] and mix it with the apple juice. Take the same weight of strained bee honey[75] from which the froth has been skimmed. Place the honey in a pot together with a small quantity of the rosewater and apple mixture. Add half a *dirham* of saffron, half a *dirham* of pepper,[76] a *dirham* of ginger and two *dirhams* of cloves. Boil everything until the strength has been extracted from the ingredients, then strain and store until needed,[77] at which time add[78] double the quantity of the mixture in rain water, blend it all with the water you have boiled with the spices and pour into the pot. Place on a low fire, and stir the mixture until it thickens. Before it becomes thick, add a *qīrāṭ*[79] of pure musk.[80] Remove the pot from the fire and let the contents cool down.[81] Drink one or one and a half spoonfuls each day on an empty stomach. It is beneficial.

The third reason for the limpness of organs, and [10r.] the weakness of limbs and coitus is a weakness in the liver, which is characterized by a yellow colouring of the face, as in jaundice, the drying up of the tongue and lips, sunken eyes, emaciation and a loss of appetite.[82] When a person afflicted by this eats anything, he is unable to digest the food. When he gets up, his legs will tremble, whereas he finds it difficult to stand and is weakened. He is incapable of coitus, and when he is able to, it gives him no enjoyment or pleasure. His sperm is cold, as are the hands and feet. If a man like this engages in sexual intercourse to excess, he will be struck by one of the following three illnesses: hemiplegia, impotence or the dissipation of his innate heat, which results in sudden death[83] – may Allah protect us from that! This ailment should be treated with syrup of spikenard,[84] which heats the stomach and strengthens the liver,[85] [10v.] innate heat and potency. It has twenty-six other beneficial properties, which, if we were to mention them all, would make the book too long. As for the recipe of spikenard syrup:[86] take one *dirham* each of [spikenard,][87] cinnamon, cardamom and agarwood,[88] and half a *dirham* of cloves. Pulverize all the ingredients and, if needed, add five times the measure of water and then boil the liquid until the substances have been cooked thoroughly and half of the water remains. Afterwards, strain it, add skimmed honey in an amount equalling that of the water and cook for one hour, until everything is mixed. Add half a *dirham* of saffron dissolved in rosewater and mix. The use of this remedy will be beneficial, as we have mentioned.

The fourth cause for weakness in sexual potency, the penis and testicles, and their limpness, comes in three types.[89] Firstly, the limpness of the penis and testicles is innate and is already present in the mother's womb; secondly, [11r.] excessive sexual intercourse from a young age;[90] and, thirdly, frequent sexual intercourse above the age of forty. The first of these – weakness that is already present in the mother's womb – manifests itself in the inability to obtain an erection. In spite of this, the individual has a longing for sexual intercourse, without having any lust, but is impotent. This is to be treated with moderation over a long period of time. As for the second type – the high frequency of sexual intercourse in youth – it is characterized by the fact that the penis is erect only at the start and end of the night, only in the morning, or only in spring. This condition can be treated quickly, as will be described elsewhere, Allah willing. When the condition is caused by frequent sexual intercourse in adulthood, above the age of forty, the penis is erect only rarely, and on certain days.[91] Coitus is performed without energy and the individual either ejaculates cold sperm [11v.] or the ejaculation is accompanied by a burning sensation. Someone who suffers from this will not be able to produce offspring. The cause for this coldness lies in the back and loins; the individual is overcome with coldness.[92] This should be treated with a musk electuary, which removes the coldness and moistness[93] from his back and loins. It purifies the bladder, causes the sperm and blood in the veins to flow, and opens up blockages.[94] The person should guard against eating food that counters this action so as to ensure a speedy recovery and prevent the disease from worsening. We shall discuss the beneficial foodstuffs with which the individual can protect himself, Allah the Almighty willing. This electuary has thirty-three benefits in addition to the ones that we have mentioned.[95]

The recipe for the musk electuary is as follows: take a *qīrāṭ* of musk; two *dirhams* each of cinnamon,[96] spikenard, malabathrum[97] and Greek gentian;[98] three *dirhams*[99] each of saffron, cumin,[100] carrot[101] seeds and mastic;[102] [12r.] half a *dirham* each of agarwood,[103] cloves[104] and Turkish myrrh.[105] Crush all the ingredients, strain, and take three times the measure of the mixture in bee honey, and knead into an electuary.[106] Use one *mithqāl*[107] daily. It is beneficial, Allah the Almighty willing.

Here is another treatment: take some cockerels,[108] before they start crowing, slaughter them and collect ten *dirhams* of their gall. Add a sufficient measure of litharge[109] to enable you to knead the collected gall into a fine paste.[110] Then, leave it out in the sun so that the gall and litharge become mixed. Take care that the paste does not dry out and become hard.[111] Have a bath, and upon getting out,[112] rub the paste into the penis, armpits and buttocks. This should be done on an empty stomach. Then use with the musk electuary.[113] Cook the slaughtered cockerels, whose galls have been collected with the same weight in onions.[114] [12v.] Sprinkle radish[115] and peppergrass[116] seeds[117] on the mixture and eat it. It is beneficial, Allah the Almighty willing.

It is advisable to eat it, as required, and it lends itself to being used like *harīsa*,[118] with pullets or mutton[119] and unleavened bread, with dough made from coarse flour and chickpea water, in the manner of the sages. This is made as follows: take white chickpeas,[120] soak them, peel them, and cook them in a pot until they are done and their essence has infused the water.[121] Then, strain and remove the sediment. Collect some plump house sparrows,[122] slaughter and clean them, and cut them into pea-sized pieces. Place in a pot with the chickpea water and cook everything together with the lid on so that the steam cannot get out. Cook over a low fire so that it does not burn, that is, before you start noticing [13r.] the smell of grilled meat. Then, remove the pot from the fire and add the following ingredients:[123] five *dirhams* of ginger, two-and-a-half *dirhams* of long pepper, six nutmeg seeds and ten *dirhams* of cinnamon. All of them are pounded and set aside, then sprinkled over what we have mentioned, before eating the dish. Whenever you eat a dish like this, sprinkle these spices on. If you cannot find any sparrows,[124] use squabs in their stead. You can also eat *taqliyya*[125] with carrots and the meat of a one-year-old lamb,[126] chicken, or cockerels before they have started to crow.[127] After the carrots have been washed, peeled and cut into small pieces, cook them with the meat, as we have mentioned. Then, sprinkle the aforementioned spices[128] on and eat the mixture. This is drunk with cow's milk in which dried dates[129] have been cooked [13v.] in order to sweeten it. It can also be eaten with grilled fish[130] and white onions. If you eat it in a pottage, then add garlic.[131] It is beneficial.

Recipe for making garlic pottage:[132] take fresh Syrian garlic and peel the cloves. Take beef fat, render and strain it, and take some of the meat in which it was cooked. Pound the garlic, mix it with the fat and cook everything through. Place in a bowl[133] and forcefully whisk with the hands until it is smooth and thin. Put on a low fire until it is slightly thickened, and then add the grated garlic. Combine everything and beat the mixure until it has thickened, and then remove from the fire. Sprinkle on as much of the above-mentioned spices as required for the temperament.[134] Add half a dirham of saffron and store in a glass vessel.[135] Take three *mithqāls* of the mixture each day. It is said that [14r.] this garlic pottage removes coldness from the back and loins, clears phlegm from the stomach and chest, and superfluities from the chest, expelling all illnesses from the body, Allah the Almighty willing.[136]

One can also use roses preserved in bee-honey jam, the recipe for which is as follows: take roses and place them in a glass container in the sun. Add the honey and let both dry. Whenever the honey dries out, add some more until it reaches the required consistency. This should be eaten with unleavened bread spread with fresh clarified butter[137] and a ripe sweet apple, as we have mentioned. One should avoid eating all sour foods,[138] dairy produce and jerked meat strips[139] made from fresh beef[140] and guard against goat meat and black raisins.[141] One should only drink sweet beverages and avoid sour and bitter ones. [14v.] Master al-Ṭūsī transmitted the accounts he has heard about Hippocrates, Aristotle and others, so that those treating themselves with the foodstuffs and acidic[142] syrups we have mentioned will remain free from harm, pains and illnesses. It will remove all weakness and invigorate the individual, especially during coitus; when, Allah willing, he has sexual intercourse, he will not grow weak, his face will not change [in colour], he will never get bored and his condition will be improved.

CHAPTER 2

Description of simple foodstuffs that benefit, strengthen and restore the human body and nature.[143]

Among them, there is Persian halva,[144] the flour for which has to be very fine, moderately salted and soft. The physician Master al-Ṭūsī – may Allah the Almighty have mercy on him – recounts a report from the ancient philosophers that those who from earliest childhood

[15r.] eat dry bread without anything will not be afflicted by disease until they die. Disease is the result only of increases in humours, which are the result of various foodstuffs, including beneficial food such as roasted sheep's meat that should be well done so that it does not disturb the stomach and is quickly digested. The natural foodstuffs that are most appropriate for human nature, and more agreeable than the former two, are:[145] the meat of pigeons,[146] squabs,[147] goslings,[148] chickens,[149] pullets,[150] cockerels before they start crowing, fresh fish[151] and soft-boiled[152] chicken and goose eggs (but note that the eggs of other animals are harmful).[153] One should also eat fish roe,[154] the meat of house sparrows, their brains,[155] fresh cow's and sheep's milk,[156] half-cooked white onions, carrots, turnips,[157] [15v.] chickpeas, leek,[158] sugar, honey, clarified butter made from cow's milk,[159] almonds,[160] hazelnuts,[161] pistachios,[162] fresh ripe dates,[163] green figs,[164] grapes,[165] sweet local pomegranates,[166] sweet ripe local apples and sweet ripe quince[167] which do not contain any trace of bitterness any more. All of the things that we have mentioned strengthen sexual potency, the brain and organs. There are many others but this selection is sufficient.[168] [To strengthen sexual potency, take celery seeds, crush them, and mix them with twice their weight in sugar. Consume this mixture on an empty stomach; it is proved to be effective in *The Old Man's Return to Youth*, where it is said that one should take two *dirhams* of celery seeds and an equal amount of sugar, and to mix them with clarified butter. It should be used for three days and can be combined with anything else you like.] [169]

CHAPTER 3[170]

Description of simple remedies, a summary of medicines that are beneficial for all illnesses that are treated with them, and heighten sexual performance, increase sperm and strengthen potency.

These are the following: musk, ambergris,[171] saffron, parsnip,[172] centaury,[173] cubeb,[174] pepper, ginger, clove, [16r.] anchonium,[175] lac,[176] cinnamon, agarwood, ash tree fruit,[177] citron peel,[178] anise,[179] pistachio, pomegranate blossom,[180] long pepper,[181] costus,[182] salep,[183] red and white tar,[184] galangal,[185] pellitory,[186] lion's fat,[197] goatsbeard,[188] Greek pitch,[189] poppy,[190] carrot seeds, turnip seeds, peppergrass seeds, nutmeg,[191] mace,[192] Indian spikenard, poppy, cardamom, Armenian borax,[193] unbored pearls, shampoo ginger,[194] malabathrum, chebulic myrobalan,[195] belleric myrobalan,[196] the fruit of emblic myrobalan,[197] silk,[198] black cumin,[199] coconut[200] and galingale.[201] All these ingredients strengthen coitus and potency, increase sperm and cure illness.[202] It is especially the medicines that are beneficial that we have mentioned. Commit them to memory so you will remember when any of them are mentioned [16v.] elsewhere in the book when this is required.

CHAPTER 4

Description of compound remedies and foodstuffs that ward off illnesses, sweets that restore human temperament and remove paralysis, limpness of the limbs, and strengthen coitus and sexual potency.

Take two white onions, peel and cut them up. Cook in a small amount of olive oil[203] and water until they are done. Then cook two squabs with rock salt[204] and when they are cooked through, add the onions that have been cooked in oil, and fry everything until it is mixed well. Take a *dirham* each of cinnamon, galangal and peony.[205] Pound all of these condiments and sprinkle them on top of the cooked onions.[206] Eat with unleavened bread and drink the broth. It is very beneficial, remedies foul temperament, brightens the face, purifies the colour and blood, and strengthens [17r.] coitus. This dish has seventeen other beneficial properties in addition to the ones we have mentioned, but it would take too long to enumerate them all. The benefits will become apparent to you during use, Allah the Almighty willing.[207]

Here is another dish: take lamb meat that is neither

too fat nor too lean, that is to say, average. Chop it into small pieces and cook with an identical amount of onions until everything is cooked thoroughly. Afterwards, take a little coconut oil and pour on it [one *dirham* of][208] cardamom, a *dirham* of cinnamon, half a *dirham* of cloves and a *qīrāṭ* of musk. Pulverize these ingredients,[209] mix with coconut oil, pour on the meat in the pot, and stir until everything is mixed. Stew for a little while and then remove from the fire while keeping the lid on the vessel so that the steam does not escape. Leave for an hour to cool down and settle. This should be eaten at lunchtime. It remedies foul temperament, removes weakness, strengthens sexual potency, increases sperm and invigorates coitus, when necessary. It has many benefits that will become apparent [17v.] when it is used.[210]

Another dish: take some pullets, slaughter them, pluck,[211] wash and cut them up into slices. Sprinkle rock salt on the sides and grill on live coal, turning them over on each side, until they are cooked. Then take five *dirhams* of black cumin, three *dirhams* of goatsbeard, four *dirhams* of common ash and half a *dirham* of coconut. Pound[212] all of these and sprinkle on the meat. This dish is eaten for supper. It strengthens the principal organs, increases innate heat, removes coldness from the back and loins, expels moistness and superfluities from the body, reddens the face, and purifies the blood. It also strengthens coitus to the extent that even when one has intercourse for three days running, one need not worry about growing weak. One is able to pleasure ten slave girls and freewomen [18r.] every night, without any trouble or discomfort,[213] as stated by the ancient philosophers and physicians. They also said that one should only divulge these secrets to one's own family. Anyone who uses this recipe for longer will observe its advantages and benefits in a short period of time.

Section containing a description of sweets which, when used by human beings, restore the temperament,[214] cure paralysis, remedy limpness, strengthen the principal organs, increase innate heat, invigorate coitus and increase sperm.[215]

Take 100 *dirhams* of white skimmed bee honey and the same quantity of white onions that have been peeled and cut into small pieces. Cook the two ingredients together and add a little water until they are cooked thoroughly. Add some olive oil, stir through, transfer to a pot and heat[216] over a low fire until the mixture is semi-thickened. Strain [18v.] and wait a little while until it cools down. Then sprinkle the grounds of five *dirhams* of cinnamon, five *dirhams* of citron peel,[217] two *dirhams* of Indian agarwood and half a *dirham* of saffron on top.[218] Pulverize everything, strain through a silk cloth and add to the onions and honey. Beat the mixture with a spoon and transfer to a glass jar. Eat it every evening before going to sleep. You will see that it works wonders.[219]

Here is another recipe. Soak yellow chickpeas in water, and then peel and fry them in clarified butter until they turn red. Take care that they do not get burnt and turn black. Then, crush everything, add the same weight in ground Syrian pine[220] kernels and mix with white skimmed bee honey. Sprinkle the following ground mixture on top: half a *dirham* of saffron, five *dirhams* of citron peel, one *dirham* of cinnamon,[221] half a *dirham* of agarwood and ten [19r.] *dirhams* of cassia.[222] Crush all the ingredients and sprinkle them on the dish. Use every day before going to sleep. It is effective and you will see it works wonders. Even if you had ten slave girls you would be able to pleasure them [throughout the night][223] without any trouble or a change in temperament. It has been tried and tested.[224]

CHAPTER 5

Description of wines that restore spoiled temperaments, purify the blood, invigorate coitus and strengthen potency.

Note that a sweet or red wine is known as garnet wine. It is beneficial. A wine whose colour tends towards yellow is called Yazdi[225] wine and is sweet, white and[226] beneficial. Wine made from squeezing ripe white grapes is referred to as Rayḥānī wine and is also beneficial. However, the best kind is mixed and cooked wine.

Wine can be harmful and should be cooked down to

a third [19v.], in accordance with the customs of sages, with ingredients that are natural and provide benefits, as is known from experiments.

Here is a recipe for a *muthallath*[227] wine, according to the custom of the sages. Take any of the wines you like from the ones mentioned above and place them in a pot with three times the amount of fresh water and cook it until two-thirds of the liquid have evaporated and only one-third remains. Take the weight of 300 *dirhams* from the cooked mixture and add fifty *dirhams* of white bee honey,[228] or white sugar, and cook until the froth appears. Then take[229] two *dirhams* each of ginger and cassia, and one *dirham* each of agarwood, ambergris and Indian spikenard.[230] Pound all of these into a fine powder, strain through a silk cloth and add to the wine. Boil it for a second time for one hour over a low fire, until everything is mixed together. [20r.] Remove from the fire, wait until it cools down and store in a glass container. To use the wine, take forty *dirhams* and mix it with the same amount of water, and drink. This is beneficial, Allah the Almighty willing. It strengthens the stomach, heats the liver, brightens the face, purifies the blood, strengthens innate heat and invigorates coitus. Even if you were to have intercourse with ten slave girls, you would be able to pleasure them all without feeling tired, weakened or discomfort. Your energy will be increased. However, wait two hours before coitus and do not eat anything until afterwards. You will see the wonders it does, Allah the Almighty willing.[231]

[In his *Nuzha*, Dāwūd[232] stated that one should take one *mithqāl* of agarwood, one *qīrāṭ* of musk, three *qīrāṭs* of saffron, half a *raṭl* of honey and six *raṭls* of this wine and ten *raṭls* of fresh water, and cook everything until half of it evaporates and then throw in a small handful of sugar. This gladdens the spirit and is beneficial. It does not require anything to remedy it.][233]

[Almond syrup is also beneficial and useful. It is made by taking almonds and boiling them in hot water until all the skins are removed. Then pound them in a mortar made of marble or wood and soak them in a sufficient amount of fresh water. Afterwards, squeeze them until all the benefits are extracted and add a bit of mastic and a sufficient quantity of white sugar. Cook the mixture over a gentle flame until it thickens slightly and then remove and store.][234]

CHAPTER 6

Description of electuaries and stomachics that raise the spirits and ward off boredom, strengthen the stomach, remove[235] *phlegm and black bile, open up blockages in the brain and organs, purify the blood, dissolve foul wind, strengthen* [20v.] *the principal organs, cure headache, catarrh and innate heat,*[236] *and invigorate coitus to such a great extent that if you were to have intercourse with twenty women, these stomachics would enable you to do so tirelessly, without the member becoming weak. These substances have innumerable benefits, especially when it comes to sexual potency.*

As for the recipe for a cardamom stomachic, the author, may Allah forgive him, says:[237] take four *dirhams* each of frankincense pellets,[238] cardamom and mace; eight *dirhams* of long pepper and ginger; one *dirham* each of amber and Indian agarwood; and ten *dirhams* of saffron. Crush these ingredients as finely as kohl,[239] and strain. Then add the same amount – or half – of skimmed honey to the mixture and store. Use when necessary, and you will see that it works wonders.[240] [21r.]

The recipe for a spikenard electuary is as follows:[241] take half a *dirham* each of Indian spikenard, mace, nutmeg, cloves, black cumin, cardamom and cassia; and sixty *dirhams* of white hulled sesame seeds.[242] Crush all of these spices, except the sesame, into fine dust.[243] Pound the sesame separately and then mix it with the other grounds. Knead the mixture with half the amount of skimmed bee honey. Use when needed three *dirhams* and you will see wonders, especially during coitus.

[Description of a tried and tested extract that cheers the heart and strengthens coitus. Take one *wuqqa*[244] of good quality olive oil, half a *wuqqa* of wheat yeast, and a *raṭl* of salt. Cover everything with enough fresh water and let the mixture ferment overnight. Then, add three *raṭls* of storax and a *wuqqa*[245] of mint. Distil the mixture and store it. It is very effective.][246]

A recipe for a caltrop[247] electuary: take the prickles of the chosen amount of caltrop, cut them finely, place into a pot and boil in water until the active ingredients of the plant have been extracted. Strain the water so that the peels remain, then take out the peels and leaves. Leave the water outside in the sun on hot summer's days. Whenever it dries out, stir it [21v.] so that it becomes syrupy and remains unctuous and smooth. Take one *dirham* of the infusion and add one *dirham* of pellitory, half a *dirham*[248] of ginger, and ten *dirhams* of house sparrows' brains. Thoroughly pound the herbs and then mix with the sparrows' brains. Add the same amount of sugar and skimmed bee honey, and knead everything together into an electuary.[249] Place into a glass container and use when needed.

Whenever you wish to engage in coitus, drink two or three glasses of the *muthallath* wine whose recipe we have provided here. You will see that it works wonders, to the extent that even if you had intercourse with ten women in one night, you would be able to satisfy them all.[250]

The recipe for an electuary of *iṭrīfal*[251] has great benefits and innumerable advantages. It strengthens the intellect;[252] clears the brain from all pains and catarrh; sharpens the eyesight; increases [22r.] its brightness; opens blockages in the head and eyes;[253] improves hearing; purifies the blood; thickens and strengthens the principal organs and innate heat; strengthens potency;[254] tautens the nerves[255] and veins in the penis and testicles; heats the kidneys, bladder and sperm; and greatly invigorates coitus to the extent that one can have sex whenever one wants without growing bored, weak or limp, or suffering any harm.

The recipe is as follows:[256] take three *dirhams* each of the peel of yellow (chebulic) myrobalan, beleric myrobalan[257] and emblic myrobalan,[258] and long pepper; four *dirhams* of the peel of mace and ginger; one *dirham* of parsnip; five *dirhams* of common ash; seven *dirhams* of cassia; and twenty *dirhams* of hulled white sesame. Crush everything, strain through a thin cloth and add half the amount of white sugar [22v.] or skimmed bee honey. Knead all the ingredients and store in a glass vessel, which should be covered with a lid. Bury it in barley[259] for forty days. At need, take three *mithqāls* of the mixture and drink with water.[260] It is beneficial, Allah the Almighty willing, and has been tried and tested.[261]

CHAPTER 7

Description of suppositories that expel moistness from organs; remove coldness from the back and hip;[262] extract phlegm, yellow bile and black bile; and greatly strengthen coitus.

As for the recipe: [the author says] take five *dirhams* of white sugar, two *dirhams* of ginger and one *qīrāṭ* of pellitory and finely pound everything so that it becomes like kohl dust.[263] Add the same amount of skimmed bee honey, knead it together with the grounds into a suppository and use before going to sleep. It is beneficial, Allah the Almighty willing.

Another recipe, which is as follows, according to al-Mufīd: take the brains of three sparrows and one *qīrāṭ* of pellitory; pound the two finely [23r.] together, strain and knead with bee honey to make the medication. Take it before going to sleep. It will achieve the desired result and is beneficial.[264]

Another recipe: crush three *dirhams* each of cotton seeds[265] and colchicum,[266] and knead the grounds together with lion's fat to make the medication. Take before going to sleep with cotton. When the two are brought together, you will see its wondrous effects, especially during coitus. It is beneficial, Allah the Almighty willing.[267]

CHAPTER 8

Description of enemas which protect against joint ache, sciatica, back- and hip aches; expel foul wind; remove colic; tauten the back and strengthen coitus.

Take the testicles of two lambs, crush them and place in a pot. Add the same amount of red wheat and a handful of turnip seeds, and place everything in an earthenware pot. Pour in enough water to cover the mixture [23v.], put a lid on the vessel and leave it in a brick oven[268] overnight until it is cooked thoroughly. Remove it from the oven in the morning. Take 30 *dirhams* of the water and pour two *dirhams* of coconut oil over it. [In the absence of coconuts, walnut oil can be used.][269] Administer the enema in the morning, after bathing and on an empty stomach. Put a cushion underneath the hips so that the head is positioned low and the legs high in order for the water to penetrate the belly and flow through the bowels. You will see that it does wonders when the enema is administered twice a year, once in spring and once in autumn. It will protect from all illnesses and ailments, Allah the Almighty willing.

Here is another type of enema: take three *dirhams* each of carrot seeds, gourd[270] seeds, dill[271], onion seeds, leek seeds, cinnamon bark, ginger, pepper[272] and long pepper; a handful of peeled chickpeas and ground wheat; [24r.] a thin piece of meat; and the fat and testicles of a lamb.

Place the preparation in a pot with the lid on and leave overnight in a hot *tannūr*[273] or brick oven until everything is cooked thoroughly. Then, take it out and make an enema, which is known as the 'aperient enema'.[274] It has twenty-seven benefits. If it is administered once a year, in spring, it protects against all illnesses and ailments until the next spring, Allah the Almighty willing.

CHAPTER 9

Description of the bandages and clothing that are appropriate for human nature when they are tied tightly during the four seasons.[275]

If the bandages run counter to human nature according to the seasons, the individual may become afflicted with diseases and so it is necessary that the bandages and clothes are appropriate for the period of the year [24v.] during which they should be worn to ensure that the organs are tightened, remain strong, and that their temperament does not get spoilt.

The most appropriate bandages and clothes for spring, which is the best of all seasons because of its temperate heat and coldness, are those made of cotton since it has an average temperature and does not disturb the temperament.

As for the second season, summer, in which the heat intensifies, the bandages and waistbands should be woven out of silk and linen, or only linen, but not just silk.

In autumn, the bandages and clothes should be made out of wool, woven fabric, or patches.[276]

As for furs, they should be [25r] sable, ermine, grey squirrel, or white and black sheepskin. Bandages can also be made from camel wool or sable pelt which has to be purified in the manner known in Turkish as *kamar qashāq*.[277] Anyone who proceeds in this way will be protected from a weakening of the principal organs, ache in the joints, palpitations, colic, and various other illnesses,[278] Allah the Almighty willing.

CHAPTER 10

Description of the conditions of coitus and how to conduct it so as to as to avoid weakness, harm, premature old age and grey hair.[279]

Know that having sexual intercourse standing up harms human beings and causes palpitations, pleurisy, sciatica, pneumonia, gout and headache[280] – may Allah protect us from all of this![281] These are all dangerous diseases [25v.] that are difficult to treat. Most of them occur as a result of having coitus standing up. Some people do not heed these words, claiming that they have always had intercourse standing up, without being afflicted by any of these illnesses. However, we say that these illnesses caused by coitus while standing up occur either immediately, or result in a weakness of the innate heat or of the temperament. How can those who subscribe to this view say that they are free from these illnesses when they may occur gradually? We say that this only applies to those who perform sexual intercourse standing up to excess, not once or twice in their lifetime, out of passion or love in their youth. Perhaps protection against this kind of pain [26r.] and harm is offered by great innate heat and strength of the principal organs. Some of these people also experience harm due to a lack of knowledge about themselves or about their strength. This should suffice for the intelligent.

As for coitus when the man is standing sideways, it is also extremely harmful and causes heart and liver pains, colic and urinary incontinence.[282] Allah protect us from this! Sexual intercourse on the right-hand side, in particular, is more harmful than that on the left.[283]

Coitus from behind, with the woman lying on her stomach, causes bladder pain, inhibited urination,[284] urine dribbling or a burning sensation when urinating, gall pains with blood and pus in urine, or both, whether urinating or not. Allah protect us from that! [26v.]

An intelligent man should be wary of engaging in coitus in the above-mentioned harmful positions, so as to avoid the illnesses we have described.

These illnesses can be cured as follows: take ripe black nightshade[285] and squeeze the juice out. Then take ripe juniper,[286] extract the juice from it by cooking and add the same amount of cane sugar.[287] Mix both liquids together and cook the mixture over a low fire. Use in a quantity of one spoonful on an empty stomach, and one spoonful in the evening before going to sleep. It is beneficial, Allah the Almighty willing.[288]

Know that the best and most appropriate position for coitus is when the woman is lying flat on her back.[289] Put a thin cushion underneath her hips, with the woman then lifting her thighs by herself, rather than the man doing it since this will cause him hardship [27r.] during coitus and be harmful. The man should be on all fours until he is close to ejaculating, at which point he places his knees on the floor and lies down on the woman, who embraces him with both arms and legs, clutching him tightly to her chest until ejaculation has been completed and the sperm goes straight to the uterus. The man should not get up so that the sperm is not wasted since this will lead to non-conception, while also causing harm to the man. Coitus that takes place in this manner and under the conditions that we have just described, leads to the benefits that we have mentioned and protects the man against the illnesses listed.[290]

CHAPTER 11

Description of the medicines that are rubbed on the penis in order to thicken and harden it and making it stand up without any limpness.[291]

Especially if a man [27v.] is unable to ingest hot substances, he is treated with medicines that are rubbed onto the penis. Take identical measures of narcissus bulbs,[292] pellitory and seedless red raisins, and crush them with one quarter the amount of coconut until everything is finely ground. One hour prior to coitus, wash the penis with hot water, massaging it vigorously when doing so. Then, rub the mixture onto the penis. You will see that it works like fire and will make the penis thick, powerful and sturdy, as required.

According to another preparation, you should take half a *dirham* of cottonseed kernels, two and a half *dirhams* of galingale, half a *dirham* of Syrian carob kernels and one *qīrāṭ* of coconut. Crush all the ingredients, add the water of grapes or Rāziqī[293] raisins, and cook over a low fire until everything is mixed and the water has thickened. Remove the decoction from the fire and rub on [28r.] the penis, when required.[294]

Another recipe, which works on those whose organs and penis are limp, leaving them impotent after coitus or when they have not had it, or for whatever other reason. This is treated by[295] taking ten *dirhams* of goat gall and pellitory, which is finely ground and mixed with the galingale oil. Leave it outside in the sun for three days, until everything has been mixed together. Add one and a half *dirhams* of pounded coconut, combine well and then store the mixture. Rub the decoction on the penis several times a day for three days prior to coitus. It will restore and strengthen the penis. Galen stated that it improves the condition of those who treat themselves by using this preparation; it stiffens the limp penis and restores youth to old age, [28v.] whereas those who use it in their youth will never become impotent, and are able to perform like a twenty-year-old. This is how the situation is resolved.[296]

Description of the properties of sweet basil or galingale oil, as well as other oils.[297]

If you want to make an aromatic oil, choose any one you like. For instance, take either sweet basil or galingale and crush it. Put the ground substance in a flask, pour on double the measure of good olive oil and cover with a lid secured with wax so that the container becomes airtight. Hang it outside in the hot sun for forty days during summer. The sun should shine on it without interruption from sunrise until sunset. Afterwards, strain the mixture through a fine-meshed sieve or a thin cloth, and store. This is the way and method oil of aromatics such as galingale or sweet violet is extracted.

As for oil of kernels, such as [29r.] pistachio oil, almond oil, hazelnut oil, cottonseed oil, walnut oil and others, and pomegranate blossom[298] oil and the such, these are made differently. They are extracted as follows: take the desired quantity of kernels and pound them until you obtain something resembling fine grounds. Take a tinned copper tray and place it over hot ashes on the fire.[299] Wet your hands with tepid water and beat the grounds on the plate. Fold and roll until all the oil has been extracted. Proceed in this fashion for all kernels.[300]

CHAPTER 12

Description of the medicines that are rubbed on the penis so that it is lengthened and strengthened, as you desire.

Know that the penis consists of many veins and that it becomes longer during coitus and by massaging it. However, this is not similar to what happens when using an ointment, which is [29v.] stronger due to the medicines it contains, as mentioned by Plato, Aristotle, Hippocrates and Galen, who have written about this phenomenon based on their knowledge and experiments.[301]

Muḥammad al-Dāmghānī[302] and the Imam al-Rāzī[303] – may Allah the Almighty have mercy on him – reported from Plato the following about lengthening the penis.[304] Take the root of a caltrop plant over one year old, clean it with water, dry, pound it fine, and then strain through a fine-meshed sieve. Get into the bath, massage the mixture into the penis and wash it with hot water until it grows red. Then, put the crushed caltrop root on the penis. Afterwards, rub it with an ointment made from galingale oil mixed with half a *dirham* of ground coconut. If you comply with this recipe and apply the ointment onto the penis three times while in the bath, until it rises above the surface of the water, you will be astonished by its lengthening. It will only be effective [30r.] for ten days, but you may repeat the procedure.

Here is an unusual and strange recipe, which is one of the secrets of the wise, and doubles the length of the penis. Take fresh moist sheep dung and dry ambergris in an amount that is required for rubbing the penis, as well as one *qīrāṭ* of musk. Pound it and mix vigorously with two *dirhams*[305] of very finely crushed coconut. Get into the bath and forcefully massage your penis with the galingale oil until your member becomes red. Then rub the ingredients mixed with the sheep dung on the penis in the way that a ring is coated, and wrap it into a cloth from dawn till dusk. Afterwards, remove the cloth and wash the penis. You will see a wonder, since the penis will have grown twice in size. This effect only lasts for twenty days, and must be repeated.

CHAPTER 13

Description of medicines that are rubbed in between the fingers [30v.] *and toes in order to invigorate coitus and stiffen the penis so that one never becomes weak, tired or limp, no matter how much one engages in sexual intercourse.*

Take house sparrows before they have acquired their flight feathers, tie them up with a string and hang them from the entrance of a beehive. Then, agitate the bees so that they start stinging the sparrows. Once the birds have been stung several times, take them down quickly and slaughter them, making sure not to let their blood drip on the floor, but to collect it in a container. Put them in a pot and pour over the above-mentioned aromatic oil until the birds are submerged in it. Cover the pot and place on a fire until the sparrows are fully cooked. Then, remove them, strain the water with a cloth until the essence of the birds has infused the oil. Then finely pound a *qīrāṭ* of resin spurge[306] until it has the texture of kohl, and mix very well with the oil. Put the oil into a flask and seal. Place in the hot sun for three days. If required, pour some of the oil on a cotton cloth [31r.] and rub between your fingers and toes. You will see a wonder as you will be able to engage in coitus as much as you like without ever becoming weak, limp or tired. Your penis will not go to sleep either and will remain standing until you wash it several times with cold water.

Another recipe: take 100 small and large black ants and put them in a flask. Pour on five *dirhams* of blue liquorice oil, seal the flask and hang in the hot sun for twenty days. Then, vigorously pound everything until the mixture has fermented. At the time it is needed, take one *qīrāṭ* of Indian agarwood, crush it finely, put it in ten *dirhams* of hot water and wash the penis, hands, feet and armpits with the water. Take one drop – or another small quantity – from the flask, [31v.] without the water, and rub it on your fingers, teeth, armpits and elbows. Wait one hour before coitus. Even if you were to engage in coitus with ten women during the night, you would not be incapacitated or weakened.

CHAPTER 14

Description of pills, which, when used by a man, provide great pleasure during coitus.

Take a *dirham* of mastic, one and a half *qīrāṭs* of musk, half a *dirham* of cloves, five *dirhams* of sugar and half a *dirham* of coconut. Pound everything as finely as kohl powder, place in a flask, pour oil over it, covering the grounds, and hang in the sun for three days until everything has mixed with the oil. Then add the same amount of white skimmed bee honey and thicken the mixture. Mould pills of one *dirham* in weight each. When needed [32r.] for coitus, place one pill in your mouth and you will see the wonders it does.

Another type of recipe: roast pistachio kernels over a fire, making sure that they do not get burnt. Once they are roasted and dried, crush an amount equalling one *dirham* and add one *dirham* of cloves, one *qīrāṭ* of musk, and one *dirham* of ambergris. Pound everything as finely as kohl and stir in the pistachio oil remaining from the roasting until it turns into a paste, and leave it out in the sun for three days. Make the pills with sugar or skimmed bee honey, in the usual manner, and store. Each pill should weigh one *dirham*. When needed, put one pill in your mouth and then have sexual intercourse. You will see a miracle.

CHAPTER 15

Description of the position during coitus that provides great pleasure to both the man and woman, as stated by the ancient philosophers and physicians [32v.] *who gained knowledge of this from their experiments.*

Take one *dirham* of cinnamon, half a *dirham* of pellitory

and one *qīrāṭ* of cardamom, and pound everything as finely as dust. Afterwards, mix it with Rāziqī grape juice and rub the preparation onto the whole penis. Wait one hour and wash the penis with hot water. Put half a *dirham* of cassia in your mouth and chew it. Take some of the saliva and rub it on the penis before engaging in coitus. Both the man and woman will experience wondrous rapture, without either of them suffering any disturbance.

Another type of preparation: take one *qīrāṭ* each of cubeb, pellitory, cassia, ginger and coconut. Pound everything together and knead with thick bee honey. Put some of the mixture in your mouth and then rub some of the saliva on your penis prior to coitus. You will see the wonder of indescribable rapture experienced by both the man and the woman.

CHAPTER 16

Description of medicines which, if inserted by women, lead to a narrowing of their wombs and vaginas, increasing their heat and pleasure.[307]

[33r.] Take two *dirhams* of pellitory, five *dirhams* of goatsbeard, sixteen *dirhams* of undiluted wine, as well as myrtle berries,[308] and crush everything. Place in a pot, immerse in water, and boil over a fire until one-third of the water and some of the wine have evaporated. At that point, the woman should stand over the steam seven times, after which the pot is removed, and its contents stored. When needed, the woman moistens a cloth with the decoction and inserts it [into her vagina]. This will make the vagina narrower and hotter than a virgin's.[309]

Another preparation: take equal parts of undiluted wine, pomegranate peels and pellitory.[310] Crush everything and cook in undiluted aged wine.[311] The woman then moistens a woollen cloth with it and inserts for one hour. This will make the vagina as narrow and hot[312] as a virgin's.[313]

Another one: take equal measures of acorn,[314] safflower, galingale, rosemary[315] and houseleek.[316] Coarsely pound and mix them all together [33v.], then boil and strain. Afterwards, strain the weight of five *dirhams* of pellitory onto the mixture and boil everything over a high fire. Remove it and, at need, the woman takes two or three portions, as a result of which her vagina will be as narrow and hot as a virgin's.

CHAPTER 17

Description of medicines that, when inserted by a woman, prevent pregnancy for as long as she uses them and make her vagina as tight and hot as a young girl's.

Take bear gall and mix thoroughly with Rāziqī grape juice. If the woman puts a very small amount of the mixture inside [her vagina], she will not conceive and will remain like a young virgin.

According to another recipe, take one *mithqāl* of cow gall and the same amount of wolf gall, place in a pot and immerse in sesame oil. When a woman soaks a piece of cotton or wool in the mixture and wears it inside her vagina, she will become like a young virgin, and will never conceive.

Another one: anyone who takes pitch[317] and rubs it on his penis at the time of [34r.] coitus, will experience the greatest pleasure and the woman will not be able to conceive, unless she receives treatment.[318]

CHAPTER 18

Description of the medicines that result in a woman becoming pregnant, if Allah the Almighty wills it.

Take half a dirham each of Indian agarwood and fresh myrtle leaves, one *qīrāṭ* of musk, and pulverize everything. Then, wrap the mixture in a fine cloth and place in a pot. Pour over a little aged wine and boil over a low fire until the essence of the ingredients has infused the wine. Then, strain with water and transfer to a flask. When needed, the woman inserts a piece of wool [soaked in it]. She will be like a young virgin and it will make her conceive, Allah the Almighty willing.

Another recipe: take green oak apples,[320] Mekkan lemon-grass,[321] two *dirhams* of each, and one *dirham* of fresh dates.[322] Pound everything finely and boil in wine until the essence of the ingredients has been released, and then store.[323] When necessary, a woman inserts a piece of wool [soaked in it]. This will make her conceive, [34v.] Allah the Almighty willing.

Another one: take four *dirhams* of crushed[324] camphor[325] peel, two *dirhams* of red alum,[326] one *dirham* of galingale, four and a half *dirhams* of pounded green oak apples and half a *qīrāṭ* of Mekkan soil. Coarsely crush all of these, except the oak apples, and then boil in wine as usual, strain its water and store. When it is needed, the woman soaks a piece of wool in the decoction and inserts it, while lying down on her back for one hour prior to coitus. She will be like a young virgin, and conceive, Allah the Almighty willing.

Another recipe: take goatsbeard, pound and crush it to extract its juice. Then, take green oak apples, pomegranate peels, Indian agarwood and citron peel, half a *dirham* each; four *dirhams* of red alum; and one *dirham* of galingale. Pound everything and cook in aged wine until the essence of the substances has infused the wine. When [35r.] the woman inserts it, she will become like a young virgin and conceive, Allah the Almighty willing.

Another recipe: take cardamom, half a *dirham*; gum

Arabic[327] and black cumin, one *qīrāṭ* of each; Isfahani kohl and citron peel,[328] half a *dirham of* each. Pound everything together and boil in aged wine, until the essence of the substances has infused the wine. When needed, the woman puts some on a piece of cloth and inserts it. She will become like a young virgin, untouched by a man, and conceive, Allah the Almighty willing.

This completes the book, thanks to Allah, His assistance and His granting of success. Praise be to Allah for everything and may Allah bless our Master Muḥammad, his family and companions and grant them salvation until the Day of Judgement, He is the Lord of the Worlds. In the Name of Allah, the merciful the compassionate.[329] (1208)[330]

Notes

1. [C] addition: 'This is the book of sexual stimulants and the sultan's potions written by the most erudite shaykh, freeborn and endowed with great understanding, holder of blessings, Nāṣir [*sic*] al-Dīn al-Ṭūsī, may Allah have mercy on him and all Muslims. Amen. Amen. Amen.' In [B], the title is missing.
2. The folio numbers in square brackets are based on [A].
3. [C] addition: 'and the one we seek assistance from, praise be to Allah, who demonstrates His love for all beings. Prayers and peace upon the finest of the human race, Master Muḥammad, the messenger of clear verses, upon his family and companions, and exaltations upon those who follow them.'
4. This character, commonly endowed with the epithet *al-ḥakīm* ('the wise') was known for his wisdom. The thirty-first *sūra* of the Qur'ān is named after him.
5. Qur'ān 31:12. The Qur'ān translations are those of M. Pickthall, *The Meaning of the Glorious Koran.*
6. Qur'ān 57:29.
7. See Introduction.
8. See Introduction.
9. This is how the name appears in all three manuscripts, rather than the more correct 'Naṣīr'.
10. *al-adwiya al-mufrada* or *al-basīṭa* (< Greek φάρμακα ἁπλᾶ). In Islamic medicine, drugs (*adwiya*, sg. *dawā'*) were divided both according to origin (vegetable, animal, mineral) and to composition ('simple' vs 'compound'), which, of course, went back to the Greek tradition. See *EI*[2], s.v. 'adwiya' (B. Lewin).
11. *al-adwiya al-murakkaba* (< Gr. φάρμακα σύνθετα). The most famous treatises dealing with the 'compound drugs' were those by Sābūr Ibn Sahl (d. 869), Amīn al-Dawla Ibn al-Tilmīdh (d. 1165) and al-Rāzī. *EI*[2], s. vv. 'Aḳrābādhīn' (B. Lewin), 'Sābūr b. Sahl' (O. Kahl); Ibn Sahl [O. Kahl 2003]; *GAL*, I, 269, 642.
12. The passage 'obstructions ... sexual potency' is abridged in [C] to: 'on medicines beneficial for the temperaments, weakness of the organs, etc.'
13. *ja/uwārishāt*, sg. *ja/uwārish* (with *ja/uwārishn* being a common variant in medical texts), from the Persian *jawārish* (Pahlavi *guwārish*), meaning 'whatever is used in the dressing of meat, or assists in digestion', F. Steingass 1892: 376; I. Fellmann 1986: 198 –200.

14. The description of this chapter appears as follows in [C]: 'The description of electuaries and stomachics that are beneficial for the stomach and the removal of yellow bile, phlegm, black bile, and the brain; to open blockages in the organs; reduce foul wind; and strengthen the innate heat.'
15. *ashyāf* (sg. *shiyāf*) – this term generally denoted eye medicines, collyria, but was also sometimes applied to 'suppositories'; Ibn Janāḥ 2020: No. 27; E. Lev and Z. Amar 2008: 568; E. Lane 1863–74: IV, 1619.
16. [C] omits reference to yellow and black bile.
17. The passage 'lungs ... all functions' is omitted in [C].
18. The phrase 'in order not to upset human nature and cause illness' is omitted from [C], which simply has 'to restore <human> nature'.
19. [C] omits the reference to impotence.
20. [C]:'on other benefits related to sexual potency and increasing lust [of medication] to rub on the penis'.
21. 'They are useful during coitus, strengthen it and prevent impotence resulting from frequent intercourse' is reduced to 'to strengthen coitus' in [C].
22. The description of Chapter 15 in [C] is as follows: 'description of what happens to the man and the woman in terms of pleasure during coitus and the frequency of it'.
23. The passage 'if used by women ...' is as follows in [C]: 'if women use it, their cheeks will become red and their vaginas will improve'.
24. [C]: 'description of medicines that prevent pregnancy and tighten the vaginas'.
25. [C]: 'description of drugs for conception and other benefits, Allah the Almighty willing'.
26. [B]: 'the index of the book and chapters.'
27. Qur'ān 3:173.
28. The passage 'which we have presented ... student' is as follows in [C]: 'In order to make it easier for those who need it to obtain information without difficulty, in the Name of Allah who provides assistance and to Whom you pray. Know that He grants us success.'
29. The passage 'praise be to Him ... pairs' is as follows in [C]: 'Through His beneficence and generosity Allah has created animals and brought them into existence out of nothing. He has created them in pairs and given them souls as they need and yearn for each other as a pair.'
30. This phrase is omitted from [C].
31. Qur'ān 17: 70. This is only part of the verse, the remainder of which reads: 'and [We] have made provision of good things for them, and have preferred them above many of those whom We created with a marked preferment.'
32. The previous sentence and the part until 'no more awful cause' is missing from [C].
33. The notion of sperm (*minan*) in Islamic medicine went back to the Greek (Galenic) tradition, and women were also thought to have sperm. There was a correlation between the amount of sperm and sexual potency in men. The concept of sperm was discussed by a number of authorities, both medical and philosophical, including Ibn Sīnā (1999, II: 726ff.), D. al-Anṭākī (1999: 174ff.) and al-Ṭabarī (1928: 266). Also see B. Musallam 1983: 43–52; D. Jacquart and F. Thomasset 1988: 52–6; E. Anwar, in S.

Joseph and Nağmābādī 2003: 31ff.; de Lacy 1992; J. Dugan, 'Preventing Ciceronianism: C. Licinius Calvus' Regimen for Sexual and Oratorical Self-Mastery', *Classical Philology*, 96:3, 2001, 400–28.

34. ʿAlī Ibn Abī Ṭālib (600–61), cousin and son-in-law of the Prophet Muḥammad, and the fourth of the so-called 'Rightly Guided Caliphs' (*al-khulafāʾ al-rāshidūn*). The conflict surrounding the succession to the Prophet pitted two sides of the Muslim community against each other, with ʿAlī's supporters considering him the only rightful heir to the Prophet, and thus the first caliph. This disagreement gave rise to the split between sunni (< *sunna*, 'sayings and deeds of the Prophet') and shīʿī (< *shīʿat ʿAlī*, 'the party of ʿAlī').
35. Instead of ʿAlī, [C] has 'Prince of the Believers' (*amīr al-muʾminīn*), the title reserved for caliphs.
36. The preceding part of this sentence appears as follows in [C]: 'He who knows the circumstances and conditions of coitus is not harmed by it, but benefits from it.'
37. cf. al-Kātib 1977: 48–50.
38. cf. *ibid.*, 48.
39. The remainder of this paragraph and the whole of the next are mising from [C].
40. [D] adds 'as long as the principal organs remain free from pain, the body will not weaken, especially if it has medicines ...'
41. al-Ṭūsī's phrase *lā rāda li-qaḍāʾihi wa lā mānīʿ li-ḥukmihi* is a variant on the more common *lā rāda li-qaḍāʾihi wa lā muʿaqqab li-ḥukmihi wa lā ghālib li-amrihi*, which is a quote from *al-ʿAqīda al-Ṭaḥāwiyya*, by Imam Abū Jaʿfar al-Ṭaḥāwi (d. 935).
42. This sentence is omitted from [C].
43. Addition in [D] and [E].
44. Gr. Παλλάδιος; in the text, the name is transliterated as *Pallāṭiyūs*. This sixth-century Greek author was active in Alexandria, and is known to have written commentaries on some of Hippocrates' and Galen's works. Palladius was also quoted by al-Rāzī.
45. *Arisṭū* – this is somewhat confusing, as this is the usual rendition in Arabic texts of 'Aristotle' (alongside the more narrow transliteration *Arisṭūṭālīs*, which appears earlier in the sentence).
46. The last two sentences appear as follows in [C]: 'These organs are strengthened by medicines, electuaries, syrups, unguents, and by taking precautions against harm to ensure that the limbs remain safe from defects and illnesses.'
47. This section is missing from [E].
48. 'the most temperate' is omitted from [C].
49. For similar comments, see Ibn Lūqā 1973: 24 (trans. 16); Ibn Māssa 1971: 7–8 (though he is also favourable towards autumn, provided the nights and days are of equal length). In addition to seasons, frequency of sexual activity was also linked to age (al-Tīfāshī 1970: 13–6).
50. 'If this is the case' is omitted from [C].
51. Part of the sentence ('does not make the body sluggish ...') is missing from [C].

52. The last two sentences appear as follows in [C]: 'Coitus outside spring are harmful except if it is done with medication, [in which case] it does not cause any harm, Allah the Almighty willing.'
53. In [C], 'wheat-coloured skin, with either strong or limp flesh' is reduced to 'with strong flesh'.
54. [C]: 'and coitus does not harm them' (for 'Those who fall into this category are eager for sexual intercourse').
55. The last two sentences are missing from [C].
56. 'of and slight lean build' is omitted from [C].
57. cf. Ibn Lūqā 1974: 24. [D] adds 'and who have a choleric temperament'.
58. According to al-Suyūṭī (n.d.: 24), sexual intercourse was harmful to those with choleric and melancholic temperaments (even if they practised it only once a year!), whereas phlegmatics and sanguines were endowed with a great capacity for coitus and should have intercourse two or three times a week (though not twice in one day or night). Ibn Sīnā (1999, II: 728) held that coitus was beneficial for the melancholic.
59. The whole passage on white-skinned individuals is missing from [C].
60. The first part of the sentence is as follows in [C]: 'weakness of the limbs arises from weakness for coitus and its signs are vertigo, weak eyesight and sunken eyes.'
61. [D] has 'vigour' instead of ecstasy.
62. [D] adds that 'sugar syrup expels moistness'.
63. This sentence is as follows in [C]: 'Its treatment consists of sugar syrup, which dissolves superfluities, strengthens coitus and increases sperm; it has a number of benefits.'
64. *zanjabīl* (< Gr. ζιγγίβερι) – hot (in the third degree) and dry (in the second degree), only the root was used of this plant, which is also mentioned in the Qur'ān (76:17). In medicine and pharmacology, it was considered beneficial for digestion and as a sexual stimulant (especially in a conserve, *zanjabīl murabbā*). E. Lev, Z. Amar 2008: 174–5; al-Bīrūnī 1973: 206ff.; Ibn Sīnā 1999, I: 455–6, II, 734; al-Rāzī 1955–69, XX, 569–73; al-Tīfāshī 1892: 13, 14; Ibn Lūqā 1974: 16 (trans. 23); *Kitāb* (Tunis No. 20648[09]): fol. 87; al-Shayzarī, *al-Īḍāḥ*, fol. 3; D. al-Anṭākī 1952: I, 180; Ibn al-Bayṭār 1874: II, 167–8, Ibn al-Jazzār 2004: 126–7; al-Dhahabī 1987: 185; al-Suyūṭī n.d.: 14; A. Dietrich 1988: II, 306; Ibn al-Quff [H. Kircher 1967]: 195.
65. *qirfa* (*Cinnamomum zeylanicum*) – the dried rolled bark of the cinnamon tree, which some authors credited with aphrodisiacal qualities. See al-Tīfāshī 1892: 14; *Kitāb* (Tunis No. 20648[09]): fol. 87; al-Shayzarī, *al-Īḍāḥ*, fol. 3; al-Rāzī 1955–69, XXI: 270; Ibn Sīnā 1999: I, 643, II, 734; al-Bīrūnī 1973: 398; Ibn al-Bayṭār 1992: 230; A. Dietrich 1988: II, 127–8; J. Leibowitz and S. Marcus 1974: 233; Ibn Sahl [O. Kahl 2003]: *passim* ('canella', *Canella winterana*). For a discussion of the terminology relating to 'cinnamon', see E. Lev and Z. Amar 2008: 143–6. Also see the notes below on *salīkha* and *dār ṣīnī infra*.
66. 1 *dirham* = 3.125 grammes; W. Hinz 1970: 3; *EI*[2], s.v. 'dirham' (G. C. Miles); S. D. Goitien 1967–88: II, 267 (3.5 grammes).
67. *qāqulla* (from the Akkadian *qāqullu*) – in Arabic medicine and pharmacology, a distinction was made between 'large (male) *qāqulla*' (*haylabū*; *Amomum subulatum Roxb.*) and 'the small *qāqulla*' (also known

by the Persian borrowings *hāl* or *hīl*; *Elettaria cardamomum*). Hot and dry, this aromatic spice was used in cooking and as a digestive, anti-emetic, to relieve obstructions in the liver and kidneys, and as a remedy for colds. It should not be confused with *qāqullā* (saltwort, *Salsola fruticosa*), which was sometimes also known as *qilī* (the etymon for the English *alkaline*). Some authors claimed it had aphrodisiacal properties. Ibn al-Bayṭār 1955–69: IV, 2; Ibn al-Jazzār 2004: 15, 21; D. al-Anṭākī 1952: I, 253–4; Ibn Sīnā 1999: I, 642–3; al-Tīfāshī 1892: 14; *Kitāb* [Tunis No. 20648(09)]: fol. 87; al-Bīrūnī 1973: 299 (trans. 263); Ibn Wāfid 2000: 83ff.; A. Dietrich 1988: II, 425–6, 488; Ibn Janāḥ 2020: No. 280.

68. *qaranful* (*Syzygium aromaticum*) – this herb (the unopened flower buds of evergreen trees from China and India) had a wide range of applications and was used in perfumes, cooking as well as medicine for all manner of ailments. In Arab pharmacology, it was said to strengthen and gladden the heart, to improve eyesight, breath, digestion and sexual potency, as an anti-emetic and to treat diabetes. When taken by women, cloves could either aid or prevent pregnancy. According to Maimonides, it was an ingredient in an aphrodisiac pill for stimulating erection and increasing sexual pleasure. *EI*[2], s.v. 'ḳaranful' (E. Ashtor); Ibn Jazla, ff. 169v.–170r.; E. Lev and Z. Amar 2008: 151–2; A. Dietrich 1988: II, 394; D. al-Anṭākī 1952: I, 255; Ibn al-Bayṭār 1874: IV, 7ff, *idem* 1992: 229–30; Ibn al-Jazzār 2004: 73; al-Kindī (M. Levey 1966): Nos. 3, 106, 152, 213, 225–6; al-Bīrūnī 1973: 302; Ibn al-Quff (H. Kircher 1967): 314–5; al-Suyūṭī n.d.: 15; Ibn Sīnā 1999: I, 642.

69. *za'farān* (*Crocus sativus*) – in addition to its uses in cooking, saffron (which was considered hot and dry) was said to have a number of medicinal properties (for example, as a stimulant for the nervous system, digestive, anaesthetic, diuretic and emmenagogue, and as an ingredient in collyria), as well as being an aphrodisiac. It is for this reason that, according to one hadith, the Prophet forbade the wearing of clothes dyed with saffron (or warras) for pilgrims who were in a state of ritual purity (*muḥrim*), and thus debarred from sexual activity. Some scholars, such as al-Qazwīnī, warned that high doses of saffron were poisonous. The spice was also sometimes known as *ghumr*, *jasād*, *rayhaqān*, *jādī* or even *kurkum* (which, in fact, denotes turmeric). *EI*[2], s.v. 'za'farān' (D. Waines / F. Sanagustin); E. Lev and Z. Amar 2008: 270–3; al-Bīrūnī 1973: 202-4 (trans. 166–8); Ibn Wāfid 2000: 146–7; al-Dhahabī 1987: 184–5; Ibn al-Bayṭār 1874: II, 162–3; Ibn al-Jazzār 2004: 78–9; Ibn Sīnā 1999: I, 464; D. al-Anṭākī 1952: I, 178–9; al-Tīfāshī 1892: 14; *Kitāb* [Tunis No. 20648(09)]: fol. 87; al-Kātib 2002: 36; al-Shayzarī, *al-Īḍāḥ*, fol. 3; *Risāla* [Cairo 362]: p. 5; Maimonides [M. Meyerhof 1940]: No. 135; E. Lev *and* Z. Amar 2008: 270, 272–3; al-Qazwīnī 1849: 250; A. Dietrich 1988: II, 107–8; Ibn al-Quff [H. Kircher 1967]: 193–4.

70. [C]: 'caradamom ...': 'cloves and cardamom, two *dirhams* each; pour freshwater on until everything is covered and boil over a fire until the essence of the medicines has infused the water. Strain and throw away the dregs. Add thirty-three *dirhams* of sugar, boil over a fire until everything is mixed and then remove it before use.'

71. [C]: 'During coitus, there is weakness of the heart, which manifests itself during forceful movement, walking and anger in ...'

72. [B]: '... heart and nerve palpitations, and when the nerves have subsided they will become weak and limp. If there is excess in these ailments during coitus the person will die. These ailments should be treated with apple syrup, which expels them, strengthens the heart ...'; [C]: 'the person's colour will change and this harms him during coitus. This should be treated with apple syrup as this expels ailments, strengthens the heart, removes superfluities from the stomach, heats up and increases sperm. It has many benefits and its recipe is as follows: take an apple segment, peel it and throw ...'

73. *tuffāḥ* (*Malus sylvestris* [*Pyrus malus*], *Rosaceae*) – the Syrian and Isfahani apples were traditionally considered the best varieties. In medicine, apples, which were cold and dry, were used (mainly the skin) to relieve intestinal pains, as a lactation inducer and antidote (especially the juice from the leaves) against poisons (notably scorpion bites). The mere smell of apples was said to be able to strengthen the heart and brain. As a treatment of eye diseases, apples were cooked in water, or even breast milk. Ibn Wāfid 2000: 123–4; *EI*[2], s.v. 'tuffāḥ' (A. Dietrich); E. Lev & Z. Amar 2008: 335–6; A. Dietrich 1988: I, 86–7; II, 175–6, 631–3; al-Dhahabī 1987: 137; Ibn al-Bayṭār 1874: I, 138–9; D. al-Anṭākī 1952: I, 96; Ibn Sīnā 1999: I, 691–2; Ibn Sahl [O. Kahl 2003]: Nos. 255, 279, 318, 327; al-Bīrūnī 1973: 115–6 (trans., 91).

74. *mā' al-ward* – in addition to its primary uses in cosmetics (for example, as a deodorant) and cooking, rosewater (usually distilled from the damask rose) had a number of medical uses, mainly in ophthalmic treatments such as ophthalmia and cataract, as well as against migraine and nausea. Frequent application to the hair allegedly accelerated grey hair growth. It was considered cold and dry in the first degree. EI2, s.v. (F. Sanagustin); D. al-Anṭākī 1952: I, 339; Ibn al-Bayṭār 1874: IV, 136; Ibn al-Jazzār 2004: 9–10; Ibn al-Quff [H. Kircher 1967]: 332–3; al-Dimashqī 1866: 195–8; E. Lev & Z. Amar 2008: 264–6.

75. *'asal naḥl muṣaffā* (strained of its wax and impurities) – the healing properties of honey are referred to on numerous occasions, both in the Qur'ān (16:68–9) and hadith, whereas 'rivers of purified honey' are one of the beneficences to be enjoyed in Paradise by the elect. In medicine and pharmacology, honey – which was hot and dry – was used as a diuretic and laxative, and a powerful antidote against poisons (as well as rabies). It also appears in compounds for the treatment of eye diseases (esp. cataract). According to Maimonides ([F. Rosner 1984]: 168), honey water helped erection. In cooking, honey was, of course, the core ingredient in a host of sweet dishes, pastries, syrups, etc., as well as being a preserving agent. In botany, the term *'asal al-naḥl* also denoted lemon balm (*Melissa officinalis*). *EI*[2], s.v. 'naḥl' (F. Viré); E. Lev & Z. Amar 2008: 185–7; A. Dietrich 1988: II, 238; al-Bīrūnī 1973: 264–6 (trans. 225ff.); Ibn Wāfid 2000: 164–5; Risāla [Cairo 362]: p. 6; al-Kātib 2002: 36; al-Dhahabī 1987: 258; al-Suyūṭī n.d.: 12–3; Ibn Sīnā 1999: I, 619–20; D. al-Anṭākī 1952: I, 236–7; Ibn al-Bayṭār 1874: III, 121–3; Ibn al-Quff [H. Kircher 1967]: 274–6.

76. [B] and [D] call for 'long pepper', while [C] has 'black cardamom'. Pepper (*fulful*) – both black and white – was considered hot and dry, and was used extensively in medicine: for instance, in the treatment of bladder stones,

gum and throat inflammation, joint aches, as well as being an effective digestive, carminative and aphrodisiac (arousing desire, stiffening erection and increasing sperm). Other terms for pepper included *ḥabb Hindī* ('Indian seeds') and *bābārī* (< Gr. πιπέρι). E. Lev and Z. Amar 2008: 236–9; A. Dietrich 1988: II, 305–6; al-Dhahabī 1987: 224; al-Suyūṭī n.d.: 14; ; Ibn al-Bayṭār 1874: III, 16–20; Ibn al-Jazzār 2004: 183, 195–6; Ibn Sīnā 1999: I, 626–7, II, 734; al-Rāzī 1955–69: XXI, 235–9; al-Ṭabarī 1928: 395–6; al-Bīrūnī 1973: 292; al-Tīfāshī 1892: 14; Ibn Lūqā 1974: 16 (trans. 23); *Kitāb* [Tunis No. 20648(09)]: fol. 86b.; al-Shayzarī, *al-Īdāḥ*, fol. 3; *Risāla* [Cairo 362]: fol. 3r.

77. [D] adds 'and another variety is when you take equal quantities of apple juice and rose water.'

78. 'thin piece of cloth ...', [C]: 'strain then mix with the same measure of rosewater, add the weight of both in skimmed honey and boil over a fire. Sprinkle on it half [a *dirham*] of saffron and cardamom, a *dirham* of ginger, two *dirhams* of cloves, strain, and then take ...'

79. 1 *qīrāṭ* = 0.195 grammes. Originally denoting the weight of a carob seed, it was one-sixteenth of a *dirham* and equalled four *sha'īra*, whereas its canonical (Iraqi) variant was one-twentieth of a *mithqāl*. L. Chipman 2009: 91; W. Hinz 1970: 27.

80. *misk* – considered hot and dry (in the third degree), musk was highly prized because of its rarity. It was used to strengthen the internal organs, to heighten the senses, in the treatment of headaches, muscle spasms, palpitations and a gloomy disposition, as a diuretic, emmenagogue, abortifacient, aperient, carminative and antidote (*tiryāq*) against venomous stings and bites. Its reputation as a powerful aphrodisiac was based on the fact that it is produced by a gland in the male musk deer (*Moschus*) to attract the female during the mating season. It was also recommended as a remedy for colds and as a deodorant. Arab scholars believed that the best musk came from a species of gazelle indigenous to China and Tibet (Ibn Wāfid, Ibn al-Baytār). The medicinal uses of musk were pioneered by al-Rāzī. In cooking, musk was used as an aromatic (*ṭīb*), whereas it was a key ingredient in perfumes as well. *EI*[2], s.v. 'misk' (A. Dietrich); E. Lev & Z. Amar 2008: 215–17; Ibn Wāfid 2000: 156–7; al-Dhahabī 1987: 259–61; Ibn al-Bayṭār 1874: IV, 155–7; Ibn al-Jazzār 2004: 61; Ibn Sīnā 1999,: I, 553, II, 735; D. al-Anṭākī 1952: I, 297–8; al-Shayzarī, *al-Īḍāḥ*, fol. 3r.; *Kitāb* (Tunis No. 20648[09]): fol. 86v.; al-Tīfāshī 1892: 14; al-Rāzī 1955–69: XXI, 516; H. Schindler and H. Frank 1961: 288–92; Ibn al-Quff [H. Kircher 1967]: 346–7.

81. The passage 'blend it with the water ...' appears as follows in [C]: 'boil everything over a fire, sprinkle a *qīrāṭ* of musk on it, remove and use.'

82. This sentence has the following variant in [C]: '[it is useful] as has been mentioned. The signs are a weak liver, yellow face, dry tongue and lips, emaciation and a weak appetite.'

83. 'When a person...' is as follows in [C]: 'He cannot digest [food] and does not have the strength for coitus. When he does engage in sexual intercourse, he does not experience any pleasure, while his sperm and limbs are cold. In addition, he flees coitus and baulks at it, lest he be afflicted by hemiplagia and a drop in innate heat because of it.'

84. *sunbul* (*Nardostachys jatamansi*) – one of the basic aromatic spices (*afwāh*, sing, *fūh*), it was synonymous with *nārdīn* (also *nardīn*) in Arabic botanical and pharmacological works. There were three principal varieties: : Indian (*sunbul, sunbul al-ṭīb*), *sunbul al-ʿaṣāfīr* and *nārduṭākhus*; Greek *(sunbul rūmī, Nardostachys jatamansi)*, which Ibn Sīnā equates with *nardīn*; and wild *(sunbul barrī, Asarum europaeum)*. The Indian variety was considered the most powerful; it was beneficial for the liver and stomach, colds, skin conditions, haemorrhoids, uteral tumours, to sweeten the breath, as a diuretic, abortifacient, and a sexual stimulant. E. Lev & Z. Amar 2008: 289–93; Ibn Wāfid 2000: 75–6; Ibn al-Bayṭār 1874: III, 36–8; Ibn al-Jazzār 2004: 26–7; D. al-Anṭākī 1952: I, 328; al-Rāzī 1955–69: XXI, 579–82; *Kitāb* [Tunis No. 20648(09)]: fol. 87; al-Shayzarī, *al-Īḍāḥ*, fol. 3; A. Dietrich 1988: II, 91; Ibn al-Quff [H. Kircher 1967]: 220–1; Ibn Sīnā 1999: I, 575, 602–3; Ibn Janāḥ 2020: Nos. 600–2.

85. This is missing from [B].

86. 'strengthens the liver ...'; [C]: 'it increases coitus and there are other benefits, which would take too long to explain. The recipe is as follows ...'

87. Addition in [D].

88. *ʿūd hindī*, which also appears as *aghālūgh(/kh)un* (< Gr. ἀγάλοχον), *ʿūd liyyā*, *(y)alanjūj* and *alanj*, was used to make the breath smell sweet (by chewing on it), as a carminative, diuretic, to strengthen the stomach, to relieve obstructions and to cure liver defects and dysentery, all of which are also indications for *ʿūd* (*vide post*). Indian agarwood was considered the best variety of *ʿūd*, with Ibn Wāfid equating both with *bakhūr*. A. Dietrich 1988: II, 105–106 (Nos. 19, 20); Ibn Wāfid 1987: 166–7; Ibn Sahl [O. Kahl 2003]: Nos. 58, 65, 254, 265, 293; Ibn al-Bayṭār 1874: III, 143; D. al-Anṭākī 1952: I, 51, 241–2; al-Tīfāshī 1892: 14; *Kitāb* [Tunis No 20648(09)]: fol. 86v.; al-Shayzarī, *al-Īḍāḥ*, fol. 3r.; al-Qazwīnī 1849: 260; al-Dhahabī 1987: 220; al-Bīrūnī 1973: 52 (trans. 34).

89. The last three sentences are as follows in [C]: 'Add half a *dirham* of saffron dissolved in rosewater, remove and then use when needed. It is beneficial, as we have mentioned. As for the limpness and weakness of the penis, this comes in three types.'

90. The notion that a lack of moderation in sexual intercourse was harmful to health goes back to Galen; see for instance, P. de Lacey 1994: 138–41.

91. 'without having any lust ...', [C]: 'and there is no treatment for it. The second sign is that the penis is erect at the end of the night. This is remedied by the following medication and electuaries. The third sign is ...'

92. 'ejaculates cold sperm ...', [C]: 'and his sperm is cold, whereas the ejaculation is accompanied by a burning sensation, without lust. This is due to coldness in the person's back.'

93. 'and moistness' is omitted in [C].

94. *sudad* (sg. *sudda*), lit. 'obstruction', or more specifically in this context 'a thing that obstructs the passage of the humours, and of the food, in the body' (E. Lane 1863–74: III, 1329).

95. 'food that counters this action ...', [C]: 'bad bitter food in order to get rid of this illness. This electuary has thirty-three benefits.'

96. *salīkha* (*Cinnamomum cassia*) – hot and dry, the spice was an important simple and was said by Islamic medical authorities to strengthen the

stomach, liver, womb and to relieve obstructions. The information for women was, somewhat contradictory; on the one hand it was said to strengthen the womb, provided a woman sits in a decoction of the herb, whereas it was also an emmenagogue and abortifacient. In erotological literature it is frequently mentioned as an aphrodisiac. The term was often used interchangeably with *dār ṣīnī* (see below). In erotological literature it is frequently mentioned as an aphrodisiac. A. Dietrich 1988: II, 96–7; E. Lev & Z. Amar 2008: 143ff.; Ibn Lūqā 1974: 16 (trans. 23); J. Leibowitz & M. Shlomo 1974: 233; Ibn al-Bayṭār 1874: III, 25–6; Ibn al-Jazzār 2004: 135–6; *idem* ([G. Bos 1997]: 246, 265, 294, 307; al-Tīfāshī 1892: 14; D. al-Anṭākī 1952: I, 196; Ibn Sīnā 1999: I, 603–4, 643; al-Rāzī 1955–69: XXI, 4ff.; al-Bīrūnī 1973: 226–8 (trans. 186-7); al-Ṭabarī 1928: 319; Issa Bey 1930: 49 (No. 3); Ibn al-Quff [H. Kircher 1967]: 228–9.

97. *sādaj* (a dialectal variant of the more common *sādhaj*) was said to be hot and dry in the second degree. A Persian borrowing, it was often wrongly equated with spikenard (*sunbul*) and sometimes appears as *sādaj hindī*. The identification of the plant is somewhat uncertain and has been said to be a member of the *Stratiotes* family (*Stratiotes aloides* or *Pistia stratiotes*), a cinnamon (*Cinnamonum citriodorum* [*Laurecae*]) or a laurel (*Laurus malabathrum*). In medicine, it was used as a diuretic, to strengthen the stomach or, in an unguent, for the treatment of tumours (especially in the eyes), and to combat flatulence. In view of its fragrance, it was also said to sweeten the breath (when chewed). See A. Dietrich 1988: II, 94–6; E. Lev & Z. Amar 2008: 444–5; Ibn al-Jazzār 2004: 97–8; Ibn Sīnā 1999: I, 585–6; Ibn Wāfid 2000: 76; D. al-Anṭākī 1952: I, 185; al-Rāzī 1955–69: XXI, 6; Ibn al-Bayṭār 1874: III,2; E. Lev & Z. Amar 2008: 444–5; F. Steingass 1892: 639; Ibn Sahl ([O. Kahl 2003]: No. 366 ('laurel', *Laurus malabathrum*); al-Ishbīlī 1995: I, 259 (who states that *sādhaj hindī* is the term used in al-Andalus for *rand hindī*), 382 (= *nārdīn nahrī*); Dioscorides 2000: 17.

98. *janṭiyāna* (< Gr. γεντιανή, *Gentiana lutea*) was used as a fortifier, emmenagogue, abortifacient, and to treat digestive problems (appetite, gas, diarrhoea). A. Dietrich 1988: II, 344–5; D. al-Anṭākī 1952: I, 109; al-Rāzī 1955–69: XX, 230–2; Ibn al-Bayṭār 1874: I, 170–1; Ibn al-Quff [H. Kircher 1967]: 142–3.

99. [C]: 'one *dirham.*'

100. *kammūn* (*Cuminum cyminum*) – considered hot and dry, the seeds of this plant (whether wild or cultivated) were a highly popular aromatic for cooking, whereas in medicine it was used as a digestive, carminative, eructative, diaphoretic, emmenagogue, aphrodisiac (with Maimonides adding that it stiffened the penis) and a cure for urinary, intestinal and eye diseases. Several varieties occur in the literature (Persian, Syrian, Kermani, Nabataean), whereas the term was also used as a generic to denote other plants: *kammūn rūmī/armanī* ('Byzantine/Armenian cumin' – caraway), *kammūn ḥulw* ('sweet cumin' – aniseed). The variety known as black cumin is referred to in Arabic as *ḥabba sawdā'* (see below). Confusingly, the Persian *zīre siyāh* ('black cumin') refers to caraway (Ar. *karāwiyā*; *Carum carvi*). *EI*², s.v. (G. S. Colin); Ibn Janāḥ 2020: Nos. 139, 441, 443; E. Lev & Z. Amar 2008: 159–60; A. Dietrich 1988: II, 408ff.; al-Dhahabī 1987: 235; Ibn al-Jazzār 2004: 160–1; D. al-

Anṭākī 1952: I, 275; Ibn al-Jazzār 2004: 149; al-Tīfāshī 1892: 14 (though elsewhere [31], he claims that it has a diminishing effect because it cuts the flow of sperm); al-Rāzī 1955–69: XXI, 332–5; Ibn al-Bayṭār 1874: IV, 81–2; Ibn al-Jazzār 2004: 149; Ibn Sīnā 1999: I, 523–4; Ibn al-Quff [H. Kircher 1967]: 328–9.

101. *jazar* (also sometimes referred to as *dawqū, aṣṭūfūlin*) – the varieties used included the red (*aḥmar* or *bustānī,* 'cultivated'), yellow (*aṣfar* or *barrī,* 'wild') and white (*abyaḍ*). In the medical tradition, carrots (including its seeds) were used against kidney pains, palpitations, cough, as a diuretic, carminative and emmenagogue. According to Ibn Jazla, the best variety was the sweet red winter carrot. Both the wild carrots and carrot jam (*jazar murabbā*) were thought to be aphrodisiac, though al-Kindī prescribed it to cure sexual addiction. E. Lev & Z. Amar 2008: 127–8; Ibn Wāfid 2000: 142; Ibn Sīnā 1999: II, 734; Ibn Jazla, fol. 54r.; al-Kindī [M. Levey 1966]: Nos. 207, 221, 226; al-Rāzī 1955–69: XX, 226–8; Ibn al-Bayṭār 1992: I, 221–3; al-Dhahabī 1987: 148; D. al-Anṭākī 1952: I, 105–6; Dietrich 1988: II, 286, 402; Issa Bey 1930: 69; Maimonides [F. Rosner & S. Muntner 1970]: 21:80.

102. *maṣṭi/akā* (< Gr. μαστίκη) – the aromatic resin of the pistachio tree (*Pistacia lentiscus*), which came in a number of varieties: white (Greek) and black (Nabataean). It was also known as *'ilk al-anbāṭ,* 'gum of the Nabataeans' and *arā.* Medicinally, it was thought to strengthen the stomach, liver and intestines, to improve the appearance of the skin, to treat ulcers and tumours, as well as being an eructative, expectorant, analgesic (especially for toothache and stomach pains) and carminative. E. Lev & Z. Amar 2008: 203–5; Ibn al-Bayṭār 1992: IV, 448–50; Ibn Janāḥ 2020: Nos. 83, 476, 715; Ibn al-Jazzār 2004: 62; Ibn Sīnā 1999: I, 553–4; al-Suyūṭī n.d.: 15; Ibn Wāfid 2000: 154–6; al-Tīfāshī 1892: 14; al-Dhahabī 1987: 261; *Kitāb* [Tunis No. 20648(09)]: fol. 87r.; Maimonides [M. Meyerhof 1940]: No. 232; Ibn al-Quff [H. Kircher 1967]: 340–1.

103. *'ūd* (also *'ūd ḥabb, 'ūd bukhūr*) – literally means 'wood', 'rod' or 'stick' and refers to (chips of) agarwood (grown in India, China and Yemen), or its resin extracts. It was variously thought to strengthen the heart and senses, in addition to the uses already mentioned for *'ūd hindī* (see above). In cooking, it was used for fumigating receptacles before putting food in them. According to Maimonides it arouses the lust for coitus, stiffens the penis and increases sexual pleasure, whereas al-Tīfāshī stated it arouses women's lust and desire for coitus. E. Lev & Z. Amar 2008: 97–8; Ibn al-Jazzār 2004: 65; Ibn Wāfid 1987: 166–7; al-Tīfāshī 1970: 32; Ibn Sahl [O. Kahl 2003]: Nos. 206, 292 ('lignaloes'); A. Dietrich 1988: II, 105; al-Dhahabī 1987: 220; Ibn Sīnā 1999: I, 614–5; Issa Bey 1930: 10.

104. 'cloves' is omitted in [C].

105. *murr* (lit. 'bitter') – the resin extracted from the bark of trees growing in the south of the Arabian Peninsula (as well as northern Ethiopia and Somalia), myrrh (whose Arabic etymon refers to its taste) was used, for instance, against stomach complaints, coughs and colds, as an anthelminitic, abortifacient, theriac, breath sweetener, embalming agent and aphrodisiac. Ibn al-Bayṭār quotes Ibn al-Jazzār when recommending making a paste of myrrh and Palestinian olive oil to rub on the big toe of the man's right foot, which would allow the man to continue having

intercourse for as long as the substance remained on his toe. E. Lev and Z. Amar 2008: 221–4; al-Rāzī 1955–69: XXI, 500–4; Ibn Jazla, fol. 209r.; Ibn Sīnā 1999: I, 565; al-Bīrūnī: 345 (trans. 304); al-Kindī [M. Levey 1966]: 333–4 (No. 283); Ibn al-Bayṭār 1992; IV, 430–33; Ibn al-Jazzār 2004: 85–6; D. Antākī 1952: I, 293–4; A. Dietrich 1988: II, 110; Ibn al-Quff [H. Kircher 1967]: 338–9. For a detailed discussion of the origins and trade of the substance, see N. Groom 1981.

106. Instead of 'strain ...' [C] has: 'Crush ...'; [C]: 'and bee honey equalling three times the total amount. Then boil everyting over a fire and turn into an electuary.'

107. 1 *mithqāl* = 4.464 grammes; W. Hinz 1970: 4.

108. *duyūk* (sg. *dīk*) – in the Arabic tradition, the rooster appears often in literature, and was thought to be highly sensual (as well as conceited). The voice of the rooster was considered very attractive and allegedly alleviated pains in those who heard it. According to a hadith, Allah also liked the sound of the rooster's voice, whereas the Prophet used to keep a white rooster in his house. In medicine, the bile, brain, comb and blood were used in remedies for colics, fevers and those with cold temperaments. According to Maimonides, rooster testicles were very effective in increasing sperm. EI2, s.v. 'dīk' (L. Kopf); Ibn Sīnā 1999: I, 436–7; Ibn al-Jazzār 2004: 209; Maimonides [F. Rosner 1984]: 167; al-Ṭabarī 1928: 432–3; al-Kātib 1977: 274.

109. The Arabic *murdāsank* is a (miswritten) calque of the Persian *murdāsang*. In Arabic, it was also known as *martak* and *mu/ardāsanj*. A by-product of separating silver from lead, litharge (which was considered cold and dry in the second degree) was used in the treatment of various dermatological conditions (scrofula, vitiligo alba, abscesses, swollen sores), eye diseases, haemorrhoids, and as a deodorant. E. Lev & Z. Amar 2008: 440, 553; Ibn Sīnā 1999: III, 285, 559–60; W. Lane 1863–74: III, 1028; Ibn al-Bayṭār 1874: IV, 150; Ibn al-Jazzār 2004: 89; al-Kindī [M. Levey 1966]: 334–5; al-Suyūṭī n.d.: 14; Ibn al-Quff [H. Kircher 1967]: 336–8; Maimonides [M. Meyerhof 1940]: Nos. 239. 256.

110. 'sufficient to enable you to knead the collected gall into a fine paste' is missing from [C].

111. This sentence is missing from [C].

112. The reference to the bath is missing from [C], which simply states 'in the morning'.

113. The last two sentences are as follows in [C]: 'Eat the musk electuary after coming out of the bath.'

114. *baṣal* – a number of varieties of onion are mentioned in the literature (red, white, long, etc.). It was considered hot and moist, and both the vegetable and its seeds are mentioned as an appetizer and anti-emetic but most often as a sexual stimulant, to increase sperm (including its motility), and as a remedy for impotence. Al-Nafzāwī [J. Colville 1999] recommended 'ground onion seeds, sifted or strained and mixed with honey; a spoonful to be taken on an empty stomach' (66), while one individual was able to keep an erection for thirty days and thirty nights by eating meat with lots of onions and drinking onion juice with honey (81). According to Ibn al-Quff, pouring onion juice in the ear was a remedy for tinnitus (*ṭanīn*

fī 'l-udhun), while rubbing it in the eyes increased vision. On the other hand, onions can also cause headaches, whereas excessive consumption leads to forgetfulness and haemorrhoids. In cooking, it was (and still is) a staple in both North African and Near Eastern dishes. D. al-Anṭākī 1952: I, 76; Ibn Sīnā 1999: I, 390–2, II, 734 ('especially when grilled'); Ibn al-Bayṭār 1874: I, 96; Maimonides [F. Rosner 1984]: 167; Ibn Lūqā 1974: 13, 16 (trans. 19, 20, 23); *Kitāb* [Tunis No. 20648(09)]: fol. 87r.; *Risāla* [Cairo 362]: p. 3r.; Ibn Māssa 1971: 8, 9 (trans. 10, 11); al-Tīfāshī 1892: 13, 14; Ibn Lūqā 1974: 16 (trans. 23); al-Kātib 2002: 36; al-Dhahabī 1987: 129–30; A. Dietrich 1988: II, 297–8; Ibn al-Quff [H. Kircher 1967]: 100–1; E. Lev & Z. Amar 2008: 230–1.

115. *fujl* (also *fajl*) – hot and dry, it had a wide variety of medical applications, ranging from clearing of obstructions in the liver to improving eyesight, combating arthritis, as an emetic, digestive, appetizer, eructative, antidote (against scorpion bites), and to trigger hair growth. It was also thought to increase sperm, and assist in coitus. In cooking, it was eaten both raw and cooked. However, some physicians (including Maimonides) considered it a harmful food. E. Lev & Z. Amar 2008: 257–9; A. Dietrich 1988: II, 260–1; al-Dhahabī 1987: 223–4; al-Rāzī 1955–69: XXI, 218–22; Ibn Sīnā 1999: I, 672–3, II, 734; Ibn al-Bayṭār 1874: III, 156–8; D. al-Anṭākī 1952: I, 248; al-Suyūṭī n.d.: 12; al-Tīfāshī 1892: 14; *Kitāb* [Tunis No. 20648(09)]: fol. 87r.; Ibn al-Quff [H. Kircher 1967]: 295–6; Maimonides [F. Rosner & S. Muntner 1970]: 15:6, 21:80, 22:45.

116. *rashād* (also known as *ḥurf*, *Lepidium sativum*), 'garden cress', sometimes appears under the name *thuffā'*. Aside from being an appetizer, anthelmintic, emmenagogue, abortifacient (when the woman inserts the seeds into the vagina) and carminative, the herb (or rather its seeds), was also thought to increase the lust for coition. There was often terminological confusion between this herb and cardamom because of the similarity in the Greek etyma κάρδαμον and καρδάμωμον, respectively. Cardamom became known as *qardamānā*, which was used interchangeably with *karawiyā barrī* ('wild caraway'). E. Lev and Z. Amar 2008: 172-4; A. Dietrich 1988: II, 15, 301ff.; Ibn Janāḥ 2020: Nos. 519, 361, 1030; Ibn al-Jazzār 2004: 206–7; al-Kātib 2002: 36; Ibn al-Bayṭār 1874: II, 15–7; *Kitāb* [Tunis No. 20648(09)]: fol. 87; *Risāla* [Cairo 362]: p. 5; al-Shayzarī, *al-Īḍāḥ*, fol. 3; al-Qazwīnī 1849: 278; Ibn Sīnā 1999: I, 476–7, II, 734; al-Bīrūnī 1973: 156 (trans. 125); al-Rāzī 1955–69: XX, 319–23; Ibn al-Quff [H. Kircher 1967]: 162.

117. [C] has 'ginger' instead of 'turnip seeds'.

118. In the modern Near and Middle East, *harīs(a)* (from the verb *harasa*, 'to beat, crush') usually refers to a dish (stew) of meat and bulghur (cracked wheat). In North Africa – especially Tunisia – it is a chilli paste. In medieval times, *harīsa* was a meat porridge, made with wheat or rice. D. Newman 2020: Nos. 67, 315; *idem* 2023: Nos. 97, 188.

119. The rest of the sentence is omitted from [C].

120. *ḥimmiṣ* (also *ḥimmaṣ*, *ḥummuṣ*), *Cicer arietinum* – the varieties used are white, red and black, all of which were said to cause bloating and thus difficult to digest, but highly nutritious. Roasted chickpeas are less bloating than fresh chickpeas, while drinking water immediately after eating them increases their bloating effect. The water in which chickpeas

are cooked with cumin, cinnamon, and dill is beneficial for phlegmatic illnesses, bloating, and back pain. Chickpea flour was reportedly useful against testicular tumours, scabies and freckles, and a soup of the flour and milk was said to be beneficial for people with dry lungs and weak voices. They were widely known as a diuretic, emmenagogue and powerful aphrodisiac, often linked to the bloating effect which also manifests itself in the veins; this stimulates desire and increases semen. This property is allegedly strongest when chickpeas are soaked in water and eaten raw on an empty stomach. According to al-Tīfāshī, chickpeas (and eggs) were particularly effective in increasing sexual potency because they combined three basic qualities: creating coarse winds, nutritional, and moderate in heat. If one does not wish to engage in sexual activity after eating chickpeas, so al-Samarqandī tells us, one should eat them with thyme, salt, and pennyroyal. A. Dietrich 1988: II, 253; al-Samarqandī 2016: 51–2; al-Dhahabī 1987: 160; Ibn Jazla, fol. 74r.; Ibn Sīnā 1999: II, 734; al-Suyūṭī n.d.: 9; al-Ṭabarī 1928: 432–3; Ibn al-Bayṭār 1874: II, 302; D. al-Anṭākī 1952: I, 28; al-Tīfāshī 1892: 13, 14; *Risāla* [Cairo 362]: fol. 3r.; al-Kātib 2002: 36; al-Qazwīnī 1849: 279; al-Bīrūnī 1973: 163 (trans.129–30); al-Rāzī 1955–69: XX, 356–9.

121. [C]: 'in which it has been cooked.'

122. *ʿaṣāfīr* (sg. *ʿuṣfūr*) – hot and dry, the bird was widely held to increase sperm and potency (especially their brains). According to several hadiths, the Prophet even forbade its killing. al-Tīfāshī 1892: 14; al-Dhahabī 1987: 217; Ibn Jazla, fol. 154r.

123. 'Cook over a low fire ...'; [C]: 'If it starts smelling, remove from the fire and boil with ...'

124. '(...) cinnamon ...'; [C]: 'six walnuts and ten *dirhams* of cinnamon. Mix everything together and eat by sprinkling on your food. It is beneficial as we have mentioned.'

125. This is a dish associated with Mamluk Egypt and made with meat, onions, raisins, and various aromatics (mastic, cinnamon, pepper, coriander) served with a sauce. D. Newman 2020: No. 83.

126. *shīshak* – the one-year-old lamb is among the meats mentioned by Maimonides ([R. Rosner 1984]: 171) as being beneficial for coitus.

127. [E] omits the section after 'it is advisable' until this point.

128. *abāzīr* (*abzār*, sg. *bizr*), refers to spices and condiments, whether dried or fresh, and some scholars (e.g. al-Rāzī) included vinegar and *murrī* (a liquid fermented sauce); there were overlaps with another generic term for spices, *tawābil* (sg. *tābil*). According to al-Qumrī (10th), *tawābil* are 'things that season (*yuṭayyib*) the pot, such as salt, vinegar and saffron', while *abāzīr* refers to fresh ones like coriander, mint, and dry ones like coriander seeds, cumin, caraway, etc. (1991: 86). For a full discussion, see D. Newman 2020: lii–iv; idem 2023: 51–2.

129. *Tamr* – denotes the last stage in the growth of the fruit of the date palm (*nakhla*, *Phoenix dactylifera*), as well as dried dates. The fruit has been a staple in the Middle Eastern diet for millennia and is highly praised in Muslim culture. Ibn Waḥshiyya called it 'Adam's sister' and thought it was more useful even than the olives. It is mentioned several times (nineteen in total) in the Qur'ān, usually as a beneficence granted by Allah to humanity

(for example, 6:99; 6:141; 16:11; 16:67; 18:32) and occurs in a large number of hadiths praising the date palm as being the most blessed of trees; the Prophet Muhammad is said to have had dates as one of his meals every day, while 'a family which has no dates will be hungry'. In addition to its flesh (either whole or in a paste), the stones were also used in various applications. Dates were recommended for a variety of illnesses and conditions (for insance, diarrhoea, colic, poisons), including to increase sexual lust and potency, and to increase semen. Ibn Sīnā 1999, I: 691–2; Ibn al-Bayṭār 1992: I, 191–2; Ibn Jazla, fol. 49v.; Lev & Amar 2008: 397–8; Lane 1863– 74: I, 316; Ibn Waḥshiyya 1993–8: II, 1339; al-Dhahabī 1987: 138–42; *EI²*, s.v. 'nakhla' (F. Viré); D. Waines, 'date palm', in J. Mcauliffe 2001–6: I, 494–5.

130. 'cow's milk...'; [C]: 'fresh cow's milk.'

131. *thūm* – hot and dry, it came in two varieties: *barrī* ('wild') and *bustānī* ('cultivated'). Medicinally, it was used to relieve flatulence, for various dermatological conditions and as an emmenagogue. Though some authors stated garlic had a negative effect on coitus (as well as the breath), others recommended it as a remedy for impotence. In the *Kama Sutra*, garlic root mixed with white pepper and liquorice and drunk with sugared milk enhances virility. E. Lev & Z. Amar 2008: 412–4; Ibn Lūqā 1974: 16 (trans. 23); *Risāla* [Cairo 362]: fol. 2a (who claimed it was very effective when drunk with milk and honey); Ibn al-Bayṭār 1874: I, 151–3; Ibn al-Jazzār 2004: 202–3; D. al-Anṭākī 1952: I, 101–2; al-Dhahabī 1987: 144–5; al-Suyūṭī n.d.: 13; Ibn Sīnā 1999: I, 695–6; A. Dietrich 1988: II, 298; al-Bīrūnī 1973: 125; Ibn al-Quff [H. Kircher 1967]: 130–2; Issa Bey 1930: 9 (No. 15); A. Daniélou 1994: 499.

132. The preceding passage, 'you can also eat *taqliyya* ...' is missing from [C], which simply has: 'and cook the carrots with the meat or the chicken and sprinkle on top. The recipe for the broth is as follows.'

133. The manuscript has the misspelling *sukūrruja* for *suku/arruja* (< Persian *sukraja*, 'saucer'), which was used 'to put sauces and the like to excite the appetite and to aid digestion' (E. Lane). It came in two sizes (six ounces and three ounces, or four *mithqāls*), though as a measure, it often equalled 125 grams. E. Lane 1863–74: IV, 116; W. Hinz 1970; L. Chipman 2009: 91.

134. The preceding five sentences are omitted from [C], which has: 'Throw the grated garlic on, cook over a low fire and sprinkle the above-mentioned spices on top.'

135. 'in a glass vessel' is omitted from [C].

136. This entire sentence and the remainder of the chapter are omitted from [C].

137. *samn*, with *zubd* denoting butter made from churned milk. In medicine, *samn* (often mixed with honey), on its own, was used as an antidote against poisons and snake bites, or (in an unguent) to treat haemorrhoids, for instance. In addition, it figures as an ingredient in many medical preparations for a variety of ills. In cooking, *samn* was the most-frequently used oil in the Near, with fresh butter being a rarity. *EI²*, s.v. '*samn*' (J. Ruska –[D. Waines]); Ibn Sahl [O. Kahl 2003]: *passim*; al-Dhahabī 1987: 192–3; al-Suyūṭī n.d.: 9, 13; Ibn Sīnā 1999: I, 602; E. Lev & Z. Amar 2008: 132–4 ('sour cream').

138. The Arabic *ḥawāmiḍ* (the plural of *ḥāmiḍ*) refers to sour dishes, notably vinegar and fruit stews, and were contrasted with so-called 'plain' dishes (*sawādhij*) and fried ones (*qalāyā*); al-Baghdādī 1964. The author's advice is predicated in the belief that sour foods have a cooling and drying effect on the body; al-Warrāq 1987: 20.

139. *qadīd* – according to a thirteenth-century Andalusian recipe the meat was cut into thin long strips and marinated in sour vinegar and salt. Afterwards it was rubbed with pepper, coriander, cumin, caraway and *murrī* (rotted barley condiment) and left so that it could absorb the spices. Then it was dried out in the sun for a couple of days. It could be eaten cold or fried. A similar dish was *namaksūd*, a Persian borrowing translating as 'rubbed salt', which meant salted beef. Unlike *qadīd, namaksūd* was put into the pickle as a whole or divided into two pieces only. Al-Rāzī (1881: 2–5) held that *qadīd* benefits the body, in that it safeguards against nausea caused by greasy food and excess consumption of wine, but when one eats too much of it, it causes indigestion and thirst (alleviated by either oxymel or *jullāb*). See D. Newman 2023: No. 466, notes 74–5.

140. [E] has 'jerky made from beef and poultry'.

141. *zabīb* – which also denoted currants, were used extensively in cooking but were also thought to have beneficial medicinal properties. The seed, juice, as well as wine based on it (which was said to be lighter than that made from grapes), were all used in remedies. Raisins were recommended, for instance, to strengthen the stomach and liver, and as a remedy for cough, ulcers and tumours. When eaten to excess, raisins (which are hot and moist in the first degree) were thought to burn the blood, which could be countered by green cucumbers. Ibn Jazla, fol. 111r.; E. Lev & Z. Amar 2008: 176–80; Ibn Wāfid 2000: 59–62; *Risāla* [Cairo 362]: p. 4; al-Dhahabī 1987: 282–4; Ibn Sahl [O. Kahl 2003]: s.vv. 'raisin', 'raisin-seed', 'raisin water', 'raisin wine'; *EI*[2], s.v. 'zabīb' (D. Waines); M. Steinschneider 1900: 74; Ibn al-Quff [H. Kircher 1967]: 203–4; al-Suyūṭī n.d.: 11. Also see the note below on *'inab*.

142. [D] has 'non-acidic.'

143. 'and nature' is omitted from [C].

144. A dessert typically made with wheat flour, rosewater, saffron and honey, and garnished with pistachios and almonds. See D. Newman 2020: No. 142.

145. The preceding passage is considerably shorter in [C]: 'Among them Persian halva, which is made from fine flour, clarified butter, bee honey and eaten with dry bread and ...'

146. *ḥamām* – like other poultry, it was said to be very moist. Pigeon blood was used to stop nasal bleeding and in remedies for paralysis. It was recommended to prepare them with verjuice and coriander or vinegar and to eat them with cucumber. Ibn Jazla, fol. 75v.; Ibn Sīnā 1999: I, 492; al-Samarqandī 2016: 92–3.

147. *afrākh* (sg. *firākh*) – their medicinal properties were similar to those of chickens (*dajāj*); see note below.

148. *iwazz* (sg. *wazz*) – goose blood and fat were used in electuaries for the treatment of ear diseases, as an emmenagogue or to stem excessive menstrual bleeding. Al-Ṭabarī 1928: 433.

149. *dajāj* – considered cold and moist, its properties were praised in a number of hadiths, as it was thought to be beneficial to the mind, to relieve stomach inflammation and increase sperm. Ibn Sīnā 1999: I, 436–7; al-Dhahabī 1987: 184–5; Ibn al-Jazzār 2004: 209.

150. *farārīj* (sg. *farrūj*) – their medicinal uses were thought to be identical to those of chickens, including benefits for coition and as a sperm booster, while the best ones are those that start clucking. It was said that they could provoke quinsy, unless cooked doused in vinegar; Ibn Jazla, fol. 163r.; al-Tīfāshī 1892: 14; Ibn Sīnā 1999: II, 734.

151. *samak* (pl. *asmāk*) – generally considered cold and moist, fish were recommended in the treatment of, for instance, arthritis, whereas a number of them (for instance, eels) were aphrodisiacs. Ibn Sīnā 1999: I, 605–7, II, 734.

152. *birisht*, which is a term used in ECA. It is a borrowing from Persian, *nīm birisht*, 'poached egg (half-boiled)' (F. Steingass 1892: 1445). Hard-boiled eggs were said to be harmful as they are difficult to digest and cause colic and stones (both in kidney and bladder); Ibn al-Quff [H. Kircher 1967]: 97–8.

153. This is a rather strange comment as eggs (considered cold and moist) from most poultry were generally held to be beneficial. Their ability to increase potency (and sperm) is often mentioned in the literature. According to Ibn al-Quff, the best eggs were those from young, black hens. Ibn Sīnā 1999: II, 734; Maimonides [F. Rosner 1984]: 167; al-Tīfāshī 1892: 14; M. al-Fallātī [BN 5662]: fol. 83r.; al-Dhahabī 1987: 135; Ibn al-Quff [H. Kircher 1967]: 97–9; al-Suyūṭī n.d.: 11.

154. The reference to soft-boiled eggs and the harmfulness of other types of eggs is omitted from [C].

155. *admigha* (sg. *dimāgh*) – various animal brains, such as those of bulls, veal, camel and sheep, were used medicinally in the treatment of, for instance, ulcers, tumours, sciatica, colic, as well as being endowed with aphrodisiacal qualities. According to Ibn al-Bayṭār (1992: 209), the best brains were those of birds and quadrupeds (chiefly the camel). Sparrows' brains are also mentioned by al-Kātib (2002: 36), who recommends using the brains of birds when they are sexually excited (1977: 280), and by Ibn Sīnā (1999: II, 734), alongside those of pullets, ducks and squabs to enhance coitus. Also see Ibn al-Quff [H. Kircher 1967]: 347–8; by Ibn Sīnā 1999: I, 573, 635.

156. *laban* (also *laban ḥalīb* or *ḥalīb*) – milk was considered particularly useful for hot and cold temperaments and had a number of medicinal applications,; for instance in the treatment of stomach complaints, ulcers and coughs (especially donkey and goat's milk), and as an emmenagogue. Physicians warned, however, about the fact that milk was difficult to digest, causing flatulence and colic. It was considered a potent aphrodisiac (even the sour variety), with fresh milk and butter being prescribed to strengthen the erection. Some recommended breastmilk in medical treatments (e.g. al-Kindī). Al-Kindī [M. Levey 1966]: Nos. 9–11, 28, 37, 40, 46, 96, 127, 140, 142, 166, 170, 178, 180, 258; Ibn Sīnā 1999: II, 546–50, II, 732; E. Lev & Z. Amar 2008: 132–4; Ibn al-Bayṭār 1874: I, 157–9, IV, 93–100, 132–4; al-Kātib 2002: 36; D. al-Anṭākī 1952: I, 103.

157. *lift* (*Brassica rapa*) – also commonly known in Arabic as *s<h>aljam* (from the Persian *shalgham*). The literature mentions wild (*barrī*), garden (*bustānī*) and small varieties. It was thought to generate sperm, arouse appetite, and act as a diuretic. In culinary texts, turnips are among the most pickled vegetables. D. Newman 2020: Nos. 191–209; A. Dietrich 1988: II, 257–9, 621–2; Maimonides [F. Rosner 1984]: 167; Ibn al-Bayṭār 1992: III, 48–90; D. al-Anṭākī 1952: I, 198, 283; al-Dhahabī 1987: 199–200; Ibn al-Quff [H. Kircher 1967]: 230–1; Ibn Sīnā 1999: I, 679–80. Ibn Jazla, fol. 138r.

158. *kurrāt* (for *kurrāth, Allium ampeloprasum);* in addition to the commonly used *kurrāth shāmī* ('Syrian') – sometimes confusingly known as the 'Andalusian' variety – and *Nabaṭī* ('Nabataean'; also *kurrāth al-jabal,* 'mountain l.'), the leek varieties mentioned include *kurrāth Fārisī* ('Persian l.'). Some authors equated *kurrāth Rūmī* ('Greek leek') with elecampane (*rāsan*). The term *kurrāth al-ḥayya* ('snake leek') is not a leek but a type of garlic, which occasionally is even equated (wrongly) with gentian. Medically, leeks were used as a diuretic, anthelmintic, in the treatment of ulcers, swellings, colic, haemorrhoids, headaches, asthma (when eaten with barley water), and as an aphrodisiac. Maimonides recommended it to prevent the growth of pubic and armpit hair. According to Ibn Lūqā (1974: 14), Syrian leek was one of the substances that could 'loosen the sperm if it was solid, make it more fluid, soluble and eager to be expelled'. Al-Tīfāshī stated the benefit of leek for increasing female sperm and coital vigour (1970: 22). E. Lev *&* Z. Amar 2008: 433–4; al-Jazla, fol. 185v.; A. Dietrich 1988: II, 296–7, 299; Ibn al-Bayṭār 1874: IV, 61–3; Ibn Sīnā 1999: I, 532–3; D. al-Anṭākī 1952: I, 271; al-Rāzī 1955–69: XXI, 383–8; al-Kindī [M. Levey 1966]: Nos. 29, 148; al-Bīrūnī 1973: 315; Maimonides [M. Meyerhof 1940]: No. 198; al-Kindī [M. Levey 1966]: Nos. 29, 148; Ibn Janāḥ 2020: Nos. 436–38.

159. 'clarified butter' is omitted from [C].

160. [E] adds that it should the oil of almonds, etc. The Arabic *lawz* (*Prunus amygdalus*) usually refers to 'sweet' almonds (*lawz ḥulw; Prunus dulcis* var. *dulcis*), as opposed to the bitter variety (*murr*; *Prunus dulcis* var. *amara*). In addition to being used fresh, almonds were also roasted and salted (*mamlūḥ*), which were said to satisfy false hunger. Almond conserve (*lawz murabbā*) was made by boiling them with *dibs* (date molasses). Both sweet and bitter almonds were used to make almond oil, which was often used for frying. In cooking, almonds, predominantly the sweet type, were used extensively in both savouries and sweets, as an ingredient and/or thickener, usually pounded and sometimes previously toasted. They are often used to decorate dishes, in which case they are left whole or cut in half. Almonds were often toasted. One variety of the almond confection known as *lawzīnaj*, required almond paste and is the direct ancestor of our modern marzipan. In the medical tradition, almonds were recommended to cleanse the intestines, clear obstructions, for the chest, bladder, kidneys, skin diseases, and as a laxative (when eaten with figs), and to increase semen (when eaten with twice- or thrice-cooked sugar, known as *ṭabarzad* and *fānīd*, respectively). The bitter variety was used to relieve blockages (esp. in the liver), and cure uteral pains and renal calculus.

E. Lev & Z. Amar 2008: 91–4; A. Dietrich 1988: II, 187–8; Ibn Jazla, fol. 199r.–v.; Maimonides [F. Rosner 1984]: 167 ('peeled dried almonds'); al-Samarqandī 2016: 148–51; Ibn Wāfid 2000: 92–3; Ibn al-Bayṭār 1992: IV, 386–87; 111–2, III, 86; Ibn al-Jazzār 2004: 118–9; Ibn Sīnā 1999: I, 544–5; D. al-Anṭākī 1952: I, 284; al-Dhahabī 1987: 252–3; al-Suyūṭī n.d.: 9; al-Bīrūnī 1973: 334–5; D. Newman 2023: 126, note No. 92.

161. *bunduq* (> Gr. Ποντικόν) – also known as *jillawz* (< Persian *j/galūz*), hazelnuts (*Corylus avellana*) originally hailed from Turkey and in medicine were used, for instance, to cleanse and strengthen the intestines, improve memory, and treat palpitations, urinary infections and epilepsy. The so-called 'Indian hazelnut' (*bunduq hindī*) was another name for betel nut (*fawfal*), though some scholars equated it with the nickernut (*rata, aṭmāṭ*). Hazelnuts were said to strengthen the brain, serve as an antidote against scorpion stings, as well as being a sexual stimulant. Bizarrely, it was held that hazelnuts applied to the fontanelle of a blue-eyed child, can remove the blueness. Hazelnuts were also said to cause bloating, gas and headaches, all of which could be alleviated by fennel. A. Dietrich 1988: II, 189–90; Ibn Jazla, fol. 42v.; E. Lev & Z. Amar 2008: 416–7; al-Dhahabī 1987: 134; al-Tīfāshī 1892: 14; Maimonides [F. Rosner 1984]: 167; Ibn Sīnā 1999: 734; Ibn al-Bayṭār 1992: I,162–63; Ibn Sīnā 1999: I, 406–8; Ibn Wāfid 2000: 140–1; D. al-Anṭākī 1952: I, 85; al-Rāzī 1955–69: XXI, 383–8; al-Bīrūnī 1973: 101–2; Maimonides [M. Meyerhof 1940]: No. 43; Ibn al-Quff [H. Kircher 1967]: 114–6; Maimonides [M. Meyerhof 1940]: No. 335.

162. *fustuq* (also *fustaq* < Gr. πιστάκια) – hot and dry (more so than walnuts and almonds), pistachios (*Pistacia vera*) were used to unblock obstructions in the liver, as an anti-emetic, while they were thought to be beneficial for chest and lung ailments, to strengthen the stomach and to invigorate coitus. A. Dietrich 1988: II, 188; Ibn Jazla, fol. 164r.; E. Lev & Z. Amar 2008: 468–70; Maimonides [F. Rosner 1984]: 167; *idem* [M. Meyerhof 1940]: No. 301; al-Dhahabī 1987: 224; al-Tīfāshī 1892: 14; Ibn Sīnā 1999: 734; Ibn al-Bayṭār 1992: III, 222; Ibn Wāfid 2000: 80; D. al-Anṭākī 1952: I, 249–50; al-Rāzī 1955–69: XXI, 214; al-Bīrūnī 1973: 289.

163. *ruṭab* – hot and moist, it comes in two varieties, 'one that cannot be dried and spoils soon if not eaten; one that dries, and is made into *'ajwa*' (E. Lane 1863–74: III, 1101). This type of date was believed to benefit those with cold stomachs, and to increase semen and soften the bowels. However, it is harmful to the throat and voice, and causes headaches. Ibn Jazla, fol. 107v.; Ibn Wāfid 2000: 84–5; al-Dhahabī 1987: 179.

164. *tīn* (*Ficus carica*) figs were generally considered the most nutritious of all fruit. A number of varieties were identified but the fresh, peeled white (or yellow) type was thought to be the best. Both the fruit and the leaves were used in medicine. Its applications included as a diuretic, appetizer, antidote against poisons, laxative, anti-cough treatment, and to relieve obstructions. Figs (especially fresh ones) were also thought to increase semen, increase fertility and were, therefore, often considered an aphrodisiac. The fruit appears in the title of a Qur'ānic *sūra* (95) as well as in a large number of hadiths, the most famous of which is that the Prophet considered it descended from paradise. Ibn al-Bayṭār 1992: I, 200–202; al-Tīfāshī 1892: 14; *idem* 1970: 31 (trans. 46), 35 (trans. 51); D. al-Anṭākī

1952: I, 99–100; Ibn Wāfid 2000: 176–9; al-Dhahabī 1987: 143; al-Ṭabarī 1928: 381; al-Qazwīnī 1849: 251–2; Ibn al-Quff [H. Kircher 1967]: 122–3; A. Dietrich 1988: II, 192–3.

165. *'inab* (*Vitis vinifera*) – hot and moist, the best quality was said to come from Jurjan. The juice of sour unripe grapes was known as *ḥisrim*, a frequently encountered ingredient in the culinary literature. The fruit is given great prominence in Islam (on a par with the date); it occurs a number of times in the Qur'ān, where it is listed as one of the fruits of paradise (2:266, 6:99, 16:67, 17:91, 23:19; 36:34; 80:28). Even wine made from it (and from dates) is said to be good nourishment (Qur'ān 16:69), though the relevant verse was later superseded by others prohibiting intoxicating substances (4:46; 5:92). In Arabic literature, too, there are numerous references to the grape, particularly in relation to wine of course, which is the object of a genre in poetry known as *khamriyyāt*. Grapes were used in a variety of ways (fresh, dried, vinegar, its lees as fertilizer). In pharmacology and medicine, the fruit, leaves, juice and wine of grapes were used for the stomach, as a diuretic, against vaginal ulcers and eye ailments, as an anti-emetic for pregnant women, as well as being an aphrodisiac. It was held to be good for the chest and lungs, and its astringent properties help stop bleeding, whereas old wine was used in the treatment of impotence. *EI*[2], s.vv. 'khamr' (A. J. Wensinck-J. Sadan), 'karm' (L. Bolens-Cl. Cahen); E. Lev *&* Z. Amar 2008: 176–80; Maimonides [F. Rosner 1984]: 167; al-Tīfāshī 1892: 14; Ibn al-Bayṭār 1992: III, 192, IV, 56–7; Ibn Wāfid 2000: 59–61; D. al-Anṭākī 1952: I, 270; Ibn Sīnā 1999: I, 615–6, 622–3; al-Rāzī 1955–69: XXI, 318–22; al-Qazwīnī 1849: 263–5; al-Kindī [M. Levey 1966]: No. 121; al-Dhahabī 1987: 219; al-Suyūṭī n.d.: 11; P. Heine 1982: 111–2.

166. *rummān* (*Punica granatum*) – the sweet variety of the fruit is mentioned several times in the Qur'ān, including as one of the fruits of paradise (6:99; 6:144; 55:68). Both the sweet and sour varieties frequently appear in the culinary literature. In medicine, both the fruit (especially the juice) and peel were used in the treatment of diarrhoea, fevers, cough, stomach and liver ailments, against coughs, to curb yellow bile, as a diuretic and anaphrodisiac (because of its acidity). E. Lev *&* Z. Amar 2008: 248–50; Ibn Wāfid 2000: 119–20; Ibn al-Bayṭār 1992: II, 439–42; al-Tīfāshī 1892: 31; D. al-Anṭākī 1952: I, 169–70; al-Dhahabī 1987: 179–80; Ibn Sīnā 1999: I, 666–7; al-Suyūṭī n.d.: 12; al-Qazwīnī 1849: 290–1; al-Rāzī 1955–69: XX, 512–9; A. Dietrich 1988: II, 170–1; al-Kindī [M. Levey 1966]: Nos. 36, 38, 42, 55, 59, 77, 86, 91; Ibn al-Quff [H. Kircher 1967]: 187–8. Also see the note on *'jullanār'*, below.

167. *safarjal* (*Cydonia oblonga*) – considered cold and dry, both the sour and sweet varieties of the quince were used in medicine, mainly to strengthen the stomach, digestive, appetizer, anti-emetic, against headaches, and to prevent hangovers. Its juice was thought to be beneficial for shortness of breath and asthma, to quench thirst and to strengthen the stomach. When eaten before meals, it prevents constipation. Syria was renowned for quince (though its original birthplace was Babylon), with the best variety being allegedly found around Aleppo. Ibn Wāfid 2000: 123–4; Ibn Jazla, fol. 121r.; al-Rāzī 1955–69: XXI, 10–3; Ibn al-Bayṭār 1874: III, 17; al-Kindī [M. Levey 1966]: Nos. 166, 173; al-Bīrūnī 1973: 357; D. al-Anṭākī 1952: I,

189–90; al-Dhahabī 1987: 189–91; Ibn Sīnā 1999: I, 607–8; A. Dietrich 1988: II, 176–7; E. Lev & Z. Amar 2008: 255–7; R. Degen 1978; Issa Bey 1930: 64.

168. 'which do not contain ... is sufficient' – [C]: 'all of these are beneficial to strengthen the brain and organs.'

169. The enclosed passage is included in the margin of [D] (fol. 15v.). The reference is to al-Tīfāshī's book, which contains one recipe including celery (1892: 24) that is very different from the one cited here. Elsewhere (*ibid.*, 51), it states that 'celery stimulates sexual desire to the extent that a nursing mother should be prevented from eating it because it spoils her milk by increasing sexual desire.'

170. This entire chapter is omitted from the [C], whereas the content of [A] Chapter 4 corresponds to Chapter 3 in [C], which thus lacks a Chapter 4.

171. *'anbar* – the term denotes grey amber (or ambergris, the secretion of the sperm whale's gall-bladder), so named to distinguish it from yellow amber (fossilized tree resin). Both have been used in perfumes (Ibn al-Bayṭār called it 'the king of scents') and medicines, but only the latter was (and still is) prized as a gemstone. The ancient Greeks knew it as *elektron*, which gave the word 'electricity', initially denoting static electricity because of (yellow) amber's capacity to attract other materials after friction. Islamic scholars were unsure about the origins of ambergris but distinguished between the various types. Ibn al-Quff stated that the best kind was fatty and grey, whereas the black one was of the lowest quality. In the medical tradition, ambergris was said to be hot and dry, and was used to strengthen the brain and senses. It was especially beneficial for old men and those with a cold disposition. E. Lev & Z. Amar 2008: 331–3; Ibn Wāfid 2000: 164–5; *EI*[2], s.v. 'anbar' (J. Ruska/M. Plessner); Ibn al-Bayṭār 1992: III, 183–84; Ibn al-Jazzār 2004: 73–4; Ibn Sīnā 1999: I, 613–4; al-Qazwīnī 1849: 245; al-Ya'qūbī 1892: 366ff.; Ibn al-Quff [H. Kircher 1967]: 276–7.

172. *shaqāqul* (*Pastinaca schekakuli*) also appears under the following names in the literature: *shaqāqil, jamjam, shaḥmīla, fīlla, ḥashqāl, ḥurṣ al-Nīl*. This vegetable was thought to be highly beneficial for coitus, increasing lust and potency, and assisting erection, especially when used in a conserve mixed with honey. E. Lev & Z. Amar 2008: 462; Ibn Wāfid 2000: 96; Ibn al-Jazzār 2004: 31–2; Ibn Sīnā 1999: I, 675–6, II, 734; Maimonides ([F. Rosner 1973]: 21:72); *idem* ([F. Rosner 1984]: 176; al-Tīfāshī 1892: 13, 14; *Kitāb* [Tunis No. 20648(09)]: fol. 86v.; al-Shayzarī, al-Īḍāḥ, fol. 2r.; R. Muschler 1912: 468; M. Steinschneider 1900: 91.

173. *qanṭāriyūn* (also *qanṭūr<i>yūn*). This genus contains some 600 species; the ones that are most commonly referred to in Arabic pharmacology are the 'small (*ṣaghīr, daqīq*) and 'great' (*tūmāghā, kabīr, jalīl, ghalīẓ*) centaury (*Centaurium minus/maximus*), the former of which was also known as *'arbaz* (< Syriac *'arbzaz*). Medicinally, it was used in the treatment of cramps, sciatica, backache, liver and spleen obstructions, and as an emmenagogue. A. Dietrich 1988: II, 348ff.; *idem* 1991: 152ff. (note No. 9); E. Lev & Z. Amar 2008: 377–8; Ibn al-Jazzār [G. Bos 1997]: 140, 204; Ibn Sīnā 1999: I, 645–6; D. Antākī 1952: I, 263; Ibn Sahl [O. Kahl 2003]: Nos. 38, 45; al-Kindī [M. Levey 1966]: No. 241; Ibn al-Bayṭār 1874: IV, 33–4; Maimonides [M. Meyerhof 1940]: No. 333; Ibn al-Quff [H. Kircher 1967]: 310.

174. *kabāba* (also *kubāba, kabbāba*; *Piper cubeba*) – hot and dry, it was also known as *ḥabb al-ʿarūs* ('seed of the bride') because of its aphrodisiac strength, according to al-Idrīsī. In addition to its aromatic qualities, it was used in the treatment of gingival ulcers, to open blockages in the liver and kidneys, to expel kidney and bladder stones, whereas the saliva of a man chewing cubeb pleases women during intercourse. It was also said to be useful against hoarseness. E. Lev & Z. Amar 2008: 393; Ibn al-Bayṭār 1992: IV, 303–304; Ibn Jazla, fol. 184r.–v.; Ibn Janāḥ 2020: No. 490; Ibn al-Jazzār 2004: 30–1; Ibn Sīnā 1999: I, 519–20, II, 746; al-Kindī [M. Levey 1966]: Nos. 69, 77, 91, 102, 106; al-Rāzī 1955–69: XXI, 391; D. Antākī 1952: I, 255.

175. *Abū Zaydān* – this was also used by al-Tīfāshī (1970: 33/ trans. 48) in a recipe aimed at arousing the lust for coitus in women to such a degree that they would go out on the street to look for it.

176. *lakk* – considered hot and dry (in the second degree), this resinous excretion of a number of insects left on trees was also used in the treatment of palpitations, jaundice, dropsy, liver aches, to release obstructions (in the stomach and liver) and as an emmenagogue (especially when prepared in a honey syrup). In addition, it was thought to cause weight loss, and was used in red dye and ink. E. Lev & Z. Amar 2008: 193; Ibn al-Quff [H. Kircher 1967]: 330–1; Ibn Sīnā 1999: I, 539; Ibn al-Bayṭār 1992: IV, 385; Ibn Wāfid 2000: 153–4.

177. *lisān ʿuṣfūr* (*lisān al-ʿuṣfūr, lisān al-ʿaṣāfīr*, 'sparrows' tongue') – the fruit of the *dardār* tree, it was said to be very potent, and was recommended for the treatment of ulcers and palpitations, as a diuretic, carminative, theriac, purgative, but especially to increase sexual desire and potency (stiffness of erection). E. Lev & Z. Amar 2008: 340–1; Ibn al-Bayṭār 1992: IV, 384; Ibn Janāḥ 2020: No. 505; Ibn Sīnā 1999: I, 541, II, 734, 735; *Kitāb* [Tunis No. 20648(09)], fol. 86v.; *Risāla* [Cairo 362]: fol. 3v.; al-Kātib 2002: 36; Ibn al-Jazzār 2004: 40; Ibn Jazla, fol. 197v.; Issa Bey 1930: 84, 184; Ibn Wāfid 2000: 181–2; Maimonides [M. Meyerhof 1940]: No. 212; al-Bīrūnī 1973: 157.

178. [D] also has sour orange peel as well as citron peel. The Arabic words for citron (*utrunj, utrujj, turunj* or *tuffāḥ māʾī*/'water apple') could also mean 'lemon' (*laymūn*; *Citrus limon*). Its uses in both cooking and medicine are legion, with the peel in particular, being used in preserves and in stews soured with citron pulp (*hummāḍiyyāt*). After washing the pots, cooks were recommended to wipe them down with rubbed dried citron (or sour orange) leaves to remove any odours. It was used as a fragrance, to clear blemishes and to suppress bile. It should be eaten before meals, and nothing should be had afterwards until it is fully digested. It was said that the best citron was the one grown in Susa. A. Dietrich 1988: II, 178; E. Lev & Z. Amar 2008: 147–9; Ibn Jazla, fols. 13v.–14r.; Ibn Buṭlān 1990: 94–5 (trans., 190–1); al-Tīfāshī 1892: 14; Ibn Lūqā 17 (trans. 31); *Kitāb* [Tunis No. 20648(09)]: fol. 86v.; al-Shayzarī, *al-Īḍāḥ*, fol. 2r.; Ibn al-Bayṭār 1992: I, 13–5; Ibn Wāfid 2000: 34; D. Antākī 1952: I, 37; al-Dhahabī 1987: 114–5; al-Ṭabarī 1928: 302–3; al-Bīrūnī 1973: 21–3; al-Masʿūdī 1960–79: II, 438–9; al-Qazwīnī 1849: 216–7.

179. *anīsūn* (< Gr. ἄνησσον; *Pimpinella anisum*) – in addition to the variant *yānīsūn*, it was also known as *rāzyānāj* (< Persian *rāziyānah*) *Rūmī*, 'Greek

fennel' (*Foeniculum vulgare*). Anise, which is native to Asia Minor, was said to be hot and dry. In medicine, the seeds were used as a carminative, diuretic, emmenagogue, to strengthen the stomach, and clear liver obstructions, while sniffing it cures headaches. It was also recommended as an aphrodisiac and, for women, to tighten the vagina and heal the womb. Ibn Janāḥ 2020: No. 919; Ibn al-Bayṭār 1992: I, 82; Ibn al-Jazzār 2004: 164–5; al-Tīfāshī 1892: 14; *idem* 1970: 21 (trans. 35); *Kitāb* [Tunis No. 20648(09)]: fol. 86v.; *Risāla* [Cairo 362]: fol. 3r.; al-Shayzarī, *al-Īḍāḥ*, fol. 2r.; al-Kindī [M. Levey 1966]: Nos. 114, 162, 225; al-Kātib 2002: 36; D. Antākī 1952: I, 59; Maimonides [F. Rosner & S. Muntner 1970]: 20:86; al-Ghassānī 1990: 12; A. Dietrich 1988: II, 406; Z. Amar & E. Lev 2011: 102–4; al-Dhahabī 1987: 124.

180. *jullanār* – the translation follows [D], rather than [A] which has the less likely 'cucumber' (*khiyār*). See note on *jullanār* below.

181. *dār fulful* (*Piper longum*) also appears in the literature as *fulful ṭawīl* and *falfūlaniyya*; it is the dried fruit catkins of this vine, which is closely related to the standard pepper (*Piper nigrum*) and often confused with it. It is endowed with the qualities attributed to pepper and is also considered a sexual stimulant. Ibn Sīnā 1999: I, 438–9, II, 734; Ibn al-Bayṭār 1992: IV, 227–28; Ibn al-Jazzār 2004: 130; al-Kindī [M. Levey 1966]: Nos. 108, 111, 151, 178, 216, 217, 225; al-Tīfāshī 1892: 13, 14; al-Kātib 2002: 36; Ibn Lūqā 1974: 16 (trans. 23); *Kitāb* [Tunis No. 20648(09)]: fol. 86v.; al-Shayzarī, *al-Īḍāḥ*, fol. 2r.; *Risāla* [Cairo 362]: fol. 3v.; D. al-Anṭākī 1952: I, 150; al-Bīrūnī 1973: 188; Z. Amar & E. Lev 2011: 208–9; Issa Bey 1930: 141 (Nos. 2–4); Maimonides [F. Rosner & S. Muntner 1970]: 21, 38.

182. *qusṭ* (< Gr. κόστος; *Costus arabicus*) – hot and dry, this plant was known as an aromatic and aphrodisiac by Greek and Arab physicians and pharmacologists. There were said to be three varieties: white (Arab), Indian (black) and 'clove-like' (*qaranfulī*). In addition, it was said to be beneficial for the liver, back, spleen and womb, to remove tumours and as a theriac (especially for snake bites). According to Ibn al-Jazzār (2004), it should be drunk with wine and honey in order for it to act as a sexual stimulant, whereas al-Rāzī and al-Dimashqī claimed it prevented palpitations resulting from (excessive) intercourse. See A. Dietrich 1988: II, 99–100; Z. Amar & E. Lev 2011: 157–8; Ibn al-Jazzār 2004: 125–6; Ibn Sīnā 1999: I, 648, II, 734; al-Tīfāshī 1892: 14, 18; *Kitāb* [Tunis No. 20648(09)]: fol. 87; al-Bīrūnī 1973: 307; al-Rāzī 1955–69: XXI, 262–4; al-Dhahabī 1987: 227–9; Ibn al-Jazzār [G. Bos 1997]: 83[–4] et passim; al-Kātib 1977: 283; D. al-Anṭākī 1952: I, 259; R. Dozy 1877–81: II, 344; Dioscorides 2000: 21; Ibn al-Quff [H. Kircher 1967]: 311–2.

183. [A] has the unattested *khaṭmiyat al-thaʿlab*, which may be a variant of *khiṭmī/khaṭmiyya*, marshmallow (*Althaea officinalis*), but it is far more likely that it is a misspelling for the form found in [D] and [E] – *khuṣā 'l-thaʿlab*, 'fox testicles' – which refers to orchids (also *khuṣā 'l-kalb*, 'dog testicles'), whose Greek name (οόρχις, 'testicle') also denotes their shape, as does the archaic English word 'ballockwort'. Their aphrodisiacal quality was already mentioned in ancient Greece as the plant was commonly associated with the priapic satyrs, after whom it was even named ('satyrion'). *Khuṣā 'l-thaʿlab* often referred to the tuber of the salep

(*Orchis morio*), equated by some scholars with Dioscorides' satyrion. It is hot and moist, and was said to be beneficial for treating spasms, muscle stiffness and paralysis. It was considered as effective as skink in enhancing sexual potency. Today, salep (*saḥlab*) refers to flour made from the bulbs of certain varieties of orchid which is used to make a milky porridge. Eng Soon Teoh, 'An Ancient Fantasy: Salep as Aphrodisiac', in E. Teoh, *Orchids as Aphrodisiac, Medicine or Food*, Springer, 2019, pp. 13–54; A. Dietrich 1988: II, 48–81; Ibn al-Bayṭār 1992: II, 332–3; Ibn Janāḥ 2020: Nos. 292, 664, 1035; Ibn Jazla, fol. 84v.

184. [A]: *baḍḍ*; [B]: *hinā*. It is clear that this is a misprint in [A], as *baḍḍ* is not a botanical term (Lane 1863–74, I: 213). [D] and [E] have *bahman* (Moringa). Ibn Janāḥ 2020: No. 772; Ibn Ibn Jazla, fol. 45v.

185. *khūlanjān* (also *khūlanj*; *Alpinia galanga*); it should not be confused with galingale (*Cyperus longus*). It is a member of the ginger family and its aromatic dried root is used in cooking, and in medicine against colic, as a digestive, carminative and aphrodisiac, whether drunk with milk or by chewing it. If it was chewed together with a bit of musk, it caused a powerful erection. Ibn al-Jazzār 2004: 147–8; Ibn Sīnā 1999: I, 709, II, 734; Ibn Lūqā 1974: 16 (trans. 23); al-Kātib 2002: 36; al-Tīfāshī 1892: 14; al-Shayzarī, *al-Īḍāḥ*, fol. 2r.; *Risāla* [Cairo 362]: fol. 3r.

186. *'āqir qarḥ* (more correctly *'āqir qarḥā*; *Anacyclus pyrethrum*) was used as a digestive, to control saliva flow, as well as being an aphrodisiac. According to Ibn al-Bayṭār it was a remedy for impotence when boiled down in water and then cooked in olive oil. A. Dietrich 1988: II, 422–3; al-Tīfāshī 1892: 14; al-Shayzarī, *al-Īḍāḥ*, fol. 3v.; *Risāla* [Cairo 362]: fol. 3v.. 5; al-Kātib 2002: 36; al-Bīrūnī 1973: 261; Ibn Sīnā 1999: II 734; al-Rāzī 1955–69: XXI, 191; Ibn al-Bayṭār 1992: III, 157–58; Ibn al-Jazzār 2004: 190; D. al-Anṭākī 1952: I, 235; Ibn al-Quff [H. Kircher 1967]: 272.

187. *shaḥm al-asad* – all fats were hot and moist in the first degree and were used, among other things, to ripen wounds. Among the most effective fats were those of lions, wolves and bears, but lion's fat, in particular, was thought to be an effective aphrodisiac. Ibn al-Quff [H. Kircher 1967]: 240; al-Ṭabarī 1928: 428; al-Tīfāshī 1892: 14; *Kitāb* [Tunis No. 20648(09)]: fol. 86bv.; *Risāla* [Cairo 362]: fol. 3r.; al-Kātib 2002: 36.

188. *liḥyat tays* (*Tragopogon pratensis or Tragopogon porrifolius*) is a calque of the Greek τραγοπώγων also known as '(meadow) salsify' and appears more commonly as *liḥyat al-tays*; it was used to treat ulcers, diarrhoea, and uteral discharge. Ibn al-Bayṭār 1992: IV, 378–9; Ibn Wāfid 2000:113–4; al-Rāzī 1955–69: XXI, 479–81; Maimonides [M. Meyerhof 1940]: Nos. 37, 174; D. al-Anṭākī 1952: I, 281; A. Dietrich 1988: II, 292; Ibn Janāḥ 2020: No. 501.

189. *zift rūmī* – the resin extracted from various kinds of conifers. Raw pitch (*zift raṭb*) was sometimes referred to as *qīr*, which was also applied to bitumen, while dry pitch (*zift yābis*) was known as *qār*. In fact, both denoted tar (*qaṭrān*) or pitch. Medicinally, it was thought to be beneficial for sciatica, and gout, as well as being an antiseptic. Ibn Jazla, fol. 114r.; A. Dietrich 1988: II, 118–20; Ibn Janāḥ 2020: Nos. 847, 848; Ibn al-Bayṭār 1992: II, 470–1; D. al-Anṭākī 1952: I, 140; Ibn Sīnā 1999: I, 463; Ibn al-Quff [H. Kircher 1967]: 199–200; Also see note on *qaṭrān*, below.

190. *khashkhāsh*, 'black Egypian poppy'. Medicinally, it was thought to be

beneficial as a soporific, and to treat ailments as varied as corneal ulcers and cough. In erotological literature, it is mentioned as an aphrodisiac. A. Dietrich 1988: II, 568–9; Ibn al-Bayṭār 1992: II, 328–9; Ibn al-Jazzār 2004: 199; Ibn Sīnā 1999: I, 699–701; D. al-Anṭākī 1952: I, 140; al-Ishbīlī 1995: I, 237 (*al-khashkhās al-aswad*); al-Tīfāshī 1892: 14; *Kitāb* [Tunis No 20648(09)]: fol. 86v.; al-Shayzarī, *al-Īḍāḥ*, fol. 3r.; E. Lane 1863–74: I, 70; al-Ṭabarī 1928: 376; M. Steinschneider 1900: 62 (No. 749).

191. The translation follows [D], which has *jawz al-tīb* as the 'walnuts' (*jawz*) found in the other copies is clearly a lapsus calami.

192. *basbāsa* – the covering of the seed of the nutmeg tree (*Myristica fragrans*), the spice was native to the Banda Islands (Indonesia). It only reached the Near East in the 8th century and remained a very rare spice. Its other names include *darkīsa* (< Persian) and *ṭālīsfar* (< Sanskrit). In the medical tradition, it was used against stomach ulcers, and as an aphrodisiac. Ibn Wāfid 2000: 34–5; Ibn Jazla, fol. 39r.; al-Tīfāshī 1892: 14; *Kitāb* [Tunis No. 20648(09)]: fol. 86v.; al-Shayzarī, *al-Īḍāḥ*, fol. 2v.; A. Dietrich 1988: II, 134; D. al-Anṭākī 1952: I, 74–5, 229; Ibn Sīnā 1999: I, 240; al-Bīrūnī 1973: 191; Ibn al-Bayṭār 1992: I, ; Ibn al-Jazzār 2004: 67; Maimonides [M. Meyerhof 1940]: No. 38.

193. *bawraq* ((< Persian *būrah*) – hot and dry (in the second degree), borax consists of salt and soda mined in the Egyptian desert (especially Wādi Naṭrūn). The literature mentions white, red, African and Armenian varieties, the last of which was also known by the Greek borrowing *nāṭrūn* (natron). It should be distinguished from today's borax (sodium borate), known in Arabic as *tinkār*. In cooking, it was used in (bread) baking, whereas the medical authorities recommend it as a remedy for a large number of conditions (seventy, according to al-Qazwīnī), including eye diseases and constipation. Ibn al-Bayṭār quotes al-Rāzī and others when claiming that a mixture of pounded natron and jasmine oil, or with honey, rubbed on the penis produces strong erections. Others (including al-Bīrūnī) warned about the toxicity of the borax when taken internally. Ibn Janāḥ 2020: Nos. 503, 538; Ibn Lūqā 1974: 21 (trans. 28); Ibn al-Bayṭār 1992: I, 170–1; Ibn al-Jazzār 2004: 216–7; al-Dhahabī 1987: 134; Ibn Sīnā 1999: I, 389–90, 580 (*naṭrūn*); Ibn al-Quff [H. Kircher 1967]: 106–7, 351–2; E. Lev & Z. Amar 2008: 118–20; al-Bīrūnī 1973: 80; Maimonides [M. Meyerhof 1940]: No. 51. al-Isrā'ilī 1992: 513; al-Rāzī 2000: 2957–8; al-Ghāfiqī 2014: 94r.–v. (trans., Levey 1973: 112); al-Bīrūnī 1973: 80; Ibn Jazla, fol. 44r.–v.; Renaud & Colin 1934: 42 (No. 92), 173 (No. 401).

194. *zurunbād* (or *zurunbādh*, *Zingiber zerumbet*) was also known as *'irq al-kāfūr*; considered to be hot in the second degree and moderately dry, it is a perennial aromatic plant of the ginger family. It was used very rarely in cooking. In medicine, it was thought to be an effective carminative and breath freshener, especially to counter the smell of garlic and onions. In addition, it gladdens the heart, as well as being an anti-emetic an antidote against insect bites. Ibn al-Bayṭār 1992: II, 461–2 (trans., II, 200–2), III, 65 (trans., II, 443); Dozy (1877–81: II, 119); Ibn Jazla, fols. 112v.–113r.; Ibn al-Jazzār 2004: 155; Ibn Sīnā 1999: II, 734; Ibn Janāḥ 2020: No. 206; Ibn Wāfid 2000: 146; M. Steinschneider 1900: 90 (No. 937); Ibn al-Bayṭār 2001: II, 157–8; Ibn al-Jazzār 2004: 155; Ibn Sahl [O. Kahl 1900]: Nos. 8, 25,

31, 41, 8, 49, 50, 57, 66, 232, 312, 371; al-Ishbīlī 1995: I, 273.

195. *halīlaj* (*Terminalia chebula*) – considered cold and dry, it was said to be beneficial for, among others, strengthening the stomach, removing black bile, to relieve haemorrhoids, aid digestion, dispel winds, sharpen the senses, increase memory, as well as being a remedy for leprosy, colic, headaches, vomiting and fever. Together with the other myrobalans, it was often used in electuary recipes to cure impotence. Ibn Janāḥ 2020: No. 287; Ibn Sīnā 1999: I, 447–8; Ibn Lūqā 1974: 19 (trans. 27); Ibn Wāfid 2000: 107–11; Ibn Sahl [O. Kahl 2003]: 119 (note No. 145); Ibn al-Jazzār 2004: 13–4.

196. *balīlaj* was thought to be particularly effective in strengthening the body, improving the complexion and even preventing black hair from turning grey. Ibn Jazla, fol., 41v.–42r.; Ibn Wāfid 2000: 100; Ibn Lūqā 1974: 19 (trans. 27).

197. *amlaj*, the fruit of *Phyllanthus emblica* ('Indian gooseberry') – it was said to strengthen the stomach, as well as serving as an anti-emetic and sexual stimulant. Ibn Janāḥ 2020: No. 951; Ibn Jazla, fol. 26v.; Ibn Wāfid 2000: 100–1; Ibn Lūqā 1974: 19 (trans. 27); Ibn al-Jazzār 2004: 14; E. Lev *&* Z. Amar 2008: 218ff. (Chapter 6); Ibn al-Quff [H. Kircher 1967]: 83–6.

198. [D] specifies that it should be 'raw'.

199. *ḥabba sawdā'* ('black grain'), *Nigella sativa* – hot and dry in the second or third degree, the aromatic spice was, depending on the author, also referred to as *kammūn aswad* ('black cumin'), *k. hindī* ('Indian c.'), *k. ḥabashī* ('Ethiopian c.'), *ḥabb al-baraka* ('the seed of the blessing'), or *shūnīz* (a borrowing from Persian, which could denote 'sesame', 'coriander' or 'pepper'). It was considered a remedy for a variety of ailments, including leprosy, and was thought to be useful against warts, freckles and ulcers, as well as being a diuretic, appetizer, emmenagogue, anthelmintic and carminative. However, physicians warned that the excessive use of the aromatic is fatal. According to al-Bīrūnī, droplets of nigella oil were used in cures of paralysis and tetanus. A. Dietrich 1988: II, 429–30; al-Dhahabī 1987: 150–2; al-Suyūṭī n.d.: 13; E. Lev *&* Z. Amar 2008: 362–4; Dioscorides 2000: 45 (*Melanthelaion*); al-Rāzī 1955–69: XXI, 123; D. al-Anṭākī 1952: I, 219–20; Ibn al-Quff [H. Kircher 1967]: 238; Ibn Sīnā 1999: I, 677–8; Ibn Jazla, fols. 138v.–139v.; Ibn al-Bayṭār 1992: III, 95–7; al-Bīrūnī 1973: 431–2 (trans., 363–4); F. Steingass 1894: 767.

200. *jawz hindī* (also *jawz al-Hind, nārjīl*) – it was said to be very effective as an aphrodisiac and to strengthen the erection (*in'āẓ*). It was also used as an anthelmintic, against haemorrhoids, backache and throat-ache. Confusingly, Ibn Jazla equated *nāranj* with coconut. Ibn al-Quff [H. Kircher 1967]: 135–8; al-Dhahabī 1987: 148. Ibn Jazla, fol. 57v.

201. *su'd* – (*Cyperus longus*) – also known as *su'dā*, the plant (especially its root) was used as an aromatic in cooking, with the one from Kufa being considered the best. Medicinally, it was thought to have warming and drying properties and was recommended against oral ulcers, as a diuretic, anthelmintic, emmenagogue, breath freshener, to improve memory, expel kidney stones, cure urinary stammer, and cool fevers. According to Ibn al-Quff, excessive use of the plant leads to leprosy. Ibn Wāfid 2000: 162–3; Ibn al-Bayṭār 1992: III, 20–1; Ibn al-Jazzār 2004: 102; al-Kātib 1977: 257 (who

recommends eating it together with saltwort and claims it strengthens the gums); al-Bīrūnī 1973: 220; D. al-Anṭākī 1952: I, 188; al-Shayzarī, *al-Īḍāḥ*, fol. 2v.; al-Rāzī 1955–69: XXI, 1–3; A. Dietrich 1988: II, 89; Ibn al-Quff [H. Kircher 1967]: 233-4; Ibn Janāḥ 2020: No. 651.

202. cf. Ibn Sīnā 1999: II, 734.

203. *zayt*, which as the name indicates is the juice extracted from olives (*zaytūn*, *Olea europaea*) – oil obtained from plants is referred to as *duhn*. Its use as an oil increased over time, gradually replacing sheep's tail fat for frying, and was particularly favoured in the Western Mediterranean. It is a staple in fish dishes. It was considered that the best variety is that expressed from red olives that are neither unripe nor ripe, while the oil increases in strength with age. Scholars considered young olive oil in between hot, tending towards moistness, while the old variety is in between dry and moist. It is useful against sciatica, and serves as a laxative when used with barley water. Ibn Sīnā recommended oil extracted from fresh unripe (green) olives, known as *unfāq* (< Greek *omphakion*), which is cold and dry, as it strengthens the body. Ibn al-Bayṭār referred to its use in the cure of cataracts by rubbing it into the affected eye. See EI2, s.v. 'zayt' (D. Waines); al-Dhahabī 1987: 186–8; Ibn al-Quff [H. Kircher 1967]: 182–3; Ibn al-Bayṭār 1992: II, 489 (trans., 227–8); Ibn Jazla, fol. 117r.; Ibn Sīnā 1999: I, 472–3; al-Rāzī 2000: 3105; Ibn Janāḥ 2020: No. 319.

204. *milḥ andarānī* (also *darānī*), was also known as 'Persian salt' (*milḥ Fārisī*). Medicinally, it was used to extract phlegm, sharpen the mind, and as an emetic. Ibn Sīnā 1999: I, 571–2; Ibn Janāḥ 2020: No. 568;D. Newman 2020: 3. Al-Tīfāshī used it in a recipe (boiled with alum) to warm the vagina and reduce its moistness (1970: 30).

205. *'ūd ṣalīb* – the medicinal uses of the plant were known in Indian, Chinese and Islamic medicine, where it was primarily recommended as an emmenagogue and to treat heartburn, and pains in the womb, liver and bladder. It was also known as *ward al-ḥamīr* ('donkeys' rose'). Ibn Sīnā 1999: I, 623; F. Corriente 1997: 309; A. Dietrich 1988: II, 496–7.

206. 'that have been cooked in oil and fry everything until it is mixed well. Take a dirham each of cinnamon, galangal and peony. Pound all of these spices and sprinkle them on top of the cooked onions' – [C]: 'boil until everything is mixed. Take a *dirham* each of cinnamon, galangal and peony and sprinkle on the dish.'

207. This sentence is omitted from [C].

208. Addition in [D].

209. 'Pulverize these ingredients' is missing from [C].

210. The variant in [C] of this passage ('stir until everything is mixed....') is considerably shorter: 'stir until everything is mixed, remove from the fire and drink. It is beneficial, as we have mentioned, Allah willing.'

211. The translation follows [D] rather than [A] which has the incongruous 'dry'.

212. This is a correction from [B] as the verb is missing from [A].

213. [D] adds 'without changing the temperament'.

214. [D] and [E] specify that it is 'foul temperament'.

215. The entire previous recipe up until this point is abridged in [C] to: 'cook

and throw on five *dirhams* of common ash, a *dirham* of coconut and cloves, and heat up until it becomes mixed with the rest. Remove from the fire and eat in the evening. It is beneficial, as we have mentioned. Among the sweets that restore the temperament, strengthen the principal organs, cure impotence and increase innate heat, ...'.

216. 'heat', [B]: 'boil'.

217. 'Add some olive oil ...'; [C]: 'Thicken the honey and sprinkle on it cinnamon and lemon peel (five *dirhams* each).'

218. [E] omits the agarwood and calls for a staggering five *dirhams* of saffron.

219. 'half a *dirham* of saffron...'; [C]: 'one *dirham* of saffron, remove from the fire, pour into a glass jar and eat the mixture every evening before going to sleep. You will see (it works wonders).'

220. *ṣanawbar* – considered hot and moist, it increases semen, potency and the lust for coition, as well being used to treat burns, and liver and toothaches. Ibn al-Bayṭār 1874: III, 87–9; al-Dhahabī 1987: 202; al-Tīfāshī 1892: 14; *Risāla* [Cairo 362]: fol. 3v.; al-Kātib 2002: 36; D. al-Anṭākī 1952: I, 224; Ibn Sīnā 1999: I, 490–1, 640, II, 734; Ibn Wāfid 2000: 81–2; al-Bīrūnī 1973: 249; Ibn al-Quff [H. Kircher 1967]: 253; al-Ṭabarī 1928: 383; Maimonides [M. Meyerhof 1940]: No. 317.

221. According to [D], it should be two *dirhams* of cinnamon.

222. *dār ṣīnī* (< Persian *dār chīnī*, 'Chinese wood'), *Cinnamomum* cassia, was said to be hot and dry in the third degree. In medicine, it was used, among other things, to strengthen the stomach, liver and spleen, as a diuretic, emmenagogue and antidote against scorpion poison. In erotological literature, it is often credited with aphrodisiacal properties. A. Dietrich 1988: II, 97–8; *EI²*, *Sup.*, s.v. (A. Dietrich); al-Tīfāshī 1892: 13, 14; Ibn Sahl [O. Kahl 2003]: *passim*; E. Lev *&* Z. Amar 2008: 143–4; al-Dhahabī : 173; al-Rāzī 1955–69: XXI, 490–6; Ibn al-Bayṭār 1874: II, 83–5; Ibn al-Jazzār 2004: 130–1; D. al-Anṭākī 1952: I, 149; Ibn Sīnā 1999: I, 431–3, II, 734; al-Bīrūnī 1973: 189; Ibn al-Quff [H. Kircher 1967]: 183–5; M. Steinschneider 1900: 65 (No. 792). For an overview of the variation in terms for various types of cinnamon, see J. Leibowitz *&* S. Marcus 1974: 233.

223. Addition in [D].

224. 'mix with white skimmed bee honey...'; [C]: 'pour on it the same measure of skimmed honey until everything is mixed. Sprinkle on top five *dirhams* of citron peel, half a *dirham* of saffron, stir and use one *mithqāl* daily before going to sleep. You will see the wonders it works, as has been mentioned.'

225. A reference to the Iranian city of Yazd, which has been a centre of Zoroastrian culture for many centuries. [D] has *zumurrudī* ('emerald-like'), which is also the name of a sweet pudding found in a thirteenth-century Andalusian cookery book (D. Newman 2023: No. 416).

226. [D] has the more plausible 'and it is also beneficial'.

227. In the culinary tradition, this word (meaning 'tripled') referred to dishes made with three ingredients, which,variously involved three grains or pulses, or meat, saffron, vinegar, and vegetables. In the pharmacological literature, the term denoted wine cooked down to a third. D. Newman 2023: 143, 160; Ibn Jazla, fol. 207r.

228. 'invigorate coitus...', [C]: 'and which is known as "*muthallath* wine". Take grape juice and add three times the quantity of fresh water. Boil until a

third remains and take a measure of three *dirhams* from it and fifty *dirhams* of the bee honey.'

229. 'or white sugar, and cook until the froth apears. Then take ...'; [C]: 'Then add to it ...'

230. [E] adds 'and one dirham of musk'.

231. The passage 'Crush all of these into dust...' is as follows in [C]: 'until everything is mixed. Then remove and decant into a glass vessel. If you want to use it, take a measure of forty *dirhams* of the mixture, mix with the same amount of freshwater and drink it. It is beneficial, as we have mentioned, Allah willing.'

232. This is a reference to Dā'ūd Ibn 'Umar al-Anṭākī's *Kitāb al-nuzha al-mubhija fī tashḥīdh al-adhhān wa ta'dīl al-amzija* ('The Delightful Excursion in Sharpening Minds and Regulating Temperaments'), on therapeutics.

233. This is added in the margin of [D].

234. This recipe is found only in [D].

235. [B] adds "yellow bile".

236. 'cure headache, catarrh and innate heat' is omitted from [C].

237. The passage 'to such a great extent that ...' is missing from [C], which simply has 'The recipe for the cardamom electuary is ...' .

238. *ḥaṣā lubān; lūbān* (< Gr. λίβανος), also known by its Persian name *kundur* (< Gr. χόνδρος, 'grain'), is a resin harvested from the olibanum tree. In addition to burning it for the smell, *lūbān* was recommended for a large number of ailments, such as bronchitis, stomach ulcers, diarrhoea, skin conditions, dysentery, as a digestive and to prevent the spread of tumours. However, it was also said to be highly dangerous as it can cause madness and, when taken with wine, even death. *EI*[2], s.v. 'lūbān' (A. Dietrich); E. Lev & Z. Amar 2008: 266–8; Ibn al-Bayṭār 1992: IV, 348–52; Ibn al-Jazzār 2004: 165; Ibn al-Quff [H. Kircher 1967]: 157–60; A. Dietrich 1988: II, 113–4; al-Suyūṭī n.d.: 15; Ibn Sīnā 1999: I, 515–7, II, 734; al-Rāzī 1955–69: XXI, 313–8; D. al-Anṭākī 1952: I, 275–6; al-Bīrūnī 1973: 324.

239. *kuḥl* (also known as *ithmid* and *surma*) initially was antimony sulphide (stibnite), which was pulverized and used as a cosmetic (esp. applied to eyebrows, lashes and edges of the eyelids). More often, *kuhl* denoted any eye cosmetic made from a wide variety of substances and, in some cases, a particular lead mineral, whose exact identity remains to be ascertained. The primary source of *kuḥl* was Iran. *EI*[2], s.v. 'al-kuḥl' (E. Wiedemann-[J.W. Allan]); al-Suyūṭī n.d.: 52–4.

240. According to [C], one should take one *mithqāl* after the evening meal. In [E], the recipe ends with the instructions at the end of the caltrop recipe.

241. This recipe an the next are missing from [E].

242. *simsim* (also known as *juljulān, Sesamum indicum*) – in cooking, it appears in a paste, the famous *tahina*, whereas its oil (*shīraj* < Persian *shīrah*, 'new wine') was used for deep-frying. It was considered bad for the stomach and to cause vomiting. It was also thought to increase semen and sexual potency (according to Ibn Sīnā, especially when eaten with flax and cotton seeds). Ibn Janāḥ 2020: Nos. 232, 997; Ibn Lūqā 1974: 17 (trans. 24); al-Tīfāshī 1892: 14; Ibn Wāfid 2000: 94–5; Ibn al-Bayṭār 1992: III, 40–1; Ibn Sīnā 1999: I, 604–5, II, 734; al-Rāzī 1955–69: XXI, 36–9; al-Bīrūnī 1973: 233; A. Dietrich 1988: II, 249–60.

243. This sentence is missing from [C].
244. One *wuqqa* equals approx. 2.75 *raṭls*; R. Dozy 1877–81: II, 827.
245. This is a correction of the Arabic *quffa* ('basket'), which is undoubtedly a scribal error as it does not make any sense in the context.
246. This recipe is added only in [D], fol. 20r.
247. *ḥasak* – sometimes known as *ḥimmaṣ al-amīr* ('the Prince's chickpeas'), it was said to come in a wild (*barrī*) and cultivated (*bustānī*) variety. It was used (both dried and fresh) in the treatment of tumours and kidney stones. Ibn al-Bayṭār 1874: II, 20–1; Ibn Sīnā 1999: I, 478, II, 734; Ibn Lūqā 1974; 21 (trans. 28); *Kitāb* [Tunis No 20648(09)]: fol. 86v.; *Risāla* [Cairo 362]: fol. 5r.; al-Kātib 2002: 36; al-Rāzī 1955–69: XX, 327; Ibn Wāfid 2000: 112; al-Bīrūnī 1973: 158; A. Dietrich 1988: II, 528–9.
248. [C]: 'one *dirham*'.
249. 'half a *dirham* of ginger'; [C]: 'and ginger, two *dirhams* of each; sparrow brains, ten *dirhams*. Vigorously pound everything and thicken with bee honey.'
250. 'When you wish to engage in coitus...'; [C] 'When needed, drink from the *muthallath* wine that is mentioned here and it will achieve its aim, and Allah knows best.'
251. This refers to compounds based on a number of myrobalans (*amlaj, balīlaj, halīlaj*) which come in a 'smaller' (*al-aṣghar*) and 'greater' (*al-akbar*) variety. The mixture referred to here would appear to be the 'larger', as mentioned by Sābūr Ibn Sahl, who recommended it as a treatment for a cold stomach and haemorrhoidal pains, whereas Ibn al-Jazzār recorded it as an established therapy for hernias. According to Maimonides, it strengthens the limbs, delays aging and aids coitus. This compound is distinct from *iṭrīful*, 'bitumen trefoil' (*Bituminaria bituminosa*), whose identity is obscure. Both terms would seem to go back to the Greek τρίφυλλον ('three-leaved'). A similar recipe appears in the Trotula as '*trifera saracenica*' ('the Saracen trifera), alongside a '*trifera magna*' ('greater trifera'). See Ibn al-Jazzār [G. Bos 1997]: 122; Ibn Lūqā 1974: 15 (trans. 22); Ibn Sahl [O. Kahl 2003]: 119, 120; al-Ṭabarī 1928: 480; E. Lev *&* Z. Amar 2008: 209, 219, 341, 362 (with the vowelling *iṭrīful* for the myrobalan-based compounds); al-Rāzī 2007: 310; *idem* 1955–69: XXI, 159ff.; A. Dietrich 1988: II, 461ff.; M. Ullmann 1970: 295–6, 349; W. Schmucker 1969: 48; al-Bīrūnī 1973: 255; Maimonides [M. Levey 1966]: 21:38; M. Green 2002: 134.
252. The following is ommited in [C]: 'has great benefits and innumerable advantages. It strengthens the intellect.'
253. 'its brightness opens blockages in the head and eyes'; [C]: 'intellect'.
254. [E] has 'the penis' instead of 'potency'.
255. 'strengthens the principal organs and innate heat; strengthens potency; tautens the nerves'; [B]: 'strengthens the organs'.
256. For a similar recipe, see al-Tīfāshī 1892: 15; Ibn Lūqā 1974: 19 (trans. 27).
257. [A] has the persian borrowing *balīlah* instead of *balīlaj*.
258. 'strengthens potency ...'; [C]: 'tautens the nerves and the penis; heats the kidneys, bladder and sperm; and greatly strengthens coitus. The recipe is made up of myrobalan, emblic myrobalan and belleric myrobalan.' [A] has the Persian borrowing *balīlah* instead of *balīlaj*.

259. *sha'īr* – considered (moderately) cold and dry, this cereal (or one of its derivates like meal or water), was used to remedy a number of conditions, ranging from skin blemishes to fever, bowel infections, as a diuretic and a cure for impotence. It is, however, flatulent, whereas its flour is constipating (Ibn Sīnā). Ibn Jazla said that when cooked with figs it was beneficial against phlegmatic fevers. According to Ibn Khalṣūn, barley was particularly good in summer for bilious and hot temperaments. He also recommended the white fresh variety, pounded, sieved and kneaded with salt, yeast and aniseed. Ibn Buṭlān preferred black barley due to its digestiveness. He allocated the following properties depending on the use of barley: as flour, it is drying; cooked with water it is moistening; when cooked in the oven it is neither drying nor moistening. Ibn Jazla recommended barley water with grape juice cooked over a moderate fire as it created good blood, but warned against its use by those with cold bowels. Its negative effects on the stomach can be remedied by oxymel. *EI²*, s.v. 'sha'īr' (D. Waines); Ibn Sahl [O. Kahl 2003]: e.g Nos. 20, 23, 195, 285, 290, 296351, 353, 354, 407; al-Bīrūnī 1973: 401; Ibn al-Jazzār [G. Bos 1997]: 94, 167, 170, 173, 174, 190; D. al-Anṭākī 1952: I, 215–6; A. Dietrich 1988: II, 242; Ibn al-Quff [H. Kircher 1967]: 233; al-Suyūṭī n.d.: 9. Ibn Buṭlān 1990: 78–9 (trans. 158); Ibn Jazla, fols. 137r., 187v., 204v.–205r.; Lewy 1956; Ibn Khalṣūn 1996: 157 (trans. 83); Ibn al-Bayṭār 1992: III, 83–4; D. al-Anṭākī 1952, I: 215–16; Ibn Sīnā 1999: II, 682.The same recipe is also included in the anonymous medical text that follows [A] in the binding (fol. 104).

260. The same recipe is also included in the anonymous medical text that follows [A] in the binding (fol. 104).

261. [C]: 'It is beneficial, as we have mentioned, Allah willing.'

262. 'remove coldness from the back and hip' is omitted from [C].

263. 'finely pound everything so that it becomes like kohl dust'; [C]: 'pulverize'.

264. 'Pound the two ...'; [B]: 'Pulverize, strain through a fine cloth and mix with the ingredients. Add the same amount of bee honey and use before going to sleep'; [C]: 'and cinnamon bark, clove and ginger, one *dirham* of each. Pulverize and mix with the honey. Use before going to sleep. It is very beneficial.' Abū 'Abd Allāh Muḥammad al-Ḥārithī al-Baghdādī (d. 949-1022), known as al-Shaykh al-Mufīd ('the Beneficial Sage') and Ibn al-Mu'allim ('Son of the Teacher'), was a leading Shī'ī (Twelver) theologian. See, for instance, Tamima Bayhom-Daou, Shaykh Mufid, Oxford: Oneworld Academic, 2005.

265. *ḥabb al-quṭn* - in the Islamic medical tradition, cotton (especially tree cotton, *Gossypium arboreum*, and Levant cotton, *Gossypium herbaceum*) was recommended for coughs, whereas the oil derived from it was used for sunspots and freckles. Cotton was also said to increase the lust for coitus and appears as a regular ingredient in a number of aphrodisiacs. *EI²*, s.v. 'ḳuṭn' (H. Inalcik); A. Dietrich 1988: II, 159 (Note 11); Ibn al-Bayṭār 1992: IV, 271; Ibn al-Jazzār 2004: 193; al-Kātib 2002: 36; al-Dhahabī 1987: 230; D. al-Anṭākī 1952: I, 260; Ibn Wāfid 2000: 84; al-Ṭabarī 1928: 282; *Risāla* [Cairo 362]: fol. 3r.; al-Shayzarī, *al-Īḍāḥ*, fol. 3v.; al-Rāzī 1955-69: XXI, 307; Maimonides [M. Meyerhof 1940]: No. 349.

266. *sūra/injān* (also known as 'meadow saffron'). The red and black were thought to be harmful and only the white was used in medicine. It was recommended as a laxative, antiseptic, to cure pain in the joints, gout, and

as an aphrodisiac. Ibn al-Bayṭār 1874: III, 41–2; Ibn al-Jazzār 2004: 176; al-Ṭabarī 1928: 302; D. al-Anṭākī 1952: I, 204; al-Rāzī 1955–69: XXI, 39; Ibn Wāfid 2000: 163–4; Ibn Sīnā 1999: I, 589–90 (who recommends taking it with ginger, pennyroyal and cumin to increase its aphrodisiacal potency); al-Bīrūnī 1973: 240; A. Dietrich 1988: II, 589–90; Ibn al-Quff [H. Kircher 1967]: 221–2; al-Ṭabarī 1928: 402.

267. [E] jumps from this chapter to Chapter 11.

268. *furn* (< Latin *furnus*), which also referred to the communal oven; see D. Newman 2023: 70.

269. Addition in [D].

270. *qarʿa*, also *dubbāʾ* and, more commonly, *yaqṭīn* (cf. Qur'ān 37:146) – cold and moist, it was thought to be beneficial for cough, headaches and as a soporific for people with a fever (esp. the seeds and oil). There are a number of hadiths praising the gourd, for instance because it increases the intellect and mind; indeed, the Prophet, himself, was very partial to it. When eaten with lentils, it acts as a sexual stimulant; with sour pomegranate and sumac, it is beneficial for yellow bile. A. Dietrich 1988: II, 282; Ibn al-Quff [H. Kircher 1967]: 298–9; Maimonides [M. Meyerhof 1940]: No. 332; Ibn al-Bayṭār 1992: IV, 251–53; D. al-Anṭākī 1952: I, 256; al-Rāzī 1955–69: XXI, 284–7; Ibn Sīnā 1999: I, 656; al-Ṭabarī 1928: 380; al-Dhahabī 1987: 226–7.

271. *shibitt* (absent from [C]); this herb is native to the eastern Mediterranean and both the leaves and seeds were already widely used in cooking in ancient Rome. In Islamic medicine, it was considered warming and desiccating, and useful in maturating tumours, against hiccups and gripes, as a sedative, carminative and soporific (especially its oil), as a remedy against kidney and bladder stones, and in the treatment of wounds. Its seeds were believed to stop the growth of haemorrhoids. However, dill is harmful to the stomach, kidney and urethra, which, according to Ibn Jazla, can be remedied by lemon or honey. Ibn al-Quff [H. Kircher 1967]: 236–7; A. Dietrich 1988: II, 407–8; Ibn al-Jazzār 2004: 108; al-Rāzī 1955–69: XXI, 121–3; al-Ṭabarī 1928: 380; Maimonides [M. Meyerhof 1940]: No. 363; al-Bīrūnī 1973: 391–3; Ibn Sīnā 1999: I, 678 (trans., 282–3); Ibn al-Bayṭār 1992: III, 66–7; al-Isrā'īlī 1992: 475; Ibn Jazla, fol. 132r.; Ibn Buṭlān 1992: 82–3 (trans 166-7); al-Ṭabarī 1928: 380; A. Lev 2008: 398; Dalby 2003: 117.

272. 'pepper' is omitted from [B] and [D].

273. A dome-shaped clay oven. *EI*[2], s.v. 'maṭbakh' (J. Burton-Page); D. Newman 2020: lvi.

274. 'the fat and testicles…'; [C]: 'a small amount of lamb fat and a thin piece of lamb meat; place in a pot and cover with water. Put the lid on the top and leave in the oven overnight until everything is cooked thoroughly. Then, administer an enema with it, which is called "the aperient one".'

275. In [D], after the title, this chapter consists solely of the section 'on the extraction of oils' (Chapter 11 below).

276. The translation is based on [B], which has *al-ṣūf wa 'l-mansūj wa 'l-tafkīk*, as the text in [A], *al-ṣūf al-mansūj min al-tankīk*, is clearly a misprint. The version in [C] is, simply, 'woven wool' (*al-ṣūf al-mansūj*).

277. Tu. *kemer* ('waistband') *qashāghi* ('currycomb'); J. Redhouse 1880: 722, 754 (1890: 1415).

278. This chapter is considerably shorter in [C]: 'So, you have to wear the clothes that are appropriate for the season in order to tighten and strengthen the organs. In spring the appropriate attire is made out of cotton so that the organs remain temperate and the temperament does not become foul. In summer, only flax is appropriate, whereas in autumn woven wool should be worn. As for fur, this should be sabre, ermine, squirrel, and white or black sheep. It is beneficial against the weakening of the organs and preserves the temperament.'

279. 'coitus and how to conduct it so as to as to avoid weakness, harm, premature old age and grey hair'; [C]: 'conditions and manner of coitus'.

280. The rest of this paragraph is missing from [C].

281. This position was discouraged by most authors and physicians, including Ibn Sīnā, through whom it entered the Christian European medical tradition – Ibn Lūqā 1973: 33; al-Nafzāwī n.d.: 30; al-Kātib 2002: 103–4 (trans. 1977: 305); al-Tīfāshī 1892: 66–7; D. Jacquart & C. Thomasset 1988: 132.

282. cf. al-Kātib 1977: 305 ('The side position is harmful to a man who has weakness in one of his organs <and> also makes difficult the ejaculation of the seminal fluid and causes kidney pain and a swelling in the penis').

283. The entire passage from 'These are all dangerous diseases ...' onwards, is missing from [C].

284. The passage starting here and ending in the next chapter ('... narcissus bulbs') is considerably shorter in [C]: 'a burning sensation when urinating, urinary stammer, blood in urine. A wise man should be wary of engaging in coitus in the aforementioned positions. The best position is when the woman is lying flat on her back. Put a cushion underneath her hips, with the woman lifting her thighs. The man then goes on all fours until he is close to ejaculating, at which point he lies down on the woman, who puts her arms around him until the ejaculation has been completed. The advantage of this [position] is that it provides protection against the above-mentioned ailments, Allah the Almighty willing. Chapter Twelve. Description of medicines to strengthen and thicken the penis. Take narcissus bulbs (...)'.

285. *'inab al-dhi'b* ('wolf grapes'), which is also known as *'inab al-tha'lab* ('fox grapes'). Its medicinal use was often linked to the curing of tumours in various parts of the body. When used with wine, it acts as a soporific. In erotological literature, it is considered one of the anaphrodisiacs. A. Dietrich 1988: II, 573–7; Ibn al-Bayṭār 1874: III, 135–7; Ibn al-Jazzār 2004: 115–6; Ibn Sīnā 1999: III, 297, 612–3; al-Shayzarī, *al-Īḍāḥ*, fol. 2v.; al-Bīrūnī 1973: 274–6; al-Rāzī 1955–69: XXI, 195–7; R. P. Dozy 1877–81: II, 179; D. al-Anṭākī 1952: I, 240–1; Ibn al-Quff [H. Kircher 1967]: 267–8; al-Ṭabarī 1928: 381, 401; Maimonides [M. Meyerhof 1940]: No. 297.

286. The author uses the Persian word *ardij*. The type of juniper meant here is probably *Juniperus communis*, *'ar'ar* in Arabic, while *abhal* (*abhul*) denoted the poisonous *Juniperus savina* (savin). The juniper was known to have a number of medicinal purposes and often occurs in Arab pharmacology, for instance, as a purgative, diuretic, carminative, anthelmintic, emmenagogue and abortifacient. Ibn Janāḥ 2020: No. 27; A. Dietrich 1988: II, 125–6; Ibn al-Bayṭār 1874: III, 120–1; Ibn al-Jazzār 2004:

126–7; D. al-Anṭākī 1952: I, 236; al-Rāzī 1955–69: XXI, 179; Maimonides [M. Meyerhof 1940]: No. 22.

287. *sukkar al-qand*; the latter word denotes crystallized cane sugar. Sugar was used to remedy catarrh, cough and fever, while it invigorates coitus (when taken with milk). Ibn al-Bayṭār 1992: IV, 291; M. Ouerfelli 2008: 77 *et passim*; A. Dietrich 1988: II, 238.

288. The preceding section in [D] runs as follows: 'These pains affect a person who engages in intercourse while standing, depending on how frequently he does so. If it happens rarely, there is no harm. However, intercourse while lying on one's side is extremely harmful; it can cause liver pain, heartache, paralysis, and urinary incontinence, especially if done on the right side, as it is more harmful than the left side. As for intercourse with a man's wife while he is lying down and she is on top of him, it can result in bladder pain, urine retention, dribbling, burning urine, and the disease of coldness, which is the flow of blood and pus with or without urine. God protect us from this. Therefore, a wise person should avoid these practices, as they can be causes of such diseases.'

289. cf. al-Kātib 1977: 305.

290. This paragraph is as follows in [D]: 'Know that the best position and the first one to consider is for the man to approach his wife while she is lying flat on her back. She should place a thin pillow under her lower back and lift her thighs by herself. When the man ejaculates, he should place his knees on the ground and lie on the woman, while she embraces him with her hands and legs, pressing him against her chest until the ejaculation completes inside the womb. He should not move away from her chest during ejaculation. If the semen does not enter the womb as intended, the woman will not conceive, and reproduction will cease. When intercourse is done according to these conditions, it will be beneficial and prevent the ailments we have described.'

291. [D] has 'to thicken and harden its limpness until it becomes very firm'.

292. *baṣal al-narjis* (< Gr. νάρκισσος) – hot and cold (in the second degree), it was said that the mere fragrance of the narcissus could relieve obstructions in the brain. It was also used to cleanse wounds and cure chronic joint aches. The oil was thought to be good for the nerves. Ibn al-Bayṭār 1992: IV, 476–77; Ibn al-Jazzār 2004: 80–1; Ibn Sīnā 1999: I, 575; D. al-Anṭākī 1952: I, 330; Ibn Wāfid 2000: 158; al-Rāzī 1955–69: XXI, 590–2; al-Bīrūnī 1973: 362; al-Dhahabī 1987: 267; Maimonides [M. Meyerhof 1940]: No 254; al-Ṭabarī 1928: 396.

293. This adjective refers to anything white, such as the white lily, cotton, linen, or white flaxen clothes, as well as being the name of a species of grape from al-Ṭā'if with white and long fruit. The word also denoted wine made from these grapes. Ibn Janāḥ 2020: No. 917; E. Lane 1863–74: III 1077.

294. This recipe is missing from [E].

295. The passage 'pulverize them ... This is treated by', is as follows in [C]: 'Pulverize, throw into grape water and oil, then boil over a fire, remove and rub onto the penis.'

296. The part of the sentence from 'whereas' is omitted from [E].

297. Interestingly enough, the Arabic seems to indicate that galingale (*su'd*) and

sweet basil (*rayḥān*) are one and the same thing. This section is missing from [D] here but is included instead in Chapter 10. [E] omits both this section and Chapter 12.

298. *jullanār* (< Persian *gul-i anār*, 'granate rose/blossom'), which is also sometimes referred to as 'a small seedless pomegranate', was thought to be useful against ulcers and bleeding, as well as being an aphrodisiac. It came in wild and cultivated varieties. Ibn Wāfid 2000: 184–5; Ibn al-Jazzār 2004: 117–8; A. Dietrich 1988: II, 150, 171–2; al-Tīfāshī 1892: 14; Ibn al-Bayṭār 1874: I, 164; Ibn al-Jazzār 2004: 117–8; D. al-Anṭākī 1952: I, 106; Ibn al-Quff [H. Kircher 1967]: 133. Also see note on *rummān*, above.

299. 'Take a white copper plate and place it on hot ashes'; [C]: 'Take hot ashes'.

300. 'and beat the grounds on the plate. Turn over and roll until all the oil has been extracted. Proceed in this fashion for all kernels; [C]: 'Knead the aforementioned kernels until the oil is released. Continue in the same manner with all kernels.'

301. [D] omits 'based on their knowledge and experiments'.

302. It has not been possible to ascertain who is referred to here. The name 'al-Dāmghānī' goes back to the city of Damghan, in northern Iran.

303. This is a reference to the famous physician; see Introduction.

304. The passage starting from the second sentence until this point is missing from [C].

305. [E] prescribes four *dirhams*.

306. *afrībūn*, which is a rare variant of the more common *ū/afarbiyūn* (< Gr. εὐφόρβιον), *Euphorbia resinifera* – a resin from a tree mainly found in the Atlas mountains. It was used for those with cold temperaments and in the treatment of rabies, sciatica and colic. D. al-Anṭākī 1952: I, 53; al-Tīfāshī 1892: 14, 18; Ibn al-Quff [H. Kircher 1967]: 290–2; Ibn al-Bayṭār 1874: III, 158–9; Ibn al-Jazzār 2004: 192; Ibn Sīnā 1999: I, 268–9; al-Rāzī 1955–69: XXI, 229–31; Maimonides [M. Meyerhof 1940]: No. 25; A. Dietrich 1988: II, 433–4.

307. The information in this and the next chapter may be compared with the information provided in al-Kātib 1977: 284–5; Ibn Sīnā 1999, II: 747.

308. *marsīn* (< Gr. Μυρσίνη), which is the word commonly used in Egyptian Arabic, as well as being the term in Ottoman Turkish (J. Redhouse 1880: 802). In Arabic botany, it is usually referred to as *ās* (also *marsīm*). Both the leaves and (black) berries of this evergreen shrub, which came in wild and cultivated varieties, were used for medicinal purposes (often boiled down to a syrup or in a poultice): as a diuretic, against ulcers, bleeding haemorrhoids (especially the leaves), headaches, spider bites, diarrhoea, tumours (especially hot ones, like in the testicles), hair loss and dandruff. The fruits were used to clean the teeth. According to Maimonides, myrtle oil constricted the glans of the penis, whereas al-Tīfāshī (1970: 28) recommended green myrtle leaves mixed with rosewater to make the vagina narrower and sweet smelling. Ibn Wāfid 2000: 98–9; D. al-Anṭākī 1952: I, 43–4; Ibn al-Bayṭār 1874: I, 27–30; al-Rāzī 1955–69: XX, 14–9; al-Qazwīnī 1849: 216; Maimonides [M. Meyerhof 1940]: No. 10; Ibn al-Quff [H. Kircher 1967]: 74–6; E. Lev & Z. Amar 2008: 223–5; A. Dietrich 1988: II, 172–3.

309. [E] has that the vagina will be narrower than a virgin's.

310. [D] adds 'and cloves'.

311. According to al-Rāzī (1881: 17), undiluted wine (*sharāb ṣirf*) is very good for the stomach and aids digestion. However, it is very harmful to the head because of the rising vapours of the wine and its (intoxicating) effect. He added that aged (*'atīq*) wine dries out the body but produces fewer vapours.

312. [E] adds 'and sweet'.

313. The last two sentences are missing from [C].

314. *ballūṭ* refers to both the tree and the fruit – cold and dry, it was recommended (often cooked) against diarrhoea, stomach ulcers and was thought to counter bedwetting. The term *shāhballūṭ* denoted the chestnut, which was also known as *k/qastāna* (< Gr. καστανία) or *qas/ṣṭal*. Ibn Wāfid 2000: 102–3; Ibn al-Bayṭār 1992: I, 151–52; Ibn al-Jazzār 2004: 101; Ibn Sīnā 1999: I, 408–9; D. al-Anṭākī 1952: I, 83; al-Dhahabī 1987: 133; al-Ṭabarī 1928: 383; A. Dietrich 1988: II, 166–7.

315. *kalīl*, which is a corruption of *iklīl*, as it appears in [C], and can refer to either *iklīl al-jabal* (also known as *ḥass lubān*), 'rosemary' (*Rosmarinus officinalis*), or *iklīl al-malik*, 'sweet clover' (white melilot, *Melilotus albus*). One may speculate it is the former, which was used as a diuretic, emmenagogue, to relieve obstructions and to cure cough. Ibn al-Quff recommended it against joint aches and to purify the body. Al-Kātib (1977: 272) recommends it to strengthen erection. E. Lev & Z. Amar 2008: 266–8 (*iklīl al-jabal*), 492–4 (*iklīl al-malik*); Ibn al-Bayṭār 1874: I, 50–1 (*iklīl al-malik*); Ibn al-Quff [H. Kircher 1967]: 57–8 (*iklīl al-malik*); Maimonides [M. Meyerhof 1940]: No. 7.

316. *ḥayy 'ālam* (for *ḥayy al-'ālam*) – cold in the third degree and dry in the first, was used mainly against headaches. Ibn Janāḥ 2020: Nos. 36, 350; Ibn al-Quff [H. Kircher 1967]: 144–5; Ibn al-Bayṭār 1874: II, 43; D. al-Anṭākī 1952: I, 134–5; Maimonides [M. Meyerhof 1940]: No. 162; A. Dietrich 1988: II, 595–6.

317. [E] specifies that it should be half a *dirham*. In Arabic pharmacological and botanical literature, *qa/iṭrān* refers to the substance extracted from certain conifers. Its medicinal use goes back to Antiquity when its beneficial properties were first reported, and to this day it is used to treat dermatological conditions (especially psoriasis). It was considered extremely hot and dry, beneficial for killing lice, scabies, while also sharpening eyesight. If it is applied to the penis before intercourse, it prevents pregnancy. See A. Dietrich 1988: II, 118–9; *EI*[2], s.v. 'ḳaṭrān' (A. Dietrich); M. Ullman 1970: 217; Ibn al-Bayṭār 1992: III, 80–2; Ibn Sīnā 1999: I, 647; D. al-Anṭākī 1952: I, 261; al-Bīrūnī 1973: 310–2; Ibn al-Quff [H. Kircher 1967]: 306–8; Ibn Jazla, fols. 177v–178r.; 1010 Ibn Janāḥ 2020: No. 1010.

318. 'will experience ...'; [C]: 'will prevent conception and provide pleasure to the man. Another recipe: [take] acacia and acorn, ten *dirhams* of each; oak apples and dried aubergine, fifteen *dirhams* of each. Pulverize and strain. Then, vigorously pound in a pestle. The woman inserts a piece [of cloth] soaked in it [into her vagina] for three days. You will see the wondrous result in terms of her tightness and hotness.' See also al-Kātib 1977: 311–2.

319. [E] adds 'fresh dates' as well.

320. *'afṣ*, also known as 'oak apples' – they were recommended as a 'tightening' tonic and a remedy against ulcers and festering wounds. It has also been used as a black hair-dye and to make ink. Ibn al-Quff [H. Kircher 1967]: 269–70; al-Tīfāshī 1970: 27, 28, 29, 30 (various electuaries used to improve the vagina); Ibn al-Bayṭār 1874: III, 127–8; Ibn al-Jazzār 2004: 67–9; Ibn Wāfid 2000: 187–8; D. al-Anṭākī 1952: I, 238; al-Bīrūnī 1973: 270; al-Ṭabarī 1928: 404 A. Dietrich 1988: II, 167–8; M. Hinds *&* E. Badawi 1986: 586.

321. *Idkhir* – this herb was recommended as a diuretic, emmenagogue and to treat swellings, kidney and gall stones, as well as toothache. A. Dietrich 1988: II, 100–101; al-Dhahabi 1987: 118; Ibn al-Quff [H. Kircher 1967]: 70–1; D. al-Anṭākī 1952: I, 39; Ibn al-Jazzār 2004: 148; Ibn Wāfid 2000: 47–8; al-Shayzarī, al-Īḍāḥ, fol. 2v.; Ibn al-Bayṭār 1874: I, 15–6; al-Ṭabarī 1928: 400; al-Rāzī 1955-69: XX, 6–9; al-Bīrūnī 1973: 27.

322. *balaḥ*, date 'while continuing green and small'; within the growth cycle of the fruit, it comes after the *ṭala'*, *khilāl* and before *busr*, *ruṭab* and *tamr*; E. Lane 1863–74: I, 246; Ibn Sīnā 1999: I, 393–4. See the note on *tamr*, above. for medical applications.

323. The translation follows [D].

324. The translation follows [B], [D] and [E], rather than [A], which has 'raw'.

325. *kāfūr* (< Middle Persian *kāpūr*) – cold and dry in the third degree, it is the crystalline resin of the camphor tree (*Cinnamomum camphora*). Its use has not been attested in Greek Antiquity but it was highly prized as an aromatic in pre-Islamic Persia, when it was also employed as an embalming agent. According to the Qur'ān (76:5), 'the Righteous will drink of a cup of wine mixed with camphor'. Al-Mas'ūdī traced its origin to India, while Marco Polo found that the best camphor (from Fansur) sold for its weight in gold. In cooking, it was used in a number of savouries as well as sweets, and often in conjunction with musk. It was – and still is – used extensively in perfumes, though Ibn Sīnā warned that regular use makes the hair grey. Medicinally, it was used for a wide range of applications, with al-Kindī, for instance, using it for swollen liver, complaints of the larynx, and inflammations of the mucous membrane of the mouth. Ibn Munqidh reports how Ibn Buṭlān once cleared a woman's catarrh by stuffing her hair with camphor. However, it causes insomnia, generates kidney and bladder stones, and is an anaphrodisiac, while excessive use of camphor causes kidney and bladder stones. When taken with sour apple juice, it neutralizes the effects of a scorpion stings. Ibn Sīnā 1999: I, 514–5; Ibn al-Bayṭār 1992: IV, 296–7; Ibn Buṭlān 1990: 108–9 (trans., 218–9); Levey 1966: Nos. 11, 24, 61, 77, 89, 91, 104, 152; Ibn al-Quff [H. Kircher 1967]: No. 214; Yāqūt 1866–73: III, 456; Ibn Munqidh 2003: 288 (trans. 216–7); *EI*[2], s.v. 'kāfūr' (A. Dietrich); *Encyclopaedia Iranica*, s.v. 'camphor' (Hūšang A'lam); Ibn Jazla, fol. 182r.–v.; Ibn Janāḥ 2020: Nos. 575, 850; R. Donkin 1999.

326. *shabb* (also *shabba*), potassium (potash) alum. In Islamic medicine, the mineral was used in the treatment of leprosy and ulcers, or as an astringent and coagulant. It has also been used as a dye and in cosmetics (for instance, mixed with henna, as an axillary deodorant, or depilator). Contrary to European usage, alum did not have any culinary applications in the Middle East. In erotological literature, it is an ingredient in recipes to

invigorate the vagina. Ibn al-Jazzār 2004: 217–8; Ibn Sahl [O. Kahl 2003]: Nos. 209, 389, 391; al-Tīfāshī 1970: 27, 30; Philippe Borgard et al., *L'alun de Méditerranée*, Paris: Centre Jean Bérard, 2005; Charles J. Singer, *The earliest chemical industry. An essay in the historical relations of economics and technology illustrated from the alum trade*, London: The Folio Society, 1948.

327. *ṣamgh ʿarabī* – a resin harvested from the acacia tree (*qaraẓ* or, in Morocco, *ṭalḥ*), varieties of which are found in (sub-Saharan) Africa (*Acacia Senegal, Acacia seyal*) and the Near East. The Egyptian gum was particularly prized. In cooking, it was used ground as a thickener, but was also dissolved in water and used in dishes (especially batters). Powdered gum Arabic was used in tooth-pastes. Therapeutically, it was considered cold (or warm) and dry in the second degree, and was used in remedies for cough, lung ulcers, pharyngitis and eye inflammation. It was also a basic ingredient (together with gum tragacanth, *kathīrā'*), in lochs (*laʿūq*), that is to say, electuaries meant to be licked, to which aromatics and sweeteners (sugar, molasses) were added, particularly in the treatment of ailments affecting the throat and lungs. Ibn Sīnā referred to the gum being boiled in an earthenware pot, or roasted on live coal. Ibn Wāfid 2000: 190; Ibn al-Jazzār 2004: 93; Ibn Sīnā 1999: I, 639–640, II, 734; Ibn al-Bayṭār 1992: III, 114–15; Ibn al-Quff [H. Kircher 1967]: 256–7; al-Kātib 1977: 282; Colin & Renaud 1934: 132 (No. 296); Ibn Khalṣūn 1996: 49; al-Ishbīlī 2003: 131.

328. [B] and [D] have one *dirham* of sour orange peel, and [E], half a *dirham* of sour orange peel. In [C] the passage is as follows: 'bitter orange peel, one *dirham*. Pound and boil in fine old wine. The woman puts some of it on a woollen cloth before coitus and she will become like a virgin and become pregnant with the help of Allah. This ends the Book, with the assistance of the beneficent King, on the 18th day of Rabīʿ I of the year 1334 [= 24 January 1916].

329. 'and grant them salvation until the Day of Judgement, He is the Lord of the Worlds. In the Name of Allah, the merciful the compassionate'; [B]: 'There is no strength or power save in Allah, the Supreme. [The book] has been completed with the grace and help of Allah.'

330. 03.08.1793–27.07.1794 CE. The ending in [D] is as follows: 'The book was completed with the assistance of the King, the Giver. This brief work pertains to the wondrous and beneficial compounds that are among the secrets of physicians and their useful abridgements, as they were made for the treasury of a Muslim sultan, so that it may be beneficial. It was finished by the hand of its scribe, the poor servant hoping for his Lord's mercy, the sinner drowning in his sins, Muḥammad 'Alī Ibn Ḥusayn Ibn Ḥasan al-Jazā'irī. May Allah forgive him and all the Muslim men and women, both living and dead.'

APPENDIX

List of Erotological Works

AUTHOR (C = Christian; J = Jewish)	**WORKS** ([*] = lost; [**M**] = mss only)
[ANON]	[*Untitled*] (On aphrodisiacal electuaries and pills)[1] [**M**]
[ANON]	[*Untitled*] (On aphrodisiac electuaries and talismans)[2] [**M**]
[ANON]	[*Untitled*] (Recipes for cosmetics, charms, aphrodisiacs)[3] [**M**]
[ANON]	[*Untitled*] (recipes for aphrodisiacs)[4] [**M**]
[ANON]	[*Untitled*] (on coitus)[5] [**M**]
[ANON]	[*Untitled*] (on coitus, prostitution, lesbianism)[6] [**M**]
[ANON]	[*Untitled*] (on coitus)[7] [**M**]
[ANON]	[*Untitled*] (positions for coitus)[8] [**M**]
[ANON]	*al-Īḍāḥiyya fi 'l-umūr al-nikāḥiyya* ('The Explanatory Treatise on Matrimonial matters')[9] [**M**]
[ANON]	*Bāb maʿrifat aḥwāl fi 'l-nikāḥ wa ghayrihi* ('Chapter on the Knowledge of the Concerns of Women Regarding Lawful Intercourse and Other Matters')[10] [**M**]
[ANON]	*Quṭb al-afrāḥ fi 'l-quwwa ʿalā 'l-bāh* ('The Pivot of Delights in Sexual Potency')[11] [**M**]
[ANON]	*Madhhab al-muḥibbīn wa iʿtiqād al-ʿāshiqīn* ('School of the Beloved and Doctrine of the Lovers')[12] [**M**]
[ANON]	*Mu'akkid al-maḥabba bayna 'l-muḥibb wa man uḥibbuhu* ('The Certainty of Love Between the Beloved and He Who Loves Him')[13] [**M**]
[ANON]	*Jāmiʿ al-masarrāt fī-mā li 'l-nafs min al-mufriḥāt* ('Compendium of Pleasures as Regards Things that Gladden the Soul')[14] [**M**]

AUTHOR (C = Christian; J = Jewish)	**WORKS** ([*] = lost; [M] = mss only)
[ANON]	*Kitāb al-Anyāk* ('The Book of Fuckings')[15] [*]
[ANON]	*Nubdha min kitāb fī 'l-bāh* ('Excerpt from The Book on Coitus')[16] **[M]**
[ANON]	*Irtiyāḥ al-arwāḥ fī 'ādāt al-nikāh* ('The Delight of the Souls Regarding the Customs of Lawful Intercourse')[17] **[M]**
[ANON]	*Miṣbāḥ fī asrār al-nikāḥ* ('Light on The Secrets of Lawful Intercourse')[18] **[M]**
[ANON]	*Risāla fī 'l-jimā'* ('Treatise on Lawful Intercourse')[19] **[M]**
[ANON]	*Ḍu'f al-intishār* ('On Impotence')[20] **[M]**
[ANON]	*Risāla fī 'l-jimā'* ('Treatise on Lawful Intercourse')[21] **[M]**
[ANON]	*Tuḥfat al-aṣḥāb fī mu'āsharat al-aḥbāb* ('Gift of the Friends in Relations with Lovers')[22] **[M]**
[ANON]	*Qiṣṣat Lūṭ* ('The Story of Lot')[23] **[M]**
[ANON]	*Risāla fī dhikr adwiyat al-bāh* ('Treatise on Aphrodisiacs'[24] **[M]**
[ANON]	*Kitāb al-ḥayk fī 'ilm al-nayk* ('The Book of Weaving in The Science of Fucking')[25] **[M]**
[ANON]	*Kitāb fī 'ilm al-bāh* ('Book on The Science of Coitus')[26] **[M]**
[ANON]	*al-Rawḍa al-bahiyya fī 'l-ladhdha al-bāhiyya* ('The Brilliant Garden of Coital Pleasure')[27]
[ANON]	*Risāla fī a'ḍā' al-tanāsul* ('Treatise on The Sexual Organs')[28] **[M]**
[ANON]	*Kitāb fī 'ilm al-bāh wa adwiyatihi* ('Book on The Science of Coitus and Its Medicines')[29] **[M]**

AUTHOR (C = Christian; J = Jewish)	**WORKS** ([*] = lost; [M] = mss only)
[ANON]	*al-Risāla fī 'l-jimā'* ('Treatise on Intercourse')[30] **[M]**
[ANON]	*Risāla fī waṣf al-nisā' wa ādāb al-jimā'* ('Treatise on the Description of Women and The Rules of Conduct for Coitus')[31] **[M]**
[ANON]	*Kitāb al-īḍāḥ fī 'ilm al-nikāḥ* ('Book of Elucidation on the Science of Lawful Intercourse')[32]
al-Aqfahsī, Shihāb al-Dīn [d. 1406 – Egypt]	*Raf' al-janāḥ 'ammā huwa min al-mar'a al-mubāḥ* ('The Raising of the Wings as Regards the Lawful Woman')[33]
Badr al-Dīn, Ibn Sālim Ibn Muḥammad Ibn Ṭābi' al-Ṣiddīq	*Nuzhat al-abṣār wa 'l-asmā' fī akhbār dhawāt al-qinā'* ('The Delight of the Eyes and Ears in the Stories of Veiled Women')[34] **[M]**
al-Baghdādī, Abū 'Abd al-Raḥmān [14th c. – Egypt]	*Kitāb al-zahr al-anīq fī 'l-baws wa 'l-ta'nīq wa 'l-hayj wa 'l-shahīq wa mukhālafat al-zawj wa mutā'at al-'ashīq* ('The Elegant Blossom on Kissing and Embracing, Arousal and Sighing, Defying the Husband and Obeying the Lover')
al-Fallātī, Muḥammad Ibn Muḥammad Tuqur [d. 1741 – Sudan]	*Mu'āwanat al-ikhwān fī mu'āsharat al-niswān* ('Assistance of the Brothers in the Association with Women')[36] **[M]**
al-Ghazlāwī, Muḥammad Ibn 'Umar [17th c.]	*Yāsamīn al-rawḍ al-'āṭir fī nuzhat al-khāṭir* ('Jasmine of The Scented Garden in The Excursion of Desire')[37] **[M]**
al-Ḥawrānī, 'Abd al-Raḥīm [14th c. – Bilād al-Shām]	*Kashf asrār al-muḥtalīn wa nawāmīs al-ḥayyālīn* ('Uncovering the Secrets of Swindlers and the Laws of Tricksters')[38] **[M]**
al-Ḥimṣī, al-Muẓaffar Bin Nāṣir Bin 'Alī al-Qurayshī [d. 1215 – Bilād al-Shām]	*Maqāla fī 'l-bāh* ('Treatise on Coitus')[39] **[M]**

AUTHOR (C = Christian; J = Jewish)	**WORKS** ([*] = lost; [M] = mss only)
Ḥunayn Ibn Isḥāq (C) [809–873 – Iraq]	*Kitāb asrār al-falāsifa fi 'l-bāh* ('Book on the Secrets of the Philosophy of Coitus') **[M]**[40]
Ibn 'Ādī, Yaḥyā [893–974]	*Kitāb fi manāfi' al-bāh wa maḍārrihi wa jihāt isti'mālihi* ('Book on The Benefits and Disadvantages of Coitus and The Ways of Practising it')[41] **[M]**
Ibn Bukhtīshū', Jibrā'īl Ibn Jūrjiūs (C) [d. 827 – Persia]	*Kitāb fi 'l-bāh* ('The Book on Coitus')[42] [*]
Ibn Falīta al-Yamanī, Aḥmad Ibn Muḥammad Ibn 'Alī Abū al-'Abbās [d. 1331 – Yemen]	*Rushd al-labīb ilā mu'āsharat al-ḥabīb* ('An Intelligent Man's Guide to Intercourse with A Loved One')[43]
Ibn Ḥājib al-Nu'mān, Muḥammad Ibn 'Abd al-Azīz [d. 1031]	*Kitāb al-qiyān* ('The Book of Dancing Girls')[44] **[M]**
Ibn Hishām, Abū Ahmad [13th century]	*Maḥāsin al-nisā'* ('The Beauties of Women')[45]
Ibn Ishāq, 'Alī [mid-14th c.]	*Kitāb fi 'ilm al-bāh* ('Book on The Science of Coitus')[46]
Ibn Kannān, Muḥammad Ibn 'Īsā al-Khalūtī [1663–1740 – Bilād al-Shām]	*Nuzhat al-nufūs wa daftar al-'ilm wa rawḍat al-'arūs fi 'umūr al-nikāḥ wa ghayrihi* ('The Excursion of Souls, the Register of Knowledge, and the Bride's Garden on the Matters of Marriage')[47] **[M]**
Qusṭā Ibn Lūqā [C] [820–912 – Bilād al-Shām]	*Kitāb fi 'l-bāh wa mā yuḥtāju ilayhi min tadbīr al-badan fī isti'mālihi* ('The Book on Coitus and which Regimen is Required to Practise It')[48]

AUTHOR (C = Christian; J = Jewish)	**WORKS** ([*] = lost; **[M]** = mss only)
	Kitāb fi 'l-bāh ('The Book on Coitus')[49]
Ibn Mandawayh, Abū 'Alī [d. 1019 – Persia]	*Risāla fī asbāb al-bāh* ('Treatise on The Reasons for Coitus')[50] **[M]**
Ibn Marzūq, Shams al-Dīn Abu 'Abd Allāh [d. 472/1080 – Tunis]	*al-Intibāh li-mu'ālajat al-bāh* ('Vigilance Regarding the Treatment of Coitus')[51] **[M]**
Ibn Māssa, 'Īsā (C) [9th c. – Persia]	*Masā'il fi 'l-nasl wa 'l-dhurriyya wa 'l-jimā'* ('Questions about Progeny, Offspring and Coitus')[52]
Ibn Maymūn (Maimonides) [J] [1135–1204 – al-Andalus]	*Fi 'l-jimā'* ('On Coitus')[53]
Ibn al-Qaṭṭā' [1041–1121 – Sicily]	*Kitāb al-nikāḥ fi 'l-lugha* ('The Book on The Language of Lawful Intercourse')[54]
Ibn Raḥmūn, Sallāma [J] [d. 1136 – Egypt] doctor|	*Maqāla fī khiṣb abdān al-nisā' bi-Miṣr 'inda tanāhī al-shabāb* ('Treatise on The Fertility of Egyptian Women's Bodies upon The Expiration of Youth')[55] [*]
Ibn Raqīqa, Maḥmūd Ibn 'Umar al-Shaybānī, Sadīd al-Dīn [1169–1238 – Bilād al-Shām]	*Kitāb mūḍiḥat al-ishtibāh fī adwiyat al-bāh* ('The Clarification of Doubts about Aphrodisiacs')[56] **[M]** *Kitāb al-farīda al-shāhiyya wa 'l-qaṣīdah al-bāhiyya* ('Book of the Rare Pearl and the Ode on Coitus')[57] [*]
Ibn Riḍwān [ca 998– ca 1061 – Egypt]	*Maqāla fi 'l-bāh* ('Treatise on Coitus')[58] [*]
Ibn Sīnā [d. 1037 – Persia]	*Urjūza fi 'l-bāh* (Poem on Coitus)[59] **[M]** *Asrār al-jimā'* ('The Secrets of Intercourse')[60] **[M]**

AUTHOR (C = Christian; J = Jewish)	**WORKS** ([*] = lost; [M] = mss only)
Ibn Sulaymān, Aḥmad	*Zahr al-bustān fī maʿrifat aḥwāl al-bāh fī 'l-insān* ('Garden Flowers in the Knowledge of the Situations in which People Engage in Coitus')[61] **[M]**
Ibn al-Takrītī, Yaḥyā Ibn Jarīr [second half 11th c. – Iraq]	*Kitāb fī 'l-bāh wa manāfi al-jimāʿ wa maḍarrihi* ('The Book on Coitus, the Benefits of Intercourse and Its Harmful Effects')[62] **[M]**
al-Isrā'ilī, Samaw'āl Ibn Yaḥyā Ibn ʿAbbās al-Maghribī (J) [d. 1180 - Iraq]	*Nuzhat al-aṣḥāb fī muʿāshirat al-aḥbāb* ('The Friends' Jaunt in Coitus Between Lovers')[63] *Kitāb fī 'l-Bāh* ('The Book on Coitus')[64] [*]
al-Jāḥiẓ, Abū ʿUthmān [781–868 – Iraq]	*Mufākharāt al-jawārī wa 'l-ghulmān* ('Boasts of Girl and Boy Slaves')[65] *Kitāb al-ʿurs wa 'l-ʿarā'is* ('The Book of Marriage and Brides')[66] **[M]**
al-Jildakī, Īdmar Ibn ʿAlī ʿIzz al-Dīn [d. 1342 – Egypt]	*Kitāb durrat al-ghawāṣṣ wa kanz al-ikhtiṣāṣ fī ʿilm al-khawāṣṣ* ('The Diver's Pearls and The Specialist Treasure regarding The Science of Properties')[67] **[M]**
al-Kātib, Abū 'l-Hasan ʿAlī Ibn Naṣr al-Samnānī (floruit 10th c., Bagdad)	*Jawamiʿ al-ladhdha* ('The Encyclopedia of Pleasure')[68] *Kitāb kīmiyā' al-bāh* ('Book on the Chemistry of Coitus')[69] * *Al-Nafā'is fī ʿilm al-nikāḥ wa 'l-ʿarā'is* ('Precious Accounts of the Science of Lawful Intercourse')[70] [*] *Al-Munākaḥa wa 'l-ashyā' allatī tuqawwī al-bāh wa tuḍʿif* ('Lawful Intercourse and Things That Strengthen and Weaken Sexual Potency')[71] **[M]**

AUTHOR (C = Christian; J = Jewish)	**WORKS** ([*] = lost; [**M**] = mss only)
Khān, Muḥammad al-Ṣādiq Ḥasan [d. 1878]	*Nashwat al-sakrān min ṣahbā' tidhkār al-ghizlān* ('The Intoxication of the Drunkard on the Wine of the Commemoration of Youths')[72]
Khān, Fatḥ 'Alī Ibn Ḥakīm, Ḥikmat Allāh Khān (12th c., India)	*Risāla fi 'l-bāh* ('Treatise on Coitus')[73] [**M**]
al-Khaṭīb, Abū Naṣr	*Kitāb akhbār al-nisā'* ('Book on The Stories about Women')[74] [**M**]
al-Khuwārizmī, Abū Bakr [d. 993, Persia]	*Kitāb fi 'l-bāh* ('The Book on Coitus')[75] [**M**]
al-Kindī [d. 873 – Iraq]	*Kitāb al-bāh* ('The Book on Coitus')[76]
al-Maghribī, Ibrāhīm [first half 17th c. – Morocco]	*Ṣanf fi 'l-bāh* ('Categories of Coitus')[77] [**M**]
al-Masīḥī, 'Izz al-Dīn (C)	*al-Munākaḥa wa 'l-mufātaḥa (fī aṣnāf al-jimā' wa ālātihi)* ('Coitus and Preamble to The Categories of Coitus and Its Tools')[78] [*]
al-Mufaḍḍal, Ibn 'Umar	*Kitāb al-haft wa 'l-azilla* ('The Book of Nonsense and Slips of The Tongue')[79]
al-Mughalṭāy, al-Ḥāfiẓ [13th c.]	*al-Wāḍiḥ al-mubīn fī dhikr man ustushhida min al-muḥibbīn* ('Clarity regarding The Memory of Those Who Were Martyred because of The Loved Ones')[80]
al-Nafzāwī, Muḥammad Ibn Muḥammad [16th c. – Tunis]	*al-Rawḍ al-'āṭir fī nuzhat al-khāṭir* ('The Scented Garden in the Excursion of Desire')[81] *Tanwīr al-wiqā' fī asrār al-jimā'* ('Illumination of Coition in The Secrets of Intercourse')[82] [*]

AUTHOR (C = Christian; J = Jewish)	**WORKS** ([*] = lost; [M] = mss only)
al-Nam(a)lī, Hassān Ibn Muḥammad [9th c. – Iraq]	*Kitāb Burjān wa Ḥubāḥib* ('The Book of Burjan and Hubahib')[83] [*] *Kitāb khiṭāb al-makārī li-jāriyat al-Baqqāl* ('Address of The Muleteer to The Greengrocer's Slave Girl')[84] [*] *Kitāb bighā'* ('The Book of Prostitution')[85] [*] *Kitāb al-saḥq* ('The Book of Lesbianism')[86] [*]
al-Nawājī, Shams al-Dīn Muḥammad Ibn Ḥasan [1386–1455 – Egypt]	*Marāti' al-ghizlān fī waṣf al-ḥisān min al-ghilmān* ('The Gazelles' Pasture regarding The Description of Beautiful Boys')[87] [M]
al-Niḥillī	*Kitāb al-bāh* ('The Book on Coitus')[88] [*]
al-Qusṭanṭīnī, Maḥmūd Ibn Muḥammad [d. 1568 – Tunis]	*Kitāb adwiyat al-Bāh* ('The Book of Medicines for Coitus')[89] [M]
al-Rāzī, Muḥammad Ibn Zakariyyā' [865–925 – Persia]	*Kitāb al-bāh wa manāfi'uhu wa maḍārruhu wa mudawātuhu* ('The Book on Coitus, its Benefits, Harmful Effects and Treatments')[90] *Maqāla fīmā su'ila 'anhu fī annahu bimā ṣāra man qalla jimā'uhu min al-insān ṭāla 'umruhu* ('Treatise on Whether Engaging into Coitus with Low Frequency Increases Lifespan')[91] [M] *Risāla fī 'l-ubna* ('Treatise on Passive Sodomy')[92] [M]
al-Sā'ātī, Muḥammad Rājī al-Ḥalabī	*Rashf al-ruḍāb wa fākihat al-aḥbāb* ('The Sipping of Saliva and the Fruit of Lovers')[93]

AUTHOR (C = Christian; J = Jewish)	**WORKS** ([*] = lost; [M] = mss only)
al-Ṣafadī, Ṣalāh al-Dīn	*Law'at al-shākī wa dam'at al-bākī* ('The Complainant's Ardour of Love and the Weeper's Tear')[94]
al-Ṣaymarī, Muḥammad Ibn Isḥāq Abū al-'Anbas [827–888 – Iraq]	*Kitāb al-saḥḥāqāt wa 'l-baghghā'īn* ('The Book of Lesbians and Homosexual Prostitutes')[95] [*]
	Kitāb al-khaḍkhaḍa fī jald 'Umayra ('The Book of Masturbation')[96] [*]
	al-'Āshiq wa 'l-ma'shūq ('The Lover and the Loved One')[97] [*]
	Kitāb nawādir al-khaṣī ('The Book of Rare Anecdotes on Eunuchs')[98] [*]
	Kitāb nawādir al-quwwād ('The Book of Rare Anecdotes on Pimps')[99] [*]
	Kitāb faḍl al-surm 'alā 'l-fam ('The Book on The Superiority of The Rectum over The Mouth')[100] [*]
al-Shādhilī, 'Abd al-Qādir Ibn Aḥmad Ibn Muḥammad al-Māliki [d. 1529 – Tunis]	*Tashnīf al-asmā' bi-fawā'id al-tasmiya 'inda 'l-jimā'* ('Delighting the Ears by the Benefits of Hearing the Formula 'In the Name of Allah' during Coitus')[101] [M]
al-Shāfi'ī, 'Alā 'l-Dīn	*al-Nikāḥ* ('On Lawful Intercourse') [102] [M]
al-Shayzarī al-Ṭabarī, 'Abd al-Raḥmān Ibn Naṣr [d. 1193 – Egypt]	*al-Īḍāḥ fī asrār al-nikāḥ* ('Elucidation of The Secrets of Lawful Intercourse')[103]
al-Suyūṭī, Jalāl al-Dīn [1445–1505 – Egypt]	*al-Wishāḥ fī fawā'id al-nikāḥ* ('The Sash in the Benefits of Lawful Intercourse')[104]
	Rashf al-zulāl min al-siḥr al-ḥalāl ('The Sipping of The Pure Water of Lawful Charm')[105]

AUTHOR (C = Christian; J = Jewish)	**WORKS** ([*] = lost; [M] = mss only)
	Nawāḍir al-ayk fī nawādir al-nayk ('The Blooming of The Jungle in the Rareties of Fucking')[106]
	al-ayk fī ma'rifat al-nayk ('Jungle in The Knowledge of Fucking')[107]
	Fi 'l-jimā' wa ālātuhu ('On Coitus and Its Tools')[108]
	Shaqā'iq al-utrunj fī daqā'iq al-ghunj ('Halves of the Citron Regarding the Intricacies of Coquetry')[109]
	Nuzhat al-'umr fī 'l-tafḍīl bayn al-bīḍ wa 'l-sūd wa 'l-sumr ('The Lifelong Excursion on the Preference Between White, Black and Brown Women')[110]
	Ghāyat al-iḥsān fī khalq al-insān ('The Height of Charity in The Creation of Human Beings')[111] **[M]**
	Ādāb al-nikāḥ wa kasr al-shahwatayni ('The Rules of Conduct for Lawful Intercourse and The Breaking of the Two Passions')[112]
	Nuzhat al-julasā' fī ish'ār al-nisā' ('Jaunt of The Table Companions in The Notification of Women')[113]
	Mu'akkad al-maḥabba bayn al-muḥibb wa man aḥabba ('The Certainty of The Attachment Between The Lover and The One He Loves')[114] **[M]**
	al-Uss fī-man ra'asa bi 'l-kuss ('The Foundation in He Who Is in Charge of The Cunt')[115] [*]

AUTHOR (C = Christian; J = Jewish)	WORKS ([*] = lost; [M] = mss only)
	al-Ifsāḥ fī asmā' al-nikāḥ ('Declaration regarding the Names for Lawful Intercourse')[116] [M]
	al-Yawāqīt al-thamīna fī ṣifāt al-samīna ('Precious Stones in The Description of The Fat Woman')[117]
	Wuḍū' al-ṣabāḥ fī lughāt al-nikāḥ ('Morning Ablutions in The Language of Lawful Intercourse')[118] [M]
	al-Mustaẓrafa fī aḥkām dukhūl al-ḥashafa ('The Elegant Woman as regards Provisions for the Entry of the Glans Penis')[119] [*]
	al-Mustaẓraf fī akhbār al-jawārī ('The Delightful Book on the Stories of Slave Girls')[120]
	Nuzhat al-nadīm ('Excursion of The Boon Companion')[121]
	Nuzhat al-muta'ahhil wa murshid al-muta'ahhal fī faḍā'il al-nikāḥ ('Excursion of the Spouse and the Guide to His Wife Regarding the Virtues of Lawful Intercourse')[122]
	Mabāsim al-milāḥ wa manāsim al-ṣabāḥ fī mawāsim al-nikāḥ ('The Mouths of Wittiness and the Foot Soles of The Morning in the Seasons of Lawful Intercourse')[123] [*]
	al-Zanjabīl al-qāṭi' fī waṭ' dhāt al-barāqi' ('Cut Ginger in Coitus with Face-veiled Women')[124] [*]

AUTHOR (C = Christian; J = Jewish)	**WORKS** ([*] = lost; [M] = mss only)
	al-Īḍāḥ fī asrār al-nikāḥ ('Elucidation of The Secrets of Lawful Intercourse)')[125] *al-Kanz al-madfūn wa 'l-falak al-mashḥūn* ('The Hidden Treasure and The Loaded Star')[126]
al-Ṭabarī, 'Alī Abū 'l-Ḥasan Ibn Rabban (C) [floruit mid-9th c. – Persia]	*Kitāb al-īḍāḥ min al-simān wa 'l-huzāl wa tahayyuj al-bāh wa 'ibṭālihi* ('The Book of Elucidation Regarding the Fat and the Skinny, and Stimulation of Coitus and Its Thwarting')[127] [*]
al-Tadaghī, Abū Ṣāliḥ	*Tuḥfat al-fallāḥ fī 'ilm al-nikāḥ* ('Gift of The Peasant regarding The Science of Lawful Intercourse')[128] [M]
al-Ṭāhirī, Ibn al-Shāh (9th c. ?)	*Kitāb akhbār al-ghilmān* ('The Book of News on Catamites')[129] [*] *Kitāb akhbār al-nisā'* ('The Book of Stories about Women')[130] [*] *Kitāb al-bighā' wa ladhdhātuhu* ('The Book of Prostitution and Its Pleasures')[131] [*] *Kitāb al-khaḍkhaḍa* ('The Book of Masturbation')[132] [*]
al-Tamakrūtī, Muḥammad 'Abd Allāh Ibn Muḥammad Ibn Mas'ūd al-Dar'ī al-Tafjarūtī [10th–11th c.]	*al-Rawḍ al-yāni' fī aḥkām al-tazwīj wa-ādāb al-majāmi'* ('The Ripe Gardens in the Rules for Marrying off a Woman and the Etiquette for Intercourse')[133] [M]
Ṭayfūr, Aḥmad Ibn Abī Ṭāhir [819–893 – Iraq]	*Balāghāt al-nisā'* ('Information about Women')[134]
al-Tīfāshī, Shihāb al-Dīn Aḥmad Ibn Yūsuf [1184–1253 – Tunis]	*Nuzhat al-albāb fī-mā lā yūjad fī 'l-kitāb* ('Delights of The Hearts in Things that Cannot Be Found in Any Book')[135]

AUTHOR (C = Christian; J = Jewish)	**WORKS** ([*] = lost; **[M]** = mss only)
	Rujū' al-shaykh ilā ṣibāhi fī 'l-quwwa wa 'l-bāh ('Returning the Old Man to His Youthful Sexual Potency')[136] *Risāla fī-mā yaḥtajī ilayhi al-rijāl wa 'l-nisā' fī isti'māl al-bāh mimmā yaḍurr wa yanfa'* ('Treatise on What Men and Women Need During Coitus and Its Harms and Benefits')[137]
al-Tijānī, Muḥammad Ibn Aḥmad [13th–early 14th c., Tunis]	*Tuḥfat al-'arūs wa nuzhat al-nufūs* ('The Bride's Gift and The Delight of The Souls')[138]
al-Ṭūsī, Naṣīr al-Dīn	*Kitāb albāb al-bāhiyya wa 'l-tarākīb al-sulṭāniyya*
al-Ẓāhirī, 'Alī Ibn Muḥammad [d. 963 – Iraq]	*Akhbār al-Ghilmān* ('Stories About Boys') [139] [*] *Akhbār al-Nisā'* ('Stories About Women') [*] *al-Bighā' wa Ladhdhātuhu* ('Prostitution and Its Pleasures') [*]
Zarrūq, Aḥmad [1442–1493 – Morocco]	*al-Nikāḥ* ('Lawful Intercourse')[140] **[M]**

1. BN 3039.5, fols. 61–82 (copy dated 1075/1664–5).
2. BN 3039.13, fols. 125–127 (copy dated 1075/1664–5).
3. BN 3039.14, fols. 127–138 (copy dated 1075/1664–5).
4. Bodleian. MS. Marsh 595 (item 6, fols 88b–89a); E. Savage-Smith 2011: 434–5 (entry No. 111).
5. Gotha No. 2061 (W. Pertsch 1859–1893: III:4 [1883], 89–90), extract from a larger work.
6. Gotha No. 2062 (W. Pertsch 1859–1893: III:4 [1883], 90), extract from a larger work.
7. Gotha No. 2063 (W. Pertsch 1859–1893: III:4 [1883], 90–1), extract from a larger work.
8. Bodleian, MS. Arab. c. 85. Abridgement of *Kitāb al-anyāk* (see below).
9. Bod. MS. Marsh 530 (item 1, fols. 1a–59a); E. Savage-Smith 2011: 431–3 (No. 109).
10. Bod. MS. Arab. D. 148 (item 2, fols. 68b–70a); E. Savage-Smith 2011: 430–1 (Entry No. 108).
11. Gotha No. 2058 (W. Pertsch 1859–1893: III:4 [1883], 87–8).
12. Gotha No. 2060 (W. Pertsch 1859–1893: III:4 [1883], 89).
13. Gotha No. 2054 (W. Pertsch 1859–1893: III:4 [1883], 84–5). This is a work on aphrodisiacs (*al-adwiyya al-muqawwiyya li 'l-bāh*).
14. BN 3039.15, fol. 138ff. (copy dated 1075AH/1664–5 CE).
15. Referred to in Bodleian, MS. Arab. c. 85.
16. Damascus, al-Ẓāhiriyya, No. 7524.
17. BN 3039.11, fols. 109–110 (copy dated 1075/1664–5).
18. BN 3039.4, fols. 36–61 (copy dated 1075/1664–5).
19. BN 3039.3, fol. 30 (copy dated 1075/1664–5).
20. BN 3039.1, fols. 28–30 (copy dated 1075/1664–5).
21. BN 3039.12, fols. 111–125 (copy dated 1075/1664–5).
22. BN 3039, fols. 151–259 [3039.17], 267–268 [3039.20] (copy dated 1075/1664–5).
23. BN 1932, fols. 105–115.
24. Cairo, Dār al-Kutub, Ṭ Taymūr 362.
25. Berlin 6385 Spr. 1920.
26. A. Ihsanoglu 1984: 449; Shahid Ali library, No. 2145.
27. 'A. Hishām & 'Ā. 'Abd al-Hamīd 1999: 177–215.
28. Tunisian National Library 18248.
29. Tunisian National Library 20648 (09).
30. Aya Sofya 2938.
31. Tunisian National Library 18228 (2).
32. al-Nafzāwī n.d.: 64–84.
33. Aḥmad Farīd al-Mazīdī (ed.) Cairo: Dār al-Āfāq al-'Arabiyya, 2007, pp. 371–402. 'U. al-Kaḥḥāla n.d.: I, 214.
34. BN 3071–3 (de Slane 1883–95: 544–5).
35. Faraj al-Ḥawwār (ed.), Tunis: al-Dār al-Mutawassiṭa li 'l-Nashr, 2021; BN 3671; R. Irwin, "'Alī al-Baghdādī and the joy of Mamluk sex", in H. Kennedy (ed.), *The Historiography of Islamic Egypt: (c. 950–1800)*,

Leiden: Brill, 2000, pp. 45–57; L. Lopez-Baralt 1992: 258–60; French trans. R. Khawam, *Les fleurs éclatantes dans les baisers et l'accolement*, Paris: Albin Michel, 1973 [rev. trans. Paris: Phébus, 1989].

36. BN 5622, ff. 78b–90a. See 'U. Kaḥḥāla n.d.: XI, 132.

37. BN 3069, 3070.1 (128ff.; in this mss, the author's name is erroneously given as Muḥammad al-Nafzāwī, presumably because of the similarity in title between the two works).

38. BN 2042, 3564–6, 3612, 6146. French trans. R. Khawam, *Les ruses des femmes*, Paris: Phébus, 1994.

39. 'U. Kaḥḥāla n.d.: XII, 12; Ibn Abī Uṣaybi'a 2020: 15.39.

40. *GAS*, III, 254 (No. 25); P. Sbath 1938–40: I, 43 (No. 312). The book is quoted in al-Rāzī's *Kitāb al-Ḥāwī fi 'l-ṭibb as al-Bāh or al-Kunnāsh fi 'l-bāh* (1955–69: X, 263–295–7).

41. *GAS*, III, 304; P. Sbath 1938–40: I, 69, No. 562; Ibn Uṣaybi'a 2020: 10.20.

42. 'U. Kaḥḥāla n.d.: III, 113; *GAS*, III, 243; L. Shaykhū 1924: 224; Ibn Uṣaybi'a 2020: 8.3.

43. Aḥmad Ibn Muḥammad al-Yamanī ed., Beirut: Tāla li 'l-Ṭibā'a wa 'l-Nashr, 2002. Partial eds: Ghadhban Al-Bayati (Chaps. 1–3), unpubl. Phd. Diss. Friedrich-Alexander University Erlangen-Nürnberg, 1976; Adnan Husni-Pascha (Chap. 4), unpubl. Phd. Diss. Friedrich-Alexander University Erlangen-Nürnberg, 1975; Jalal Elias Yousif (Chap. 5), unpubl. Phd. Diss. Friedrich-Alexander University Erlangen-Nürnberg, 1977; Boulus Al-Khouri (Chap. 6, Part 1), unpubl. Phd. Diss. Friedrich-Alexander University Erlangen-Nürnberg, 1975; Abdul Hassan Abdul Khador (Chap. 6, Part 2), unpubl. Phd. Diss. Friedrich-Alexander University Erlangen-Nürnberg, 1983; Adnan Zeni (Chap. 6, Part 3), unpubl. Phd. Diss. Friedrich-Alexander University Erlangen-Nürnberg, 1978; Mohamed Zouher Djabri (Chaps. 9–11), unpubl. Phd. Diss. Friedrich-Alexander University Erlangen-Nürnberg, 1968; Elian Sabbagh (Chaps. 12–14), unpubl. Phd. Diss. Friedrich-Alexander University Erlangen-Nürnberg, 1973. English trans. A. Jarkas & S. Khawwam, *An intelligent man's guide to the art of coition by Ibn Falita Ahmad Ibn Muhammad*, Toronto: Aleppo, 1977. See S. Habib 2007: 25–31; D. Jacquart & C. Thomasset 1988: 126; *GAL, I*, 232, *GALS, I*, 415; 'U. Kaḥḥāla n.d.: II, 20, 136; A. Ihsanoglu 1984: 82; Cambridge University Library Qq. 130 (1811); Cadbury Research Library, University of Birmingham, Islamic Arabic 674 (d. 7th Dhū l-Ḥijjah 1215 AH); Gotha 2038, 2039 (W. Pertsch 1859–1893: III:4 [1883], 74–5).

44. al-Tīfāshī 1892: 2 (this is probably a reference to al-Jāḥiẓ's work); R. Burton 1885: X, 175. 'U. Kaḥḥāla n.d.: X, 173.

45. H. 'Abd al-'Aziz & 'Abd al-Ḥamīd 1999: 37–148.

46. A. Ihsanoglu 1984: 299, Tera No. 3/259 (165 pp), copy dating from 1136 AH/ 1723 CE.

47. Staatsbibliothek zu Berlin - Preußischer Kulturbesitz, Landberg 269;

Ahlwardt 1887-99: No. 6391; 'U. Kaḥḥāla n.d.: XI, 108; *GAL*, II, 299–300; *GALS*, 410–1; Ṣ. al-Munajjid 1975: 24, 168–9.

48. G. Haydar 1973; *GAS*, III, 272, No. 14; D. Jacquart & C. Thomasset 1988: 123.

49. N. A. Barhoum 1974; H. Fähndrich, *Abhandlung über die Ansteckung*, Berlin: Deutsche Morgenländische Gesellschaft, 1987. *GAS*, III, 272, No. 15; M. Ullmann 1970: 194. A. Ihsanoglu 1984: 314, Aya Sophia No 10/3729; University of Istanbul, Arabic Section No. 2/242.

50. *GAS*, III, 328; 'U. Kaḥḥāla n.d.: I, 269, XIII, 261; Ibn Abī Uṣaybi'a 2020: 11.16.

51. Tunis National Library, No. 17970; 'A. Manṣūr 1975: 408; M. Maḥfūẓ 1992: IV, 302–3.

52. Mohamed Walid Anbari, ed. 1971. This book is also known as *Maqāla fī 'l-jimā' wa mā yata'alliqu bihi* ('Treatise on Coitus and Related Matters'). See M. Ullmann 1970: 122f., 194; A. Ihsanoglu 1984: 87 (*Kitāb al-jimā' aw masā'il fī 'l-nasl wa 'l-dhurriyya wa 'l-jimā'*); *GAL* I (*Kitāb al-Jimā'*), 232, 267; *GALS*, I, 417; *GAS*, III, 257 (*Kitāb al-Jimā'*); 'U. Kaḥḥāla n.d.: VIII, 31.

53. This is the name of two works attributed to Maimonides. However, it is now generally accepted that only the shorter of the two (consisting of ten chapters) was written by Maimonides, himself; for a brief discussion, see F. Rosner, *The medical legacy of Moses Maimonides*, New York: Ktav Publishing House, 1997, 10–11; M. L. Wilensky, "Health Conduct in Intercourse Taken from Rabbi Moshe Maimon", *Proceedings of the American Academy for Jewish Research*, 56, 1990, pp. 101–110 [pp. 103–4]; S. M. Sterrn, 'Maimonides' treatise to a Prince, containing advice on sexual matters, *Maimonides comentarius in Mischam*, Corpus codicum Hebraicarum Medii Aevi, I.3 (Copenhagen, 1966), 17–21. It was written at the request of al-Malik al-Muẓaffar Taqī 'l-Dīn (d. 1191), Salāḥ al-Dīn's nephew. The shorter work is preserved in a complete Judaeo-Arabic copy (held in Granada), a Judaeo-Arabic fragment (Paris) and an Arabic-script fragment (Bodleian Library, MS. Huntington 427, item 3, fol. 61ab – E. Savage-Smith 2011: 422–4 [No. 105]). The Judaeo-Arabic text of the longer version, along with Hebrew translations (the earliest dating from 1277) of the shorter were edited and rendered into German by Hermann Kroner (*Ein Beitrag zur Geschichte der Medizin des XII. Jahrhunderts: an der Hand zweier medizinischer Abhandlungen des Miamonides auf Grund von 6 uneditierten Handschriften*, Oberdorf-Bopfingen, 1906), who concurred with M. Steinschneider (1902: 213) that both works were composed by Maimonides. For an English translation of the shorter and longer texts, see M. Gorlin, *Maimonides' On Sexual Intercourse (Fi'l-Jima). Translated from the Arabic with an Introduction and Commentary,* New York: Rambash Publishing, 1961. The Judaeo-Arabic manuscript of the shorter version was later also edited by Kroner ('Eine medizinische Maimonides-Handschrift

aus Granada. Ein Beitrag zur Stilistik des Maimonides und zur Charakteristik der hebraischen Übersetzungsliteratur. Im Urtexts herausgegeben, übersetzt und kritisch erlautert', *Janus*, 21, 1916, pp. 203–47). It was subsequently translated into Italian (U. De Martini, *Maimonides. Segreto dei segreti*, Rome: Istituto di storia della Medicina dell 'Universita di Roma, 1960), Spanish (E. Chelminiski, "Notas introductorias al 'Guia sobre el contacto sexual' de Maimonides", *An de ars medica-Mexico*, 1961, 5, pp. 240–8). The Hebrew translations were critically re-edited by Susman Muntner (*Pseudo-Maimonides and sexual life. Collection of medieval treatises*, Jerusalem: Geniza, 1965). Muntner's and Kroner's editions formed the basis for an English translation by F. Rosner (*Sex Ethics in the Writings of Moses Maimonides*, New York: Bloch Publishing Company; 1974; *idem* 1984:162–82). M. Wilenski (*op. cit.*) edited a third (spurious) Hebrew text on the topic by Maimonides. The most recent English translation/ edition is G. Bos 2018.

54. *EI2*, s.v. "Ibn al-Qaṭṭaʿ" (U. Rizzitano); *GAL*, I, 308; *GALS*, I, 540; Ṣ. al-Munajjid 1975: 142; al-Suyūṭī 2001: 125.

55. ʿU. Kaḥḥāla n.d.: IV, 237.

56. ʿU. Kaḥḥāla n.d.: XII, 185–6; Ibn Abī Uṣaybiʿa 1971: 888 (220: 15.46.

57. According to Ibn Abī Uṣaybiʿa (1971: 890; 2020: 15.46), this was a poem on sexual potency, written in what is today Silvan, eastern Anatolia (Turkey), in 615/1218, for al-Malik al-Ashraf Shāh Abū Arman Mūsā, the son of al-Malik al-ʿĀdil Abū Bakr Ibn Ayyūb; 'as he informed me, he wrote it in two days. It comprises ... lines. He also wrote an exhaustive commentary on it, expounding each item lucidly.'

58. M. Ullmann 1970: 158–159; Seymore, Jennifer Ann, *The life of Ibn Ridwan and his commentary on Ptolemy's "Tetrabiblos"*, unpublished PhD dissertation, Columbia University, 2001; Michael W. Dols, *Medieval Islamic medicine: Ibn Ridwān's treatise 'On the prevention of bodily ills in Egypt*, Berkeley: University of California Press, 1984; EI2, s.v. "Ibn Riḍwān" (J. Schacht); Ibn Abī Uṣaybiʿa 2020: 14.25.

59. M. Ullmann 1970: 195; *GALS*, I, 827; British Library 1349. This treatise is also known as *Risāla fi'l-bāh*.

60. Cairo, Dār al-Kutub, *Ṭ-ṭibb* No. 509.

61. Damascus, Ẓāhiriyya, No. 8315.

62. ʿU. Kaḥḥāla n.d.: XIII, 189; L. Shaykhū 1924: 75–6; *GALS*, I, 862; Ibn Uṣaybiʿa 2020: 10.40.

63. Aḥmad Farīd al-Mazīdī, Cairo: Dār al-Āfāq al-ʿArabiyya, 2007, pp. 7–288; Partial ed., F. Mansour (Part 2, Sections 1–5), unpubl. Phd. Diss., Universität Erlangen-Nürnberg, 1975; Partial ed., K. Hallak (Part 2, Section 6), unpubl. Phd. Diss., Universität Erlangen-Nürnberg, 1973; Partial ed., T. Haddad (Part 1, Sections 6–8), unpubl. Phd. Diss., Universität Erlangen-Nürnberg, 1976. Eng. trans., A. Jarkas & S. Khawwam, *A jaunt in the art of coition*, Toronto: Aleppo Publishing, 1978. See A. Ihsanoglu 1984: 251; Ṣ. al-Munajjid 1975:

159–60; D. Jacquart & F. Thomasset 1988: 124; *GALI*, 488; *GALSI*, 892; F. Rosenthal, 'Die arabische Autobiographie', in F. Rosenthal, G. von Grünebaum, W. J. Fischel (eds), *Studia Arabica*, I (Analecta Orientalia, 14), Rome: Pontificum Institutum Biblicum, 1937; A. Ambouba, "As-Samaw'al Ibn Yahya al-Magribī (570 H.)", *al-Machriq*, 55, 1961, pp. 89–112; L. Leclerq 1876: II, 14–17; W. Pertsch 1859–1893: III:4 (1883), 77–8.

64. M. Steinschneider 1902: 189; *GAL*, II, 643; Ibn Uṣaybiʿa 2020: 11.21.
65. Charles Pellat (ed.), Beirut: 1957.
66. A. Ihsanoglu 1984: 158–9, Ahmad III, No. 2538.
67. Berlin 4186. 'U. al-Kaḥḥāla n.d.: III, 28
68. Mss., Aya Sofia 3836 (dated 533/1139), Aya Sofia 3837 (dated 634/1236), Fatih 3729 (dated 582/1186): al-Kātib 1977: 41 (where a mss held by the Alexandria municipal library is also mentioned); A. Ihsanoglu 1984: 52. Partial ed., 2002; Beirut: Tāla li 'l-Tibāʿa wa 'l-Nashr, 2006 (under al-Qazwīnī, 'Alī al-Kātibī); English trans. A. Jarkas & S. Khawwam 1977. *GALS*, I, 945 (No. 339); Ṣ. al-Munajjid 1975: 156–8; R. Burton 1885: X, 175. This work is listed as a source by al-Tīfāshī (1892: 2).
69. Al-Kātib [S. Khawwam] 1977: 108. According to the author, the book dealt with masturbation.
70. *GALS*, II, 1032.
71. UCLA, Louise Darling Biomedical Library, MS Ar. 83 (dated 5 Jumādā I/12 August 1641); Z. Iskandar 1984: 61.
72. Constantinople: al-Jawā'ib, n.d.; Beirut: Arab Diffusion Company, 2007.
73. Khuda Bakhsh library (Patna), d. 1878; Bankipore, No. 228 [VIII], fols,138–163 (catalogue, IV, 167–8). Other copy in Rampur Library (p. 487, No. 93).
74. Ahmad III, 259 (A. Ihsanoglu 1984).
75. Istanbul University Library No. 242, Folio 63–117.
76. A. Ihsanoglu 1984: p. 314, Aya Sophia 4832 (written 568 AH/1172-3 CE.); M. Ullmann 1970: 194; *GALS*, I, 374; *GAS*, III: 245 (No. 2). G. Celentano 1979.
77. 'U. Kaḥḥāla n.d.: I, 107; *GAL*, II, 465.
78. Al-Tīfāshī 1892: 2; R. Burton 1885: X, 175.
79. 'A. Tāmir & I. Khalifa (eds), Beirut, 1960.
80. Beirut: Mu'assasat al-Intishār al-'Arabī, 1997.
81. L. A. Giffen, in J. Lowry & D. Stewart 2009: 309–21. Tunis: Maktabat al-Manār, n.d., pp. 1–64; Jamāl Jumʿa (ed.), London/Beirut: Riyad El-Rayess, 1993; F. al-Ḥawwār 2006–7: I, 35–120. Engl. trans. R. Burton 1886; J. Colville 1999. French trans. le Baron R., *Le Jardin Parfumé*, Paris: Isidore Liseux, 1886 (1906; Paris: Leopold Blondeau, 1960); re-ed., Mohamed Lasly, Paris: Philippe Picquier, 1999 (2002); R. Khawam, *La prairie parfumée ou s'ébattent les plaisirs*, Paris: Phébus, 1976 (2003, 2011; Paris: Pocket, 1993). M. Maḥfūẓ 1992: V, 39–43.
82. This work formed the nucleus of *al-Rawḍ al-ʿāṭir*.

83. Yāqūt 1936–8: II, 1474; Ibn al-Nadīm 1871–2: I, 152 (trans. B. Dodge 1970: I, 334); P. Myrne 2020: 13, 14, 61-2; R. Burton 1885: X, 175; 'U. Kaḥḥāla n.d.: IX (who states that it involves Horan-born Muḥammad Ibn Ḥasan al-Namīlī). A similar sounding *Burjān wa Janāhib* is mentioned by al-Tifāshī (1892: 2), without the name of an author. A fuller title of the work, *Burjān wa Habāhib fī akhbār al-bāh*, appears in al-Kātib's *Jawāmiʿ al-ladhdha*, with a number of quotations from it (al-Kātib 1977: 37, 219, 231–ff., 246, 275, 376).
84. Ibn al-Nadīm 1871–2: I, 152 (trans. B. Dodge 1970: I, 334).
85. *ibid.*
86. *ibid.*
87. French trans. R. Khawam, *La prairie des gazelles: éloge des beaux adolescents*, Paris: Phébus, 1989. On the author, see *EI*[1], s.v. "al-Nawādjī" (I. Krachkovskij); T. Bauer, in J. Lowry & D. Stewart 2009: 321–331.
88. al-Tīfāshī 1892: 2; R. Burton 1885: X, 175 ("al-Nahli").
89. Tunis National Library 18556. 'A. Mansūr 1975: 407.
90. 'A. Hishām & 'Ā. 'Abd al-Hamīd 1999: 149–176; Aḥmad Farīd al-Mazīdī (ed.), Cairo: Dār al-Āfāq al-'Arabiyya, 2007, pp. 291–370. *GAL* I, 270; *GALS* I, 420, No. 10; GAS, III, 285, No. 9. Mss.: A. Ihsanoglu 1984: 110 (Aya Sofia 1/3725, University of Istanbul, Arabic Section, No. 1/242); Leiden Or187 (J. J. Witkam 2006–7: I, 123; Voorhoeve, *Handlist*, 35).
91. *GAS*, III, 294. In al-Rāzī's al-Ḥāwī (1955–69: X, 263–4, 267, 298, 303, 308), there is also a reference to *Masā'il Arisṭāṭālīs fi'l-bāh* (Ibn Abī Uṣaybi'a 184: I, 69), though this is actually Aristotle's Problemata Physica. GAS, III, 51; R. Kruk 1976: 255. Ibn Abi al-Usabi'ah (1970: 557) states that it is 'a treatise being an answer to a question put to him — why does a man who restrains himself in sexual intercourse live long? Dedicated to the Emir Abū al-'Abbās Aḥmad ibn 'Alī.'
92. For a discussion of the various manuscripts, as well as an English translation of one of them, see F. Rosenthal 1978. The title of the treatise appears variously in other sources as *al-Dā' al-khafī* ('The Hidden Illness'), *Kitāb al-ubna wa 'ilājiha* ('Book on Ubna and Its Treatment'), *'ilājāt al-ubna* ('The Treatments for *Ubna*'), *Kitāb al-ubna wa 'ilājuhā wa-tabyīnuhā* ('Book on Ubna, Its Treatment and Explanation'). This is the only known extant work on the subject. The treatise is included in its entirety in al-Tīfāshī 1994: 302–308, whereas excerpts of it can be found in the medical anthology *Bustān al-aṭibbā' wa rawḍat al-alibbā'* ('The Garden of Physicians and the Meadows of the Wise') by the Damascus-born Christian (later Muslim convert) physician Muwaffaq al-Dīn Ibn Maṭrān (d. 1191).
93. ed. Jurj Kadr, Beirut: Aṭlas li 'l-Nashr wa 'l-Intāj al-Thaqāfī, 2013.
94. Muḥammad Efendi Fahmī Ḥusayn, Cairo: al-Matba'a al-Raḥmāniyya, 1341/1922. Mss: BN 3074, 4642 (de Slane 1883–95: 545, 737, with the first mss being attributed to al-Ṣāfī al-Ḥillī, an alternative title being *Risālat al-ashwāq fīmā yata'allaq bi 'l-'ushshāq*, whereas authorship

of the second mss is stated to be Zayn al-Dīn Manṣūr Ibn 'Abd al-Raḥmān, in line with Ḥājjī Khalīfa's claim); Gotha 2046–7 (W. Pertsch 1859–1893: III:4 [1883], 78–9.)

95. Ibn al-Nadīm 1871–2: I, 152 (trans. B. Dodge 1970: I, 333). This work was one of the sources for al-Kātib's *Jawāmi' al-ladhdha*. On the author, see: *EI²*, s.v. "al-Ṣaymarī" (Ch. Pellat); 'U. Kaḥḥāla n.d.: IX, 38; C. Pellat, 'Un curieux amuseur bagdādien: Abu 'l-'Anbas as-Ṣaymarī', *Studia Orientalia in Memoriam C. Brockelmann*, Halle: Universität Halle-Wittenberg, 1968, 133–7; M. B. 'Alwān, 'Abū 'l-'Anbas Muḥammad Ibn Isḥāq al-Ṣaymarī', *al-Abḥāth*, XXVI, 1973–7, pp. 35–50.

96. Ibn al-Nadīm 1871–2: I, 152 (trans. B. Dodge 1970: I, 333).

97. *ibid.* (trans. B. Dodge 1970: I, 332).

98. *ibid.* (trans. B. Dodge 1970: I, 333).

99. *ibid.*

100. *ibid.*

101. Tunisian National Library 19904.

102. BN 3039, fol. 111.

103. Muḥammad Sa'īd al-Ṭurayḥī (ed.), Beirut: Dār al-Qāri', 1986; Beirut, Dār al-Bayān al-'Arabī, 2002. Mss., BN 2776, fol. I–72; BN 3053; Berlin 6389; Gotha 2033, 2040–44 (W. Pertsch 1859–1893: III:4 [1883], 75–7); Bod. MS. Marsh 595 (item 11, fols. 92a–136a); Cambridge University Library Qq69 (E. G. Browne 1900: 19, No. 118); National Library of Medicine (Bethesda, ML) MS A89.2; Aya Sofia 3573; Fatih 5317, I, 3687–3690; Karatay Topkapi Saray No. 7296; Rabat, Maktabat Zāwiyyat al-Ḥamzāwī; Casablanca, Maktabat Mu'assasat al-Malik 'Abd al-'Azīz. A. Ihsanoglu 1984: 270–2; E. Savage-Smith 2011: 422–4 (No. 104); *GAL* I, 461,488, *GALS*, I, 832–3 (No. 3); M. Ullmann 1970: 195–6; 'U. Kaḥḥāla n.d.: V, 197; M. de Slane 1883–95: 427, 542.

104. Ḥ. Jughām 2001: 193– 228; Beirut, Tāla li 'l-Ṭibā'a wa 'l-Nashr, 2002; Damascus, Dār al-Kitāb al-'Arabī, 2001. J. Hämeen-Anttila, 'Al-Suyuti and erotic literature', in A. Ghersetti 2016: 227–40; P. Myrne 2018; R. Burton 1885: X, 174; Ṣ. al-Munajjid 1975: 171–2; W. Pertsch 1859–1893: III:4 (1883), 79–81 (Nos. 2048–9).

105. Ḥ. Jughām 2001: 129–163; Beirut: Mu'assasat al-Intishār al-'Arabī, 1997; Y. Sarkīs (1928) mentions a publication in 19th century. French translation: R. Khawam, *Nuits de noces ou comment humer le doux breuvage de la magie licite par 'Abd al-Rahmane al-Souyouti*, Paris, Albin Michel, 1972, pp. 1–94. W. Pertsch 1859–1893: III:4 (1883), 81–2 (Nos. 2049).

106. Ṭala'at Ḥasan 'Abd al-Qawī, ed., Damascus, Dār al-Kitāb al-'Arabī, n.d. This book is actually the coda (*dhayl*) to *Rashf al-Zulal.* French trans. R. Khawam, *Nuits de noces ou comment humer le doux breuvage de la magie licite par 'Abd al-Rahmane al-Souyouti*, Paris, Albin Michel, 1972, pp. 95–234. R. Burton 1885: X, 174. W. Pertsch 1859–1893: III:4 (1883), 82–3 (Nos. 2050–1).

107. Dār al-Kutub (Cairo), A. Tal'at 4532; Ḥ. Jughām 2001: 229–239.

108. F. al-Ḥawwār 2006–7: I, 35–120.
109. ʿĀdil al-ʿĀmil, (ed.), Damascus: Dār al-Maʿrifa, 1988, 1994; Muhammad Sayyid al-Rifāʿī (ed.), Damascus: Dār al-Kitāb al-ʿArabī, [2001?]. D. Rodica Firanescu, "Revisiting Love and Coquetry in Medieval Arabic Islam: Al-Suyūṭī's Perspective" in A. Ghersetti 2016: 241–59; P. Myrne 2018; Ḥ. Jughām 2001: 81–102.
110. Damascus: al-Maktaba al-ʿArabiyya, 1349/1931; ʿAbd al-Amīn Mahdī al-Tā'ī (ed.), Baghdad: Dār Ibn Nadīm, [1990]; Samīr Ḥusayn Ḥalabī (ed.), Cairo: Maktabat al-Turāth al-Islāmī 1308/1987; Beirut: Mu'assasat al-Intishār al-ʿArabī, 2005; Hammam-Sousse: Dār al-Mīzān li 'l-Nashr, 2005; Ḥ. Jughām 2001: 261–266.
111. Ḥ. Jughām 2001: 293–307.
112. Sousse/Tunis: Dār al-Maʿārif li 'l-Ṭibāʿa wa 'l-Nashr, 1990.
113. Salāḥ al-Dīn al-Munajjid (ed.), Beirut: Dār al-Makshūf, 1958; ʿAbd al-Laṭīf ʿĀshūr (ed.), Cairo: Maktabat al-Qur'ān, n.d. Ḥ. Jughām 2001: 243–50.
114. Tunis National Library, 17970.02; BN 3039, fol. 146 (without author mentioned) – ʿA. Manṣūr (1975: 421) attributes it to Muḥammad Ibn Khalīl al-Ṭawāḥnī al-Tūnisī (d. 1300).
115. *al-Wishāḥ fī fawā'id al-nikāh*, 2001: 198.
116. Mss, Cambridge, No. 2/1008.
117. Faraj al-Ḥawwār (ed.), Sousse: Dār al-Mizān li 'l-Nashr, 2003.
118. Mss, Berlin, No. 3/7061; Ḥ. Jughām 2001: 352.
119. Ḥ. Jughām 2001.
120. Ṣ. al-Munajjid (ed.), Cairo: Dār al-Kitāb al-Jadīdī, 1963; Cairo: Maktabat al-Turāth al-Islāmī, 1998. Ḥ. Jughām 2001: 251–259.
121. Ḥ. Jughām 2001: 103–127: Faraj al-Ḥawwār (ed.), Hammam-Sousse: Dār al-Mīzān li 'l-Nashr, 2003.
122. Jūrj Kadr (ed.), Beirut: Aṭlas li 'l-Nashr wa 'l-Intāj al-Thaqāfī, 2013; Mss, Cairo, No. 9424.968; Damascus Ẓāhiriyya No. 1163. P. Myrne 2018; W. Pertsch 1859–1893: III:4 (1883), 83–84 (Nos. 2052–3).
123. Ḥ. Jughām 2001: 352–3. According to al-Suyūṭī, his *al-Wishāḥ* is an abridgement of this work.
124. *Nawādir al-hayk fī nawādir al-nayk*, n.d.: 24.
125. Bibliotheca Alexandrina 7365; Rabat, Maktabat Zāwiya Ḥamzāwiyya 127; Ḥ. Jughām 2001: 165–192; F. al-Ḥawwār 2006–7: I, 121–146. This work was mentioned as a source by al-Tīfāshī (1892: 2).
126. Ḥ. Jughām 2001:323–350.
127. *GAS*, III, 239; the work is only referred to in the author's far more famous *Firdaws al-ḥikma* (1928: 113).
128. *GAL*, III, 203.
129. Ibn al-Nadīm 1871–2: I, 153 (trans. B. Dodge 1970: I, 335).
130. *ibid.*
131. *ibid.*
132. *ibid.*
133. The author's name is also sometimes written as Tamajrūtī and al-

Tamghrūtī. National Library of Medicine (Bethesda, ML) MS A89.1 (dated 1196/1782); Berlin, MS Qu. 1171 (fols. 4b–72b – dated 16 Jumādā II 1132/25 April 1720); BN, MS ar. 5573 (fols. 169a–178a); Istanbul, University Library (MS Arab. 3192, fols. 1b–70b); G. Vajda 1953: IV, 580; A. Ihsanoglu 1984: 154 (No. 133); *GALS*, II, 369: G. Schoeler: 1990: II, 152–4 (No. 157).

134. F. al-Ḥawwār 2006–7: III, 6–65. On this author, see Shawkat M. Toorawa, *Ibn Abī Ṭāhir Ṭayfūr and Arabic writerly culture: a ninth-century bookman in Baghdad*, Abingdon: Routledge, 2005.

135. Jamāl Jum'a (ed.), London: Riyad El-Rayess (Saqi Books), 1994; partial English trans. (based on the French translation by R. Khawam, *Les Délices des Coeurs*, Paris: Jérôme Martineau, 1971; (rev. eds., Phébus, 1981, 1988), Edward A. Lacey, *The Delight of Hearts: Or What You Will Not Find in Any Book*, Los Angeles: Gay Sunshine Press, 1988. See *EI*[2], s.v. 'al-Tīfāshī' (J. Ruska-[O. Kahl]); *GAL*, I, 495; *GALS*, I, 904; M. Ullmann 1970: 196–7; Ṣ. al-Munajjid 1975: 169–70; M. Maḥfūẓ 1992: I, 205–9; S. Habib 2007: 66–83; F. Malti-Douglas, 'Tribadism/lesbianism and the sexualised body in medieval Arabo-Islamic narrative', in F. Canadé Sautman & P. Shengorn 2001: 123–141.

136. Cairo: Bulaq, 1309/1892; al-Maktaba al-'Āmira al-Sharqiyya, 1322/1904: Muṣṭafā Fahmī ed. [attributed to Ibn Kamāl Pasha, Aḥmad Ibn Sulaymān]; Beirut, Manshūrāt Samar li 'l-Ṭibā'a wa 'l-Nashr, 1994; Damascus: Dār al-Kitāb al-'Arabī, 2001; in F. al-Ḥawwār 2006–7: II, 7–182. English trans., *An English Bohemian, The Old Man Young Again: Or Age-Rejuvenescence in the Power of Concupiscence*, Paris: Charles Carrington, 1898 (repr. 2009): French trans., Abdul-Haqq Effendi, *Le livre de volupté pour que le viellard recouvre sa jeunesse*, París, La Sycomore, 1979 (Paris: Minerve, 1989); Mohamed Lasly, *Le Bréviaire arabe de l'amour*, Arles: Philippe Picquier, 1998 (2002); R. Burton 1885: X, 175 ('Ahmad bin Sulayman. Surnamed Kamál Pasha'); W. Pertsch 1859–1893: III:4 (1883), 85–7 (Nos. 2055–7); Ṣ. al-Munajjid 1975: 162–6.

137. Partial ed. Hassan Mohammad El-Haw [al-Tifashi 1970]. *GAL*, I, 652; D. Jacquart & C. Thomasset 1988: 125–6.

138. Jalīl 'Aṭiyya (ed.), London: Riyad El-Rayess, 1992; Hammamet: Manshūrāt Muḥammad Būdhīnah, 1998; Beirut: Dār al-Jīl, n.d. See *EI2*, s.v. 'al-Tidjānī' (M. Plessner-[Taïeb El Achèche]); *GAL*, II, 334, *GALS*, I, 368; Y. Sarkīs 1928: 1622. Al-Tījānī is also quoted in al-Suyūtī's work (2001: 193).

139. 'U. Kaḥḥāla n.d.: VII, 202–3. None of this author's three works on the subject seems to have survived.

140. Spanish trans. L. López-Baralt 1992. Also see L. López Baralt, 'El original árabe del 'Kama Sutra español' (ms. S-2-BRAH-Madrid)', in Manuel García Martín (ed.), *Estado actual de los estudios sobre el Siglo de Oro*, Salamanca: Ediciones Universidad de Salamanca, 1974, 561–68.

References

Manuscripts

[ANON]: *Risāla fī dhikr adwiyat al-bāh*, Cairo, Dār al-Kutub, Ṭ Taymūr 362.

[ANON]: *Kitāb fī 'ilm al-bāh wa adwiyatihi*, Tunis, Dār al-Kutub, 20648(09).

[ANON]: *Taṣānīf al-aṭ'ima*, London, Wellcome, WMS Arabic 57.

al-Fallātī, Muḥammad: *Mu'āwanat al-ikhwān fī mu'āsharat al-niswān*, Paris, BNF arabe 5662.

al-Ghazlāwī, Muḥammad: *Yāsamīn al-rawḍ al-'āṭir fī nuzhat al-khāṭir*, Paris, BNF arabe 3069.

Ibn Jazla: *Minhāj al-bayān fīmā yasta'miluhu al-insān*, London, British Library, Or.7499.

Ibn Sīnā: *Asrār al-jimā'*, Cairo, Dār al-Kutub, No. 509.

al-Shayzarī al-Ṭabarī, 'Abd al-Raḥmān: *al-Īḍāḥ fī asrār al-nikāḥ*, Casablanca, Mu'assassat Malik 'Abd al-'Azīz.

Printed Works

Arabic

'Abd al-Wāḥid, Muṣṭafā (1961): *al-Islām wa 'l-mushkila al-jinsiyya*, Cairo: Dār al-I'tiṣām li 'l-Ṭibā'a wa 'l-Nashr wa 'l-Tawzī'.

Abū Nuwās (1994): *al-Nuṣūṣ al-muḥarrama. The forbidden poems*, Jamāl Jum'a (ed.), Beirut: Riad El-Rayyes. [= *al-Fukāha wa ītinās fī mujūn Abī Nuwās*, Cairo, 1898].

Anonymous (2010): *Anwā' al-ṣaydala fī alwān al-aṭ'ima*, 'Abd al-

Ghanī Abū 'l-'Azm (ed.), Rabat: Mu'assasat al-Ghanī li 'l-Nashr [= Anwā'].

Anonymous (1993): *Kanz al-Fawā'id fī tanwī' al-Mawā'id*, Manuela Marín & David Waines (eds.), Beirut/Stuttgart: Franz Steiner Verlag [= Kanz].

Anonymous (1961–62): 'Kitab al tabij fi-l-Magrib wa-l-Andalus fi 'asr al-Muwahhidin, li-mu'allif mayhul (Un libro anónimo de la Cocina hispano-magribí, de la época almohade)', Ambrosio Huici Miranda (ed.), *Revista del Instituto de Estudios Islámicos*, IX/X, pp. 15–256; English translation Charles Perry: Anonymous Andalusian Cookbook, http://daviddfriedman.com/Medieval/Cookbooks/Andalusian/andalusian_contents.htm.

al-Anṭākī, Dā'ūd (1999): *al-Nuzha al-mubhaja fī tashḥīdh al-adhhān wa ta'dīl al-amzija*, Beirut: Mu'assassat al-Balāgh.

al-Anṭākī, D. (1952): *Tadhkirat ulī 'l-ālbāb wa 'l-jāmi' li 'l-'ajab al-'ujāb*, 2 vols, Cairo.

al-Baghdādī, Muḥammad Ibn al-Ḥasan (1964): *Kitāb al-ṭabīkh*, Fakhrī al-Bārūdī (ed.), Damascus: Dār al-Kitāb al-Jadīd; English translation, Charles Perry: *A Baghdad Cookery Book*, Totnes: Prospect Books, 2005.

al-Bīrūnī (1973): *al-Ṣaydana fī 'l-ṭibb. al-Bīrūnī's book on pharmacy and materia medica*, H. M. Said & R. E. Elahie (eds), Karachi: Hamdard National Foundation.

al-Dhahabī, Shams al-Dīn (1987): *al-Ṭibb al-nabawī*, 'Ādil Abū al-Ma'ātī (ed.), Cairo: Dār al-Bashīr.

al-Dimashqī, Shams al-Dīn (1866): [*Nukhbat al-dahr fī 'ajā'ib al-barr wa 'l-baḥr*] *Cosmographie de Chems-ed-Din Abou Abdallah Mohammed ed-Dimichqui. Texte arabe, publié d'après l'édition commencé par M. Fraehn d'après les manuscrits de St-Pétersbourg, de Paris, de Leyde et de Copenhague*, A. F. Mehren (ed.), Saint Petersburg, Copenhagen: C. A. Reitzel.

Ghālib, Idwār (1986): *al-Mawsū'a fī 'ulūm al-ṭabī'a: abḥāth fī 'l-zirā'a wa 'l-nabāt wa 'l-ḥayawān wa 'l-jiyūlūjiyā*, 4 vols, 2nd edition, Beirut: Dār al-Mashriq.

al-Ghassānī, Abū 'l-Qāsim (1990): *Ḥadīqat al-azhār fī māhiyat al-'ushb wa 'l-'aqqār, Muḥammad al-'Arbī al-Khaṭṭābī*, Beirut: Dār al-Gharb al-Islāmī.

Ḥajjī Khalīfa (1835-84): *Kashf al-zunūn ʿan ʿasāmi ʾl-kutub wa ʾl-funūn*, 7 vols, ed. G. Flügel, Leipzig/London: F. C. W. Vogel.

Ibn al-Ḥashshāʾ (1941); *Mufīd al-ʿulūm wa mabīd al-humūm (wa-huwa tafsīr al-alfāẓ al-ṭibbiyya wa ʾl-lughawiyya al-wāqiʿa fī Kitāb al-Manṣūrī li ʾl-Rāzī)*, Georges Séraphin Colin & Henri-Paul-Joseph Renaud (eds.), Rabat: Imprimerie économique.

al-Ḥawwār Faraj (2006-7): *al-Jins ʿinda ʾl-ʿArab* (1997), 4 vols, Cologne: Al-Kamel Verlag.

Hishām, ʿAbd al-ʿAziz & ʿĀdil ʿAbd al-Ḥamīd (1999): *al-Nisāʾ: Thalāth makhṭūṭāt nādira fi ʾl-jins*, Cairo: Dār al-Khayyāl.

Ibn Abī Uṣaybiʿa (1882): *ʿUyūn al-anbāʾ fī ṭabaqāt al-aṭibbāʾ*, 2 vols, Cairo: al-Maṭbaʿa al-Wahbiyya.

Ibn al-Bayṭār, Abū Muhammad (1291/1874): *al-Jāmiʿ li-mufradāt al-adwiya wa ʾl-aghdhiya*, 2 vols, Būlāq; Cairo: Dār al-Kutub al-ʿIlmiyya, 1992; French trans. Lucien Leclerq, "Traité des simples par Ibn el-Beïthar", in *Notices et extraits des manuscrits de la Bibliothèque nationale et autres bibliothèques.*, 23:1 (1877), 25:1 (1881), 26:1 (1883), Paris: Imprimerie Nationale.

Ibn Buṭlān (1990): *Taqwīm al-ṣiḥḥa*, Hossam El Khadem (ed./ French translation), *Le Taqwim al Sihha (Tacuini Sanitatis) d'Ibn Butlan: Un traité médical du XIe Siècle*, Louvain: Peeters.

Ibn Buṭlān (1968): *Maqāla fī tadbīr al-amrāḍ al-ʿāriḍ alā l-ruhbān al-sākinīn fi ʾl-dayr wa min buʿd ʿan al-madīna,* Samira Yousef Jadon (ed.), *The Arab Physician ibn Butlan's (d. 1066) Medical Manual for the Use of Monks and Country People*, unpublished PhD diss., UCLA.

Ibn Janāḥ (2020): *Kitāb al-talkhīṣ*, Gerrit Bos, Fabian Käs, Mailyn Lübke & Guido Mensching (eds./English translation), *Marwān ibn Janāḥ: On the nomenclature of medicinal drugs (Kitāb al-talkhīṣ)*, Leiden: Brill.

Ibn al-Jawzī, ʿAbd al-Raḥmān (1319/1902): *Akhbār al-nisāʾ*, Cairo.

Ibn al-Jazzār, Abū Jaʿfar (2004): *al-Iʿtimād fi ʾl-adwiya al-mufrada*, Idwār al-Qishsh (ed.), Beirut: Sharikat al-Maṭbūʿāt li ʾl-Tawzīʿ wa ʾl-Nashr.

Ibn Lūqā, Qusṭā (1992): *Qusṭā Ibn Lūqā's Medical Regime for the Pilgrims to Mecca: The Risālā Fī Tadbīr Safar al-Ḥajj*, Gerrit Bos (ed.), Leiden: E. J. Brill.

Ibn Lūqā, Q. (1974): *Das Buch über die Geschlechtichkeit (Kitāb fi 'l-Bāh) von Qusṭā Ibn Lūqā. Edition und Übertragung des arabischen Textes nach der Handschrift Nr. 242 der Universitätsbibliothek Istanbul,* Najdat Ali Barhoum (ed.), Universität Erlangen-Nürnberg.

Ibn Lūqā, Q. (1973): *Kitāb fi 'l-Bāh wa mā yuḥtāju ilayhi min tadbīr al-badan fi isti'mālihi des Qusṭā Ibn Luqā. 1. Abhandeling. (Das Buch über die Kohabitation und die für ihre Ausübung notwendigen korperlichen Voraussetzungen) Edition, Übertragung und Bearbeitung des arabischen Textes auf der Grundlage der Handschrift der Universitätsbibliothek Istanbul Nr.243,* Gauss Haydar (ed.), Universität Erlangen-Nürnberg.

Ibn Manẓūr, Jamāl al-Dīn (1299/1881–1308/1890–91): *Lisān al-'Arab*, 20 vols, Būlāq.

Ibn Māssa, 'Īsa (1971): [*Masā'il fi 'l-nasl wa 'l-dhurriyya wa 'l-jimā'*] *Streitfragen über die Zeugung, Nachkommenschaft und über den Geschlechtsverkehr. Verfaßt von Isa ibn Massah. Edition, Übersetzung und Bearbeitung des arabischen Textes auf der Grundlage der Handschrift Ayasofya 3724,* Mohamed Walid Anbari (ed.), Universität Erlangen-Nürnberg.

Ibn Munqidh, Usāma (2003): *Kitāb al-i'tibār*, 'Abd al-Karīm Ushtar (ed.), Beirut: al-Maktab al-Islāmī; English translation Philip Hitti, *An Arab-Syrian gentleman and warrior in the period of the crusades: Memoirs of Usama Ibn-Munqidh,* New York: Columbia University Press, 1929.

Ibn al-Nadīm (1871–72): *Kitāb al-fihrist*, 2 vols, ed. Gustav Flügel, Leipzig: F. C. W. Vogel; English trans. Bayard Dodge, *The Fihrist of al-Nadim*, 2 vols, New York: Columbia University Press, 1970.

Ibn Qutayba, Muḥammad (1343-8/1925-30): *'Uyūn al-akhbār*, Aḥmad Zakī al-'Adawī (ed.), Cairo.

Ibn Sīnā (1999): *al-Qānūn fi 'l-ṭibb*, 3 vols, ed. Muḥammad Amīn al-Ḍannāwī,Beirut: Dār al-Kutub al-'Ilmiyya.

Ibn Wāfid al-Andalusī, al-Wazīr Abū 'l-Muṭarraf (2000): *Kitāb al-adwiya al-mufrada*, Aḥmad Ḥasan Basaj (ed.), Beirut: Dār al-Kutub al-'Ilmiyya.

Ihsanoglu, Akmāl al-Dīn (1984): *Fihris makhṭūṭāt al-ṭibb al-Islāmī bi 'l-lughāt al-'Arabiya wa 'l-Turkiyya wa 'l-Fārisiyya fī maktabāt Turkiyā,* Istanbul: Markaz al-Abḥāth li 'l-Tārīkh wa 'l-Funūn wa 'l-Thaqāfa al-Islāmīyya.

al-Ishbīlī, Abū 'l-Khayr (1995): *'Umdat al-ṭabīb fī ma'rifat al-nabāt*, Muḥammad al-'Arbī al-Khattābī (ed.), 2 vols, Beirut: Dār al-Gharb al-Islāmī.

al-Isrā'ilī, Isḥāq Ibn Sulaymān (1992): *Kitāb al-aghdhiya wa 'l-adwiya*, M. Ṣabbāh (ed.), Beirut.

al-Jāḥiẓ, Abū 'Uthmān (1938): *Kitāb al-ḥayawān*, 7 vols, Cairo: al-Maṭba'a al-Bābī al-Ḥalabī.

Jughām, Ḥasan Aḥmad (2001): *al-Jins fī a'māl al-imām Jamāl al-Dīn al-Suyūṭī*, Tunis: Dār al-Ma'ārif li 'l-Ṭibā'a wa 'l-Nashr.

Kaḥḥāla, 'Umar Riḍā [n.d.]: *Mu'jam al-mu'allifīn. Tarājim muṣannifīn al-kutub al-'Arabiyya*, 15 vols, Beirut: Dār al-Aḥyā' al-Turāth al-'Arabī.

al-Kātib, Abū 'l-Hasan (2002): *Jawāmi' al-ladhdha*, Beirut: Ṭāla li 'l-Ṭibā'a wa 'l-Nashr; English trans. Adnan Jarkas & Salah Addin Khawwam, *Encyclopedia of Pleasure by Abul Hasan 'Ali Ibn Nasr al Katib*, Toronto: Aleppo, 1977.

Maḥfūẓ, Muḥammad (1992): *Tarājim al-mu'allifīn al-Tūnisiyyīn*, 5 vols, Beirut: Dār al-Gharb al-Islāmī.

Maḥmūd Ibrāhīm (2000): *al-Mut'a al-maḥẓūra: al-shudhūdh al-jinsī fī tārīkh al-'Arab*, Beirut: Riyāḍ al-Rayyis li 'l-Kutub wa 'l-Nashr.

Manṣūr, 'Abd al-'Azīz (1975): *Tūnis. Dār al-Kutub. Al-fihris al-'āmm li 'l-makhṭūṭāt*, Tunis.

al-Mas'ūdī, 'Alī Ibn Ḥusayn (1960–79): *Murūj al-dhahab wa ma'ādin al-jawhar*, Barbier de Meynard & Pavet de Courteille (rev. C. Pellat), 7 vols, Beirut: Université Libanaise de Beirut; trans. C. Pellat: Les Prairies d'Or, 5 vols, Paris: Paul Geuthner (1962-97).

al-Munajjid, Ṣalāḥ al-Dīn (1975): *al-Ḥayāt al-jinsiyya 'inda 'l-'Arab*, 2nd rev. ed., Beirut: Dār al-Kitāb al-Jadīd.

al-Munajjid, Ṣ. (1957, 1969): *Jamāl al-mar'a 'inda 'l-'Arab*, Beirut: Dār al-Kitāb al-Jadīd.

al-Muqaddasī (1906): *Aḥsan al-taqāsīm fī ma'rifat al-aqālīm*, ed. M. J. de Goeje, Leiden: E. J. Brill.

al-Nafzāwī, Muḥammad Ibn 'Umar (n.d.): *al-Rawḍ al-'āṭir fī nuzhat al-khāṭir*, Tunis: Maktabat al-Manār; English trans. R. Burton, *The perfumed garden of the Cheikh Nefzoui. A manual of Arabian erotology (XVI. Century)*, Cosmopoli: Kama Shastra Society of London and Benares, 1886; J. Colville, *The Perfumed Garden of Sensual Delight*, London: Kegan Paul International, 1999.

al-Qazwīnī, Zakariyyā' Ibn Muhammad (1849): *['Ajā'ib al-makhlūqāt wa āthār al-bilād]* Ferdinand Wüstenfeld (ed.), *Zakarija Ben Muhammed Ben Mahmud el-Cazwini's Kosmographie. Erster Theil. 'Ajā'ib al-makhlūqāt. Die Wunder der Schöpfung. Aus den Handschriften der Bibliotheken zu Berlin, Gotha, Dresden und Hamburg*, Göttingen: Dieterischen Buchhandlung.

al-Qumrī, Abū Manṣūr (1991): *Kitāb al-tanwīr fi 'l-iṣṭilāḥāt al-ṭibbiyya*, Riyadh: Maktab al-Tarbiyya al-'Arabiyya li-Duwal al-Khalīj.

al-Rāzī, Abū Bakr Muḥammad b. Zakariyyā (2007): *Kitāb al-bāh wa manāfi'ihi wa maḍārrihi wa mudawātihi*, Aḥmad Farīd al-Mazīdī (ed.) Cairo: Dār al-Āfāq al-'Arabiyya, pp. 291–370.

al-Rāzī, A. (1982): *Manāfi' al-aghdhiya wa-daf' maḍarrihā*, Beirut: Dār Iḥyā' al-'Ulūm.

al-Rāzī, A. (1955-1969): *al-Ḥāwī fi 'l-tibb*, 23 vols, Hyderabad.

al-Saffārīnī, Ibn Aḥmad, Rashīd Ibn 'Āmir Ghufaylī (1412/1991-2): *Qar' al-siyāṭ fī qam' ahl al-Liwāṭ*, Riyadh: Dār al-Ṭaḥāwī.

al-Samarqandī, Najīb al-Dīn (2016): *Kitāb al-aghdhiya wa 'l-ashriba*, Juliane Müller (ed./German translation), Leiden/Boston: Brill.

Sarkīs, Yūsuf Ilyās (1928): *Mu'jam al-maṭbū'āt al-'Arabiyya wa 'l-mu'arabba*, 2 vols, Cairo: Maktabat al-Thaqāfa al-Dīniyya.

al-Sharīf, 'Adnān (1990): *Min 'ilm al-ṭibb al-Qur'ānī: al-thawābit al-'ilmiyya fi 'l-Qur'ān al-karīm*, Beirut: Dār al-'Ilm li 'l-Malāyīn.

Shaykhū, Luwīs (1924): *Kitāb al-makhṭūṭāt al-'Arabiyya li 'l-katabat al-Naṣrāniyya. Catalogue des manuscrits des auteurs arabes chrétiens depuis l'Islam*, Beirut: Maṭba'at al-Ābā' al-Yasū'iyyīn.

al-Suyūṭī, Jalāl al-Dīn (2001): *al-Wishāḥ fī fawā'id al-nikāḥ*, Ṭala'at Ḥasan 'Abd al-Qawī (ed.), Damascus, Dār al-Kitāb al-'Arabī.

al-Suyūṭī, Jalāl al-Dīn (n.d.): *al-Raḥma fi 'l-ṭibb wa 'l-ḥikma*, Cairo: Dār al-Kutub al-'Arabiyya al-Kubrā.

al-Ṭabarī, Abū 'l-Ḥasan (1928): *Firdaws al-ḥikma*, M. Z. al-Ṣiddīqī, Berlin: Sonne.

al-Tīfāshī, Shihāb al-Dīn (1992): *Nuzhat al-albāb fīmā lā yūjad fi 'l-kitāb*, Jamāl Jum'a (ed.), London/Cyprus: Riad El-Rayess.

al-Tīfāshī, S. (1970): *Risāla fīmā yaḥtajī ilayhi al-rijāl wa 'l-nisā' fi isti'māl al-bāh mimmā yaḍurr wa yanfa'. Abhandlung darüber, was Männer und Frauen zur Ausübung des Geschlechtsverkehrs brauchen, was dabei nützt und schadet. Die Edition des arabischen Textes auf der Grundlage der Handschrift Al-Azhar Halim 34687 und der Handschrift Dar al-Kutub Kairo Mim Tibb unter Hinzuziehung der Handschrift Paris 3056*, Hassan Mohammad El-Haw (partial ed.), Universität Erlangen-Nürnberg.

al-Tīfāshī, S. (1892): *Rujū' al-shaykh ilā ṣibāh fi 'l-quwwa wa 'l-bāh*, Būlāq.

al-Warrāq, Abū Muḥammad al-Muẓaffar Ibn Naṣr Ibn Sayyār (1987): *Kitāb al-ṭabīkh wa 'l-iṣlāḥ al-aghdhiyya al-ma'kūlāt wa ṭayyib al-aṭ'ima al-maṣnū'āt*, Kaj Öhrnberg & Sahban Mroueh (eds.), Helsinki, Finnish Oriental Society;

al-Wāsiṭī, Shams al-Dīn Muḥammad Ibn 'Umar Ghamrī (1988): *al-Ḥukm al-maḍbūṭ fī taḥrīm fi 'l-qawm Lūṭ*, Tanta: Dār al-Ṣaḥābah li 'l-Turāth.

al-Ya'qūbī, Aḥmad Ibn 'Abd Ya'qūb (1892): *[Kitāb al-buldān] Kitāb al-boldān auctore Ahmed ibn abî Jakûb ibn Wādhih al-Kātib al-Jakûbî*, (Bibliotheca Geographorum Arabicorum, VII:1), 2nd ed., ed. M. J. Goeje, Leiden: E. J. Brill.

Yāqūt al-Ḥamawī (1866–73): *Mu'jam al-buldān*, 6 vols, ed. Ferdinand Wüstenfeld, Leipzig: F. A. Brockhaus.

Yāqūt al-Ḥamawī (1936-1938): *Mu'jam al-udabā': irshād al-arīb ilā ma'rifat al-adīb*, ed. A. F. Rifā'ī, Cairo: Matba'at al-Ma'mūn.

European languages

Abu Khalil, As'ad (1993): 'A note on the study of homosexuality in the Arab/Islamic civilization', *Arab Studies Journal*, 1:2, pp. 32–34.

Ahlwardt, Wilhelm (1887-99):. Verzeichniss der Arabischen Handschriften der Königlichen Bibliothek zu Berlin, 10 vols, Berlin: A. W. Schade (I) and A. Asher & Co. (II-X).

Ali, Kecia (2006): *Sexual ethics and Islam: feminist reflections on Qur'an, Hadith and Jurisprudence*, New York: Oneworld.

Allport, Susan (2016): Publisher: The *Primal Feast: Food, Sex, Foraging, and Love*, n.p.: Open Road Integrated Media, Inc.

Al-Sammani, Hanadi (2008): "Out of the closet: Representation of homosexuals and lesbians in modern Arabic literature", *Journal of Arabic Literature*, 39:2, pp. 270–310.

Al-Sayyid-Marsot, Afaf Lutfi (ed.) (1979): *Society and the sexes in medieval Islam*, Malibu CA: Undena Publications.

Amar, Zev & Ephraim Lev (2011): "Watermelon, chate melon, and cucumber: new light on traditional and innovative field crops in the Middle Ages", *Journal Asiatique*, 299, pp.193–204.

Amer, Sahar (2009): "Medieval Arab Lesbians and Lesbian-Like Women", *Journal of the History of Sexuality*, 18:2, pp. 215–236.

Ashtiany, Julia, T. M. Johnstone, J. D. Latham, R. B. Serjeant and G. Rex Smith (eds) (1990): *The Cambridge History of Arabic Literature. 'Abbasid belles-lettres*, Cambridge: Cambridge University Press.

Babayan, Kathryn & Afsaneh Najmabadi (2008): *Islamicate sexualities: Translations across temporal geographies of desire*, New Haven Mass.: Harvard University Press.

Batten, Rosalind M. (2018): *The Arabic commentaries on the Hippocratic aphorisms: Arabic learned medical discourse on women's bodies* (9th–15th Cent.), unpublished PhD diss., University of Manchester.

Benton, John F. (1985): "Trotula, women's problems, and the professionalization of medicine in the Middle Ages", *Bulletin of the History of Medicine*, 59:1, pp. 30–53.

Bos, Gerrit (2021): *The Medical Works of Moses Maimonides: New English Translations based on the Critical Editions of the Arabic Manuscripts*, Leiden: Brill.

Bos, G., Charles Burnett & W. F. Ryan Moshe Taube (2019): *Maimonides' on Coitus*, Leiden: Brill.

Bos, G. (1997): *Ibn al-Jazzār on sexual diseases and their treatment. A critical edition of* Zād al-musāfir wa qūt al-hādir. *Provisions for the Traveller and Nourishment for the Sedentary, Book 6*, London/New York: Kegan Paul International.

Bouhdiba, Abdelwahab (1975): *La sexualite en Islam*, Paris: PUF.

Boyle, John (1963): "The longer introduction to the 'Zij-i Ilkhani' of Nasir-ad-Din Tusi", *Journal of Semitic Studies* 8:2, pp. 244–254.

Boyle, John Andrew (1961): "The death of the last 'Abbasid Caliph: a contemporary Muslim account", *Journal of semitic studies*, 6:2, pp.145–61.

Bousquet, G. H. (1966): *L'ethique sexuelle en Islam*, Paris: Desclée de Brouwer.

Brockelmann, Carl (1937–49): *Geschichte der arabischen Literatur*, 2 vols, 3 Suppl. vols, Leiden: E. J. Brill.

Browne, Edward G. (1900): A hand-list of the Muhammadan manuscripts, including all those written in the Arabic character, preserved in the library of the University of Cambridge, Cambridge: Cambridge University Press.

Bummel, Julia (1999): *Zeugung und pränatale Entwicklung des Menschen nach Schriften mittelalterlicher muslimischer Religionsgelehrter über die "Medizin des Propheten"*, unpubl. PhD thesis, University of Hamburg.

Burnett, Charles S. F. (2001): "The Coherence of the Arabic-Latin translation program in Toledo in the Twelfth Century", *Science in Context*, 14:1–2, pp. 249–288.

Burnett, C. S. F.& Danielle Jacquart (eds) (1994): *Constantine the African and 'Alī Ibn Al-'Abbās Al-Maǧūsī: The Pantegni and related texts*, Leiden: Brill.

Burton, Richard (1885–1889): *A plain and literal translation of the Arabian Nights' Entertainments, now entitled The Book of The Thousand Nights and a Night; with introduction explanatory notes on the manners and customs of Moslem men and a Terminal Essay upon the history of the Nights*, 10 vols, 7 Supp. vols, Benares: The Kamashastra Society.

Cadden, Joan (1993): *Meanings of sex difference in the Middle Ages: medicine, science, and culture*, Cambridge University Press.

Canadé Sautman, F. & P. Shengorn (2001), *Same sex love and desire among women in the Middle Ages*, New York: Palgrave.

Capezzone, Leonardo (2012): "La perfezione del triangolo. Tre soggetti d'amore dal *Kitāb al-Muwashshā di al-Washshā'*, per una rilettura dell'amor cortese arabo", *InVerbis*, 2, pp. 55–74.

Celentano, Giuseppe (ed.) (1979): *Due scritti medici di al-Kindī*, Naples: Istituto orientale di Napoli.

Cervulle, Maxime & Nick Rees-Roberts (2009): "Queering the Orientalist porn package: Arab men in French gay pornography", *New Cinemas: Journal of Contemporary Film*, 6:3, pp. 197–208.

Cervulle, M. (2008): "French homonormativity and the commodification of the Arab body", *Radical History Review*, 100, pp. 171–179.

Chebel, Malek: (1984): *Le corps en Islam*, Paris: PUF (2nd ed. 1999; 3rd ed. 2004).

Chebel, M. (1986): *Le livre des séductions suivi de Dix Aphorismes sur l'amour*, Paris: Payot (2nd ed. 1997).

Chebel, M. (1988): *L'Esprit de sérail, mythes et pratiques sexuelles au Maghreb*, Paris: Payot (2nd ed. 1997).

Chebel, M. (1995): *Encyclopédie de l'amour en Islam. Érotisme, beauté et sexualité dans le monde arabe, en Perse et en Turquie*, Paris: Payot (2nd ed. 2003).

Chebel, M. (2004): *Dictionnaire amoureux de l'islam*, Paris: Plon.

Chebel, M. (2006): *Le Kama sutra arabe, 2000 ans de littérature érotique en Orient*, Paris: Pauvert.

Chipman, Leigh (2009): *The World of pharmacy and pharmacists in Mamluk Cairo*, Leiden: Brill.

Colligan, Colette (2003): "'A race of born pederasts': Sir Richard Burton, homosexuality, and the Arabs", *Nineteenth-Century Contexts*, 25:1, 1–20.

Compier, Abdul Haq (2012): "Rhazes in the Renaissance of Andreas Vesalius", *Medical History*, 56:1, pp. 3–25.

Conrad, Lawrence I., Michael Neve, Vivian Nutton, Roy Porter & Andrew Weart (1995): *The Western medical tradition, 800BC to 1800AD*, Cambridge University Press.

Corriente, Federico (1997): *A Dictionary of Andalusi Arabic*, Leiden: Brill.

Dabashi, Hamid (1996): "Khwājah Naṣīr al-Dīn al-Ṭūsī: The philosopher/vizier and the intellectual climate of his times," in *History of Islamic Philosophy*, ed. Seyyed Hossein Nasr and Oliver Leaman, New York: Routledge, vol. 2, pp. 527–584.

Dakhlia, Jocelyne (2007): "Homoérotismes et trames historiographiques du monde islamique", *Annales. Histoire, Sciences Sociales*, 5, pp. 1097–1120.

Dalby, Andrew (2003): *Food in the ancient world from A to Z*, London: Routledge.

Dalby, A. (1996): *Siren Feasts: A history of food and gastronomy in Greece*, New York: Routledge.

Daniélou, Alain (1993): *The Complete Kama Sutra*, Rochester, VT: Park Street Press.

Davidson, Alan & Tom Jaine (eds.) (2014): *The Oxford Companion to food*, 3rd edition, Oxford: Oxford University Press.

Davidson, Richard M. (2011): *Flame of Yahweh: Sexuality in the Old Testament*, Peabody Mass.: Hendrickson Publishers.

Declich, Lorenzo (1995a): "L'erotologia araba, profilo bibliografico", *Rivista degli Studi Orientali*, LXVIII, Fasc. 3–4, pp. 249–65.

Declich, L. (1995b): "L'erotologia di Galâl ad-Dîn as-Suyūtī", *Alifba*, XVII, pp. 126–47.

Degen, R. (1978): "Al-Safarjal. A marginal note to Ibn al-Bayṭār. *Kitāb al-Jāmi' li-mufradāt al-adwiya wal-aghdhiya*", *Journal of the History of Arabic Science*, 2, pp. 143–148.

de Lacy, Phillip (1992): *Galen, On semen*, Berlin: Akademie Verlag.

De Montalvo, Soledad (1989): *Women, Food and Sex in History*, Parsippany, NJ: American Atheist Press.

De Slane, William Mac Guckin (1883–1895): *Catalogue des manuscrits arabes*, 2 vols, Paris: Imprimerie nationale.

Devereux, Robert (1966): "XIth century Muslim views on women, marriage, love and sex", Central Asiatic Journal, 11, pp. 134–40.

Dietrich, Albert (1991): *Die Dioscurides-Erklärung des Ibn al-Baitār. Ein Beitrag zur arabischen Pflanzensynonymik des Mittlealters, Göttingen: Akademie der Wissenschaften in Göttingen*, Philologisch-Historische Klasse.

Dietrich, A. (1988): *Dioscurides triumphans. Ein Anonymer Arabischer Kommentar (Ende 12. Jahrh. N. Chr.) Zur Materia Medica*, 2 vols, Göttingen: Vandenhoeck & Ruprecht.

Dioscorides, Pedanios (2000): *De Materia Medica: Being an Herbal with many other medicinal materials*, Tess Anne Osbaldeston (trans.), Johannesburg: Ibidis Press.

Dols, Michael (1984): *Medieval Islamic medicine. Ibn Riḍwān's treatise "On the Prevention of Bodily Ills in Egypt"*, Berkeley: University of California Press.

Donkin, R. A. (1999): *Dragon's brain perfume. An historical geography of camphor*, Leiden: Brill.

Dover, Kenneth Richard (1984): *Greek homosexuality*, Cambridge MA: Harvard University Press.

Dozy, Pieter Reinhart (1877–81): *Supplément aux dictionnaires arabes*, 2 vols, Leiden: E. J. Brill.

Dunne, Bruce (1998): "Power and Sexuality in the Middle East." *Middle East Reporti*, 206, 28:1, pp. 8–12.

Dunne, B. W. (1990): "Homosexuality in the Middle East: An Agenda for Historical Research", *Arab Studies Quarterly*, 12:3–4, pp. 55–82.

Duran, Khalid (1993): "Homosexuality in Islam", in *Homosexuality and World Religions*, Valley Forge, Pennsylvania: Trinity P International, pp. 181–197.

Edwardes, Allen (1963): *The jewel in the lotus. A historical survey of the sexual culture of the East*, Tandem Books.

Ekdahl Ravicz, Marilyn (2001): *Erotic Cuisine: A natural history of aphrodisiac cookery*, n.p.: Xlibris Corporation.

El Feki, Shereen (2013): *Sex and the citadel. Intimate life in a changing Arab world*, London: Chatto & Windus.

El-Masri, Y. (1962): *Le drame sexuel de la femme dans l'Orient arabe*, Paris: Lafont.

El Menyawi, Hassan (2012): "Same-sex marriage in Islamic law", *Wake Forest Journal of Law & Police*, 2:2, pp. 375–531.

El-Rouayheb, Khaled & Sabine Schmidtke (eds) (2017): *The Oxford Handbook of Islamic Philosophy*, Oxford: Oxford University Press.

El-Rouayheb, Khaled (2005): *Before Homosexuality in the Arab-Islamic World, 1500–1800*, Chicago: The University of Chicago Press.

Encyclopaedia of Islam (1960–2005), 2nd ed, 12 vols., Leiden/London: E. J. Brill.

Encyclopaedia Iranica (1982–2020), 16 vols., Leiden/London: E. J. Brill.

Farah, Madelaine (1984), *Marriage and sexuality in Islam: A translation of al Ghazzali's Book on the Etiquette of Marriage*, Salt Lake City: University of Utah Press.

Fellmann, Irene (1986): *Das Aqrābādīn al-Qalānisī: quellenkritische und begriffsanalytische Untersuchungen zur arabisch-pharmazeutischen Literatur*, Beirut/Wiesbaden: F. Steiner.

Foucault, Michel (1978–90): *The history of sexuality*, 3 vols, trans. Robert Hurley, New York: Pantheon Books.

Francoeur, Robert T. & Raymond J. Noonan (eds.) (2003): *The Continuum Complete International Encyclopedia of Sexuality*, 4 volumes, London: Bloomsbury.

Franke Patrick (2012): "Before scientia sexualis in Islamic culture: 'ilm al-bāh between erotology, medicine and pornography", *Social Identities: Journal for the Study of Race, Nation and Culture*, 18:2, pp. 161–173.

Gadelrab, Sherry Sayed (2010): "Discourses on sex differences in medieval scholarly Islamic thought", *Journal of the History of Medicine and Allied Sciences*, pp. 1–42.

Ghersetti, Antonella (2016): "Al-Suyuti, a Polymath of the Mamluk Period", *Proceedings of the themed day of the First Conference of the School of Mamluk Studies (Ca' Foscari University, Venice, June 23, 2014)*, Leiden: Brill.

Ghoussoub, Mai & Emma Sinclair-Webb (eds), (2000): *Imagined masculinities: Male identity and culture in the modern Middle East*, London: Saqi.

Giffen, Lois Anita (1971): *Theory of Profane Love Among the Arabs: The Development of the Genre*, New York: New York University Press.

Goitien, S. D. (1967–88): *A Mediterranean society; the Jewish communities of the Arab world as portrayed in the documents of the Cairo Geniza*, Berkeley: University of California Press.

Green, Monica Helen (2002): *The Trotula: An English translation of the medieval compendium of women's medicine*, Philadelphia: University of Pennsylvania Press.

Green, M. H. (1985): *The transmission of ancient theories of female physiology and disease through the early Middle Ages*, unpubl. PhD thesis, Princeton University.

Groom, Nigel (1981): *Frankincense and myrrh. A study of the Arabian incense trade*, London/New York: Longman.

Gutas, Dimitri (1998): *Greek thought, Arabic culture: The Graeco-Arabic translation movement in Baghdad and early 'Abbasid society (2nd–4th/8th–10th century)*, London: Routledge.

Habib, Samar (ed.) (2009): *Islam and Homosexuality*, 2 Vols, Santa Barbara, CA: ABC–CLIO, LLC.

Habib, S. (2007): *Female homosexuality in the Middle East: histories and representations*, London/New York: Routledge.

Hasselhoff, Görge (2002): "Maimonides in the Latin Middle Ages: an introductory survey", *Jewish Studies Quarterly*, 9, pp. 1–20.

Heine, Peter (1982): *Untersuchungen zu Anbau, Produktion und Konsom des Weins im arabisch-islamischen Mittelalter*, Wiesbaden: Harrassowitz.

Hinds, Martin & El Said Badawi (1986): *A dictionary of Egyptian Arabic, Arabic-English*, Beirut: Librairie du Liban.

Hinz, Walther (1970): *Islamische Masse und Gewichte umgerechnet ins metrische System*, Leiden/Cologne: Brill.

Hodgson, Michael G.S. (1977): *The Venture of Islam. Conscience and history in a world civilization. The Classical Age of Islam*, Chicago: Chicago University Press.

Holt, P. M. (1992): *The age of the crusades: The Near East from the Eleventh Century to 1517*, Harlow: Longman.

Hopwood, Derek (1999): *Sexual Encounters in the Middle East: the British, the French and the Arabs*, Reading: Ithaca Press.

Hospodar, Miriam (2004): "Aphrodisiac Foods: Bringing Heaven to Earth", *Gastronomica*, 4:4, pp. 82–93.

Isakander, A. Z. (1984): *A descriptive list of Arabic manuscripts on medicine and science at the University of California, Los Angeles*, Leiden: Brill.

Issa Bey, Ahmed (1930): Dictionnaire des Noms des Plantes. Cairo: Imprimerie Nationale.

Jacquart, Danielle (1996): "The influence of Arabic medicine in the Medieval West", in R. Rashed (ed.), *Encyclopedia of the history of Arabic science*, London: Routledge, III, pp. 963–984.

Jacquart, D. (ed.) (1994): *La formation du vocabulaire scientifique et intellectuel dans le monde arabe*, Turnhout: Brepols.

Jacquart, D. & Françoise Micheau (1990): *La médecine arabe et l'Occident médiéval*, Paris: Maisonneuve et Larose.

Jacquart, D. & Claude Thomasset (1988): *Sexuality and medicine in the Middle Ages*, Cambridge: Polity Press.

Jorati, Hadi (2014): "Science and Society in Medieval Islam: Nasir al-Din Tusi and the Politics of Patronage", unpublished PhD diss., Yale University.

Joseph, Suad (2003): *Encyclopedia of Women and Islamic Cultures.*

Volume 3: Family, Body, Sexuality and Health, Leiden: Brill.

Kahl, Oliver (2003): *Sabur Ibn Sahl: the Small Dispensatory*, Leiden: Brill.

Keddie, Nikkie R. & Beth Baron (1991): *Women in Middle Eastern history: Shifting boundaries in sex and gender*, New Haven/ London: Yale University Press.

Kennedy, Philip F. (2007): *Abu Nuwas: A Genius of Poetry*, London: OneWorld Publications.

Kircher, Heidi Gisela (1967): *Die "einfachen Heilmittel" aus dem "Handbuch der Chirurgie" des Ibn al-Quff*, Bonn: Rheinischen Friedrich-Wilhelms-Universität.

Kligerman, Nicole (2007): "Homosexuality in Islam: A Difficult Paradox", *Macalester Islam Journal*, 2:3, pp. 53–64.

Kraemer, Joel H. (1986): *Humanism in the Renaissance of Islam. The Cultural Revival during the Buyid Age*, Leiden: Brill.

Kruk, Remke (1976): "Pseudo-Aristotle: An Arabic version of Problemata Physica X", *Isis*, 67, pp. 251–6.

Kuru, Selim Sirri (2000): *A sixteenth century scholar: Deli Birader and his Dāfi `ül-ġumūm ve rafi`ü 'l-humūm*, unpubl. PhD diss., Harvard University.

Lagrange, Frédéric (2008): "The obscenities of the Vizier", in Babayan and Najmabadi (eds), *Islamicate Sexualities*, pp. 161–203.

Lagrange, F. (2000): "Male homosexuality in modern Arabic literature", in Mai Ghoussoub and Emma Sinclair-Webb (eds), *Imagined Masculinities: Male Identity and Culture in the Modern Middle East*, London: Saqi Books, London, pp.169–198.

Lahoucine, Ouzgane (ed.) (2006): *Islamic masculinities*, London: Zed.

Lal, Kanwar (1966): *The cult of desire. An interpretation of erotic sculpture of India*, Asia Press.

Lane, W. E. (1863–74): *Arabic-English Lexicon derived from the best and the most copious Eastern sources; comprising a very large number of words and significations omitted in the KÁmoos, with supplements to its abridged and defective explanations, ample grammatical and critical comments, and examples in prose and verse*, 5 vols, London, (vol 6–8, ed. Stanley Lane Poole, London, 1877–93).

Laqueur, Thomas (1992): *Making sex: body and gender from the Greeks to Freud*, Cambridge: Harvard University Press.

Leclerc, Lucien (1876): *Histoire de la médecine arabe*, Paris: E. Leroux.

Leibowitz, J. Joshua Otto & Shlomo Marcus (1974): *Moses Maimonides. On the causes of symptoms*, Berkeley: University of California Press.

Lev, Ephraim & Zev Amar (2008): *Practical Materia Medica of the Medieval Eastern Mediterranean according to the Cairo Genizah*, Leiden: Brill.

Levey, Martin (1966): *The medical formulary of Aqrābīdhīn of al-Kindī*, Madison: University of Wisconsin.

Lewinsohn, Richard (1959): *A History of sexual customs*, New York: Harper & Brothers.

Lewis, Bernard (1993): *Islam and the West*, Oxford: Oxford University Press.

Lindgren, Amy (2005): *The wandering womb and the peripheral penis: ender and the fertile body in late medieval infertility Treatises*, unpubl. PhD diss., University of California.

López-Baralt, Luce (1992): *Un Kama Sutra Español*, Madrid: Ediciones Siruela.

Lowry, Joseph Edmund & Devin J. Stewart (2009): *Essays in Arabic literary biography II: 1350–1850*, Wiesbaden: Otto Harrassowitz.

Mahawatte, Royce (2003): "Loving the Asian: race, gay pornography and the essentials of passion", in Pamel Church Gibson (ed.), *More Dirty Looks: Gender, Pornography and Power*, 2nd ed. London: BFI Publishing.

Malti-Douglas, Fedwa (1991): *Woman's body, woman's word: gender and discourse in Arabo-Islamic writing*, Princeton University Press.

Mande, Gabrielle (1983): *Islamische Erotik*, Fribourg: Liber.

Massad, Joseph (2002): "Re-Orienting desire: the Gay International and the Arab World", *Public Culture*, 14, pp. 361–385.

Matar, Nabil (1994): "Homosexuality in the early novels of Nageeb Mahfouz", *Journal of Homosexuality*, 26:4, pp. 77–90.

Meyerhof, M. (1940): *Un glossaire de matière médicale, composé par Maïmonide: Šarh asmā' al-'uqqār (l'explication des noms de drogues)*, (Mémoires Présentés à l'Institut d'Egypte, 41), Cairo: Imprimerie de l'Institut Français d'Archéologie Orientale.

Mimura, Taro (2020): "Ghulāms (Slave Boys) and Scientific Research in the Abbasid Period: The Example of the Amājūr Family", *Historia Scientiarum*, 29, pp. 182–197.

Mortel, Richard T. (1990): "Weights and measures in Mecca during the late Ayyubid and Mamluk periods," in R. B. Serjeant & R. L. Bidwell, *Arabian Studies*, 8, Cambridge University Press, pp. 177–85.

Murray, Stephen O. and Will Roscoe (eds) (1979): *Islamic Homosexualities: culture, history, and literature*, New York: New York University Press.

Musallam, B. F. (1983): *Sex and society in Islam: Birth control before the Nineteenth Century*, Cambridge: Cambridge University Press.

Muschler, Reno (1912): *A manual flora of Egypt*, Berlin: R. Friendländer & Son.

Najmabadi, Afsaneh (2005): *Women with mustaches and men without beards: gender and sexual anxieties of Iranian modernity*, Berkeley: University of California Press.

Myrne, Pernilla (2020): *Female Sexuality in the Early Medieval Islamic World: Gender and Sex in Arabic Literature*, London: I.B. Tauris.

Myrne, P. (2018), "Women and Men in al-Suyūṭī's Guides to Sex and Marriage", *Mameluk Studies Review*, 21, 47–67.

Newman, Daniel (2023): *The Exile's Cookbook: medieval gastronomic treasures from al-Andalus and North Africa*, London: Saqi Books.

Newman, D. (2020): *The Sultan's Feast: A Fifteenth-Century Egyptian cookbook*, London: Saqi Books.

Newman, D. (2015): "Arabic translation activity, Pre-Modern Period (8th–12th centuries)", in Martin, Richard C., Afsaruddin, Asma & Varisco, Daniel M. (eds.), *Encyclopedia of Islam and The Muslim World*, Basingstoke: Macmillan.

Nathan, B. (1994): "Medieval Arabic medical views on male homosexuality", *Journal of Homosexuality*, 26:4, pp. 37–39.

O'Boyle, Cornelius (1998): *The art of medicine: Medical teaching at the University of Paris, 1250–1400*, Leiden: Brill.

Ouerfelli, Mohamed (2008): *Le sucre. Production, commercialisation et usages dans la Méditerranée médiévale*, Leiden/Boston: Brill.

Paris, Harry S., Marie-Christine Daunay & Jules Janick (2011): "Occidental diffusion of cucumber (Cucumis sativus) 500–1300 CE: two routes to Europe", *Annales of Botany*, 108:3, pp. 471–84.

Parker, Holt N. (1992): "Love's body anatomized: the ancient erotic handbooks and the rhetoric of sexuality", in Amy Richlin (ed.), *Pornography and representation in Greece and Rome*, Oxford University Press, pp. 90–111.

Perho, I. (1995): *The Prophet's Medicine: A creation of Muslim Traditionalist scholars*, (Studia Orientalis, 74), Helsinki: Finnish Oriental Society.

Pormann, Peter E. & Emilie Savage-Smith (2007): *Medieval Islamic medicine*, Edinburgh University Press.

Rahman, Fazlur (1989): *Health and Medicine in the Islamic Tradition. Change and Identity*, New York: Crossroad.

Rasslan, W. (1934): *Mohammed und die Medizin nach den Überlieferungen*, (Abhandlungen zur Geschichte der Medizin und der Naturwissenschaften, 1), Berlin.

Redhouse, J. W. (1880): *Redhouse's Turkish dictionary: in two parts, English and Turkish, and Turkish and English*, 2 vols, London: Bernard Quaritch.

Rosenthal, Franz (1986): *The Muqaddimah. An introduction to history*, 3 vols, London: Routledge & Kegan Paul.

Rosenthal, F. (1978): "Ar-Rāzī on the hidden illness", *Bulletin of the History of Medicine*, 52, pp. 45–60.

Rosenthal, F. (1975): *The Classical heritage in Islam*, Berkeley: University of California Press.

Rosner, Fred (1995): *Šarh asmā' al-ʿuqqār. Glossary of drug*, Haifa: Maimonides Research Institute.

Rosner, F. (1984): *Maimonides medical writings: treatises on poisons, hemorrhoids, cohabitation*, Maimonides Research Institute.

Rosner, F. & S. Muntner (1970): *The Medical aphorisms of Moses Maimonides*, New York: Yeshiva University Press.

Rouhi, Leyla (1999): *Mediation and Love: A Study of the Medieval Go-*

between in Key Romance and Near-Eastern texts, Leiden: Brill.

Rowson, Everett K., (2008): "Homoerotic liaisons among the Mamluk Elite in Late Medieval. Egypt and Syria", in Kathryn Babayan & Afsaneh Najmabadi (eds), *Islamicate Sexualities*, pp. 204–238.

Rowson, E. K. (2006): "Arabic: Middle Ages to Nineteenth Century", *Encyclopedia of Erotic Literature*, I, Gaëtan Brulotte & John Phillips (eds), New York: Routledge, pp. 43–61.

Rowson, E. K. (2004): "Middle Eastern Literature: Arabic", *glbtq: An Encyclopedia of Gay, Lesbian, Bisexual, Transgender, and Queer Culture* (http://www.glbtq.com/literature/mid_e_lit_arabic.html).

Rowson, E. K. (2003): "Gender irregularity as éntertainment: Institutionalized Transvestism at the Caliphal Court in Medieval Baghdad", in Sharon Farmer and Carol Braun Pasternack (eds), *Gender and Difference in the Middle Ages*, Minneapolis: University of Minnesota Press, pp. 45–72.

Rowson, E. K. (1997): "Two homoerotic narratives from Mamluk literature: al-Safadi's *Law`at al-shaki* and Ibn Daniyal's *al-Mutayyam*," in . J. W. Wright, Jr. & Everett K. Rowson (eds), *Homoeroticism in Classical Arabic Literature*, New York: Columbia University Press, pp. 158–191.

Rowson, E. K. (1991a): "The effeminates of early Medina", *Journal of the American Oriental Society* 111, pp. 671–93.

Rowson, E. K. (1991b): "The categorization of gender and sexual irregularity in medieval Arabic vice lists", in J. Epstein & K. Straub (eds.), *Bodyguards. The cultural politics of gender ambiguity*, New York/London: Routledge, pp. 50–79.

Rüegg, Walter & H. De Ridder-Syoens (eds) (1992): *A history of the University in Europe*, Vol. 1, Cambridge University Press.

Sanders, Paula (1991): "Gendering the Ungendered Body: Hermaphrodites in Medieval Islamic Law", in Beth Baron and Nikki Keddie, eds., *Women in Middle Eastern History*, pp. 74–95.

Savage Smith, Emilie (2011): *A New Catalogue of Arabic Manuscripts in the Bodleian Library, Oxford, Volume 1: Medicine*, Oxford: Oxford University Press.

Schild, Maarten (1990): "Mujun", "Mukhannath", in Wayne R. Dynes (ed.), *Encyclopedia of Homosexuality*, New York:

Garland, pp. 848–50.

Schild, M. (1988): "The irresistible beauty of boys: Middle Eastern attitudes towards boy-love", *Paidika*, 3, pp. 37–48.

Sbath, Paul (1938-40): *Al-Fihris. Catalogue de manuscrits arabes*, Cairo: Imprimerie Al-Chark.

Sbath, P. (1932–33): "Kitāb al-Azmina. *Le Livre des temps* d'Ibn Massawaïh, *médecin chrétien célèbre décédé en 857*", Bulletin de l'Institut d'Egypte, 15, pp. 235–57.

Schindler, Herbert & Helma Frank (1961): *Tiere in Pharmazie und Medizin*, Stuttgart: Hippokrates-Verlag.

Schipperges, Heinrich (1976): *Die arabische Medizin im lateinischen Mittelalter*, Berlin: Springer Verlag.

Schipperges, H. (1964): *Die Assimilation der arabischen Medizin durch das Lateinische Mittelalter*, Wiesbaden: F. Steiner.

Schmitt, Arno (2001–2002): "*Liwāṭ* im Fiqh: Männliche Homosexualität?", *Journal of Arabic and Islamic Studies*, Vol. 4.

Schmitt, Arno & Jehoeda Sofer (eds) (1992): *Sexuality and eroticism among males in Moslem societies*, New York/London: Haworth Press.

Schmidtke, Sabine (1999): "Homoeroticism and homosexuality in Islam: A review article", *Bulletin of the School of Oriental and African Studies*, 62, pp. 260–6.

Schmucker, Werner (1969): *Die pflanzliche und mineralische Materia Medica im Firdaus al-hikma des 'Alī ibn Sahl Rabban at-Tabarī*, Bonn: Orientalischen Seminars der Universität Bonn.

Schoeler, G. (1990): *Arabische Handschriften*, Stuttgart: Franz Steiner.

Selove, Emily & Rosalind Batten (2014): "Making men and women. Arabic commentaries on the gynaecological Hippocratic Aphorisms in context," *Annales Islalogiques*, 48:1, pp. 239–62.

Serjeant, R. B. (1997): *The book of misers*, rev. Ezzedine Ibrahim, Reading: Garnet.

Serjeant, R. B. (1965): "Notices on the "Frankish chancre" (Syphilis) in Yemen, Egypt, and Persia", *Journal of Semitic Studies*, 10:2, pp. 241–252.

Sezgin, Fuat (1967–1984): *Geschichte des arabischen Schrifttums*, 9 vols, Leiden: Brill.

Shalakany, Amr A. (2008): "Islamic legal histories", *Berkeley Journal of Middle Eastern & Islamic Law*, 1, pp. 1–82.

Sharif, M. M. (1963–6): *A history of Muslim philosophy. With short accounts of other disciplines and the modern renaissance in Muslim lands*, 2 vols, Wiesbaden: Otto Harrassowitz.

Siegel, Rudolph (1976): *Galen on the affected parts*, Basel/New York: Karger.

Spies, Otto (1969): "Das erste Auftreten der Syphilis in Ägypten im Jahre 1498." *Sudhoffs Archiv Geschichte der Medizin* 52:4, pp. 382–384.

Stasolla, M.G. (2006): "Sessualità e società nel mondo islamico medievale (Baghdad, VIII-IX secolo)", in Comportamenti e immaginario della sessualità nell'Alto Medioevo, *Atti delle Settimane di Studio della Fondazione Centro Italiano di Studi sull'Alto Medioevo, LIII, 31 marzo–5 aprile 2005*, Spoleto, pp. 261–302.

Steckler, Paul (2007–8): "Brotherhood of vice: sodomy, Islam, and the Knights Templar", *Perspectives: A Journal of Historical Inquiry*, 34, pp. 13–28.

Steingass, Francis Joseph (1892): *A Comprehensive Persian-English dictionary, including the Arabic words and phrases to be met with in Persian literature.* London: Routledge & K. Paul.

Steinschneider, Moritz (1902): *Die arabische Literatur der Juden: ein Beitrag zur Literaturgeschichte der Araber, grossentheils aus hand- schriftlichen Quellen*, Frankfurt: J. Kaufmann.

Steinschneider, M. (1900): *Die Heilmittelnamen der Araber*, Frankfurt: J. Kaufmann.

Storey, C. A. (1972): *Persian literature. A bio-biographical survey*, Vol. 2:2/E, Oxford: Royal Asiatic Society of Great Britain and Ireland.

Szombathy, Zoltan (2013): *Mujūn: Libertinism in mediaeval Muslim society and literature*, Oxford: Gibb Memorial Trust.

Turner, Jack (2004): *Spice. The History of a Temptation*, New York: Vintage.

Tziallas, Evangelos (2009): *"Too dark, too hairy, too much!": Representations of Arab men and "Arabness" in contemporary gay male pornography*, Unpubl. MFA diss., York University (Canada), 2009.

Ullmann, Manfred (1978): *Islamic medicine*, Edinburgh: Edinburgh University Press.

Ullmann, Manfred (1970): *Die Medizin im Islam*, Leiden: E. J. Brill.

Uri, Johannes (1787): *Bibliothecae Bodleianae codicum manuscriptorum orientalium videlicet Hebraicorum, Chaldaicorum, Syriaocorum, Aethiopicorum, Arabicorum, Persicorum, Turcicorum, Copticorumque Catalogus. Pars Prima*, Oxford: Clarendon Press.

Vajda, Georges (1953): *Index général des manuscrits arabes musulmans de la Bibliothèque Nationale de Paris*, Paris: Bibliothèque Nationale.

Walzer, R. (ed.) (1962): *Greek into Arabic. Essays on Islamic philosophy*, Cambridge MA: Harvard University Press.

Watt, Montgomery (1972): *The Influence of Islam on Medieval Europe*, Edinburgh: Edinburgh University Press.

Wedeck, Harry E. (2022): *Dictionary of aphrodisiacs*, New York: Philosophical Library.

Weisser, Ursula (1983): *Zeugung, Vererbung und pränatale Entwicklung in der Medizin des Arabischislamischen Mittelalters*, Erlangen: Lüling.

Whelehan, Patricia & Anne Bolin (eds.) (2015): *The international encyclopedia of human sexuality*, 3 vols., London: Wiley Blackwell.

Wikan, Umi (1977): "Man becomes woman: Transsexualism in Oman as a key to gender roles," *Man*, 12, pp. 304–319 (replies, Man, 13, 1978, pp. 133–134, 322–333, 473–475, 663–671; Man, 15, 1980, pp. 541–542).

Williams, Craig A. (1999): *Roman homosexuality*, Oxford University Press.

Wright, J. W. Jr. & E. K. Rowson (eds.) (1997): *Homoeroticism in classical Arabic literature*, New York.

Yep, Stephanie (2012): *A hermeneutical consideration of Islamic jurisprudence on same-sex acts*, unpubl. PhD diss., Wake Forest University.

Ze'evi, Dror (2006): *Producing desire: changing sexual discourse in the Ottoman Middle East, 1500–1900*, Berkeley: University of California Press.

Index of Proper Names

Index of Arabic Terms

Index of English Terms

نَصيرُ الدِّينِ الطُّوسِيُّ

كتابُ البابِ الباهيَّةِ وَالتَّرَاكِيبِ السُّلْطانيَّةِ

كِتابُ البابِ الباهِيَّةِ وَالتَّراكِيبِ السُّلْطانِيَّةِ[١]

(١ظ) بسم الله الرحمن الرحيم الحمد لله رب العالمين وصلّى الله على سيّدنا محمّد خاتم النبيين[٢] وعلى آله صحبه أجمعين، **وبعد**[٣]

فإنّ الله تعالى قد أكمل النفوس الناطقة الإنسانية بمواهب إنعامه وملا معادن خواطر الحكماء بإعلامه لهم جواهر حكمته كما قال الله[٤] سبحانه تعالى[٥] ولقد أتينا لقمان الحكمة الآية[٦] فالفضل بيده كما قال الله تعالى وإن الفضل بيد الله يؤتيه من يشاء والله ذو الفضل العظيم.

ونشرع الآن في[٧] يبان سبب[٨] تأليف هذا الكتاب وكشف أسرار الحكماء وإظهار رموزاتهم في هذا الكتاب[٩] هو[١٠] أنّ خليفة الزمان سلطان قازان[١١] كان

---

١ هذا كتاب الباهية في التراكيب السلطانية تأليف الشيخ العلامة والحر الفهامة أبي البركات ناصر الدين الطوسي رحمه الله تعالي وجميع المسلمين. أمين. أمين. أمين. (ق/غ) / -- (ب)

٢ خاتم النبيين: -- (ب)

٣ الرحيم ... وبعد: + وبه نستعين الحمد لله الذي شهده بوده جميع الكائنات والصلاة والسّلام على أفضل الانام سيّد محمد المبعوث الآيات الواضحات وعلى آله وصحبه والتابعين لهم المكرمات (ق/غ)

٤ الله: -- (ق)

٥ تعالى: -- (ق/غ)

٦ الآيه فالفضل بيده كما قال الله تعالى: فالإحسان منه والفضل بيده كما قال سبحانه وان الفضل (ق)

٧ ونشرع الآن في: فصل في (ب)

٨ بيان: -- (ق)

٩ نشرع ... الكتاب: فصل في بيان سبب تأليف هذا الكتاب (ب)

١٠ في هذا الكتاب هو: وذلك

١١ قازان: فازان (ق/ب)

له ولد ذا جمال[١٢] وبهاء فحصل له في بدنه الريح[١٣] الفالج[١٤] وأبطل شقته.[١٥] فسأل[١٦] الشيخ العالم ملك (٢و) علماء العصر وأستاذ فضلاء الدهر، قطب الإسلام والمسلمين[١٧] ومربّي الملوك والسلاطين[١٨] أبو[١٩] البركات الخواجا[٢٠] ناصر الدين الطوسي رحمه الله تعالى[٢١] أن يؤلف كتابًا في الطبّ صغير الحجم كثير الفوائد لينتفع به المسلمين.[٢٢] فأجابه الى سؤاله[٢٣] وألّف هذه الرسالة وجمع فوائدها من كتب المتقدّمين والمتأخّرين[٢٤] وجعلها حاوية الفوائد نافعة وكافية[٢٥] لحفظ صحّة بدن الإنسان وسبب وقوع العلّة وعلاجها. لا يحتاج أحد بسبب مطالعتها إلى معالجة طبيب ويكتفي بها في مداوات ما يحدث من العلل والأمراض وغير ذلك من الفوائد المجرّبة والمنافع والخواصّ المنتخبة.[٢٦] ورتبتها على[٢٧] ثمانية عشر بابًا وسمّيتها[٢٨] **كتاب الباب الباهية والتراكيب السلطانية.**

---

١٢ جمال: حسن وجمال (ب)

١٣ الريح: ريح (ق)

١٤ الفالج: + بدانه خفيف ما اقدر الرفعة من المكان بعد رشيد الحلق

١٥ شقته: شقه (ب)

١٦ سأل: سألوا (ب)

١٧ المسلمين: المسك المبين (ب)

١٨ مالك ... السلاطين: الفاضل (ق)

١٩ ابو: أبا (ق)

٢٠ الخوجا: الخوجه (غ)

٢١ رحمه الله تعالى: -- (غ)

٢٢ المسلمين: -- (ق)

٢٣ فأجابه إلى سؤاله: فأجابهم إلى سؤالهم (ب)

٢٤ وجمع ... المتاخيري: -- (ق)

٢٥ وكافية: -- (ق)

٢٦ وسبب ... منتخبها: وسيتغني بها عن معالفجة الطبيب

٢٧ على: على أبواب (ب)

٢٨ سميتها: سماها (ق)

وهذه فهرسة (٢ظ) الكتاب وإليه[٢٩] المرجع والمآب.[٣٠]

الباب الأوّل في بيان تدبير[٣١] الإنسان وبيان امزجته وغير ذلك.

الباب الثاني في بيان أغذية[٣٢] المفردات وبيان[٣٣] منافعها وخواصّها وغير ذلك.[٣٤]

الباب الثالث في بيان الأدوية المفردة التي هي خلاصة الأدوية خصوصًا لتقوية الأفعال وزيادة الباه والشهوة والمنى وغير[٣٥] ذلك.[٣٦]

الباب الرابع في بيان الأدوية المركبّة لدفع الأمراض وتقوية الأفعال[٣٧] الجماع ودفع موانعه وزيادة المنى والشهوة وبيان الاغذية المركبّات[٣٨] والحلاوات[٣٩] النافعة لمزاج الإنسان والمصلح[٤٠] له ويزيل فلاجة المفلوج من بدن الإنسان ورخاوة أعضائه ويقوّي الباه.[٤١]

الباب الخامس في بيان الأشربة التي تصلح المزاج الفاسد وتصفّى[٤٢] الدم والبدن وتقوّي أفعال الجماع وتفيد فائدة (٣و) عظيمة.[٤٣]

الباب السادس في بيان المعاجين والجوارشات التي تفرح وتدفع الملال وتنفع المعدة نفعًا عظيمًا وتقويها وتزيل الصفراء والبلغم وتقطع السوداء وتنفع

---

٢٩ وإليه: إلى الله (ب)

٣٠ وإليه ... الماب: -- (ق/غ)

٣١ تدبير: تدبير بدن (ب)

٣٢ أغدية: الاغذية (ق)

٣٣ وبيان: -- (ق)

٣٤ وغير ذلك: -- (ق)

٣٥ غير ذلك: غيره (ب)

٣٦ ا لأفعال ... وغير ذلك: تقوية الشهوة وزيادة المنى والباه (ق)

٣٧ الأفعال: أفعال (ق/غ/ب)

٣٨ المركبات: المركبة (ب)

٣٩ المركبات والحلاوات: -- (ق)

٤٠ المصلح: الصلح (ب)

٤١ موانع ... الباه: وبيان الأغدية النافعة للأمزجة ورخاوة الأعضاء وغير ذلك (ق)

٤٢ تصفى: يصفى (ب)

٤٣ وتقوّى ... عظيمة: -- (ق)

الدماغ وتفتح سدد الأعضاء وتفشش[٤٤] الرياح الفاسدة وتزيلها[٤٥] وتقوّي الأعضاء الرئيسة وتدفع الصداع والنزلات وتقوّي الحرارة الغريزية وتقوّي جميع الأفعال.[٤٦]

الباب السابع في بيان الأشياف التي إذا تشيّفت بها تجذب الرياح[٤٧] والبرودات من الوسط والظهر والأعضاء وتخرجها وتزيل الرطوبات والصفراء والسوداء من المعدة والأمعاء وغيرها.[٤٨]

الباب الثامن في بيان الحقن التي تزيل وجع المفاصل وتدفع[٤٩] الأرياح الفاسدة وتخرجها[٥٠] من البدن وذات الرئة وعرق النساء ووجع الظهر وريح القولنج وتشدّ الظهر (٣ظ) والوسط[٥١] وتقوّي جميع الأفعال.[٥٢]

الباب التاسع في بيان الشدود التي[٥٣] يشدّ بها الوسط في الفصول الأربعة وما تليق من ذلك[٥٤] في كلّ فصل حتّى لا يخالف طبيعة الإنسان ولا يحصل المرض منه.[٥٥]

الباب العاشر في بيان شروطه[٥٦] وكيفيته حتّى لا يحصل منه الضرر ويقع الضعف بسبب ذلك.[٥٧]

---

٤٤ تفشش: تصفى (غ)

٤٥ تزيلها: يزيلها (غ)

٤٦ التي تفرح... الأفعال: النافعة للمعدة وازالة الصفراء والبلغم والسوداء وتنفع الدماغ وتفتح سدد الأعضاء وتفشش الرياح الفاسدة وتقوي الحرارة الغريزة (ق)

٤٧ الرياح: الأرياح (غ/ب)

٤٨ والظهر... والسوداء من: ما يزيل البرودات والرطوبات من الظهر والأعضاء و(ق)

٤٩ وتدفع: واخراج (ق)

٥٠ وتخرجها: -- (ق)

٥١ الظهر والوسط: الوسط والظهر (غ/ب)

٥٢ وذات ... جميع الفعال: -- (ق) / الشدودات (ب)

٥٣ الشدود التي: ما (ق)

٥٤ من ذلك: -- (ق) / بذلك (ب)

٥٥ حتّى لا ... منه: الاصطلاح الطبيعة (ق) / المرض منه: منه المرض أبدا (ب)

٥٦ شروطه: شروط الجماع (ب)

٥٧ حتّى ... ذلك: ومنع ضروره (ق)

الباب الحادي عشر في ذكر الأدوية التي يطلى بها على الذكر فيقويه ويطوله ويقومه.[٥٨]

الباب الثاني عشر في بيان الأدوية التي يطلى بها على الذكر فيقومه[٥٩] ويطوله كما ينبغي.[٦٠]

الباب الثالث عشر في بيان الأدوية التي[٦١] يطلى بها على[٦٢] أصابع اليدين والرجلين[٦٣] فيفيد الجماع ويقوّيه ولا يضعفه لكثرة الجماع.[٦٤]

الباب الرابع عشر في بيان الحبوب التي تمسك في الفم عند المجامعة[٦٥] فيستلذّ[٦٦] بها الفاعل.[٦٧] (٤و)

الباب الخامس عشر في بيان حالة الجماع التي[٦٨] يحصل بها لذّة عظيمة للرجل والمرأة مثل ما ذكره الحكماء.[٦٩]

الباب السادس عشر في الأدوية التي إذا استعملها النساء تحمر بها وجوهن وخدودهن كالورد الأحمر ويحصل من مجامعتهن لذة عظيمة حتّى لا يقدر أحد على مجامعتهن لحرارتهن وضيقتهن.[٧٠]

---

٥٨ بها .... ويقومه: به الذكر لتقويته وزيادة انعاظه (ق) / بها الذكر فتقويه وتشده وتغلظه وتقيمه (ب)

٥٩ فيقومه: فيقويه (غ) / فتغلظه (ب)

٦٠ في بيان ... ينبغي: في ذكر منافع آخر متعلق بالباه وزيادة الشهوة طلاء على الذكر (ق)

٦١ الادويه التي: ادويه (ق)

٦٢ على: -- (ق/غ) / بين (ب)

٦٣ اليدين والرجليون: الرجلين واليدين (ق/غ) / اليدين (ب)

٦٤ فيفيد ... الجماع: لتقوية الجماع (ق) / وتقويه ولا تضعفه كثرة الجماع (ب)

٦٥ المجامعة: الجماع (ق)

٦٦ فيستلذ: فيلتذ (ب)

٦٧ فيستلذ بها الفاعل: ويستلذ بها (ق)

٦٨ بيان التي: الأدوية التي تطلي بها الذكر حالة الجماع (ب)

٦٩ حالة الجماع ... الحكماء: ما يحصل للرجل والمرأة من لذة الجماع وكثرتها (ق)

٧٠ إذا استعملها ... ضيقتهن: إذا استعملتها بها النساء أحمرت خدودهن واستحسنت

الباب السابع عشر في بيان الأدوية التي تمنع النساء من الحبل وتبقين دائمًا كالبنات البكر.[٧١]

الباب الثامن عشر في بيان الأدوية التي إذا استعملتها المرأة لم تحبل[٧٢] بإذن الله تعالى.[٧٣]

تمت فهرست[٧٤] الأبواب وقد قدّمناها حتّى تسهل[٧٥] على طالبها إذا احتاج منها إلى شيء يسهل عليه تحصيلها من غير مشقّة ولا تعب وبالله استعين وهو حسبنا[٧٦] ونعم الوكيل.[٧٧] (٤ظ) اعلم أيّها الطالب[٧٨] وفقنا الله وإيّاك إلى طاعته إنّ الله سبحانه وتعالى خلق الحيوانات وأخرجهم من العدم إلى الوجود وخلق لهم[٧٩] أزواجًا وجعل لهم أنفسًا بحيث يحتاج ويشتاق بعضهم إلى بعض في الزوجية[٨٠] وفضل الإنسان على الجميع وفضله[٨١] بالعقل[٨٢] وزينه وكرمه.

فروجهن (ق) / استعمالتها النساء يصير كالبنات البكر في الضيق والحرارة ويحصل من مجامعتهن لذة عظيمة حتي لا يتقدى أحد على مجامعتهن لحرار وضيقهن (ب)

٧١ في بيان ...البكر: في الأدوية التي تمنع الحبل وتضيق الفروج (ق) / الحبل ... البكر: الحمل ويبقون دائما كالبكر (ب)

٧٢ تحبل: + تحبل (غ)

٧٣ في بيان... تعالى: في الأدوية التي للحبل وفوائدك آخر تاتي ان شاء الله تعالي (ق)

٧٤ فهرست الابواب: فهرسة الكتاب والابواب (غ)

٧٥ تسهل: يسهل (ب)

٧٦ حسبنا: حسبي (ب)

٧٧ الوكيل: + المقدمة (ب)

٧٨ وقد ... الوكيل: ليسهل على طالبها تحصيلها من غير مشقة وبالله المستعان وعلياه التطلا اعلم وفقنا (ق)

٧٩ وخلق لهم: خلقهم (غ/ب)

٨٠ ان الله ... الزوجية: بمنه وكرمه ان الله خلق الحيوانات واخرجهم من العدم الي الوجود وخلقهم ازواجا وجعل لهم انفاسا بحيث يحتاج ويشتاق بعضهم بعضا للزواج (ق)

٨١ على الجميع وفضله: على جميع (ق)

٨٢ بالعقل: وشرفه بالعقل (ب)

كما **قال** الله تعالى وهو أصدق القائلين[٨٣] ولقد كرمنا بني آدم وحملناهم في البرّ والبحر الآية وجعل غذائهم الطف الحيوانات وبسطنا الكلام في هذا الباب لأنّه ما تمّ شيء يكون[٨٤] سببًا لهلاك النفس أشدّ من الجماع فكلّ مرض يمكن مداواته إلّا المرض الذي يكون سببه[٨٥] كثرة الجماع فإنّه[٨٦] يطفى الحرارة الغريزية فلا يعود ينفع العلاج ولا المداواة أبدًا نعوذ بالله من ذلك[٨٧] فإنّ المنى إذا انصرف[٨٨] يخرج من الأعضاء الرئيسة وجميع (٥و) الجوارح.[٨٩]

كما قال علي رضي الله عنه[٩٠] منيك روحك ونور عينيك ومخّ رأسك مع ساقيك إن شئت فاحفظه. ومتى علمت الجماع[٩١] وجامعت كما ينبغي تحصل منه أربعة وعشرون فائدة **منها** أن[٩٢] يزيل أسقام السوداوية ويمنع العلل الصفراوية والبلغمية[٩٣] ويحصل[٩٤] الفرح والخفّة كما ذكره العلماء والحكماء المتقدّمون والأطبّاء المتأخّرون وعلموا ذلك بتجاربهم واستعمالاتهم.

وأمّا ما ذكره بعض العلماء[٩٥] أنّ الجماع رديء مضرّ[٩٦] لا ينبغي لأحد أن يستعمله، بل يتركه فهذا كلام لا أصل له، بل هذا الكلام خطأ لأنّ شرف

---

٨٣ الله تعالى وهو أصدق القائلين: تعالى (ق)

٨٤ وجعل ... يكون: فلا شيء (ق)

٨٥ يكون سببه: يحدث من (ق)

٨٦ فانه: لكونه (ق)

٨٧ فلا يعود... ذلك: -- (ق)

٨٨ إذا انصرف: -- (ق)

٨٩ وجميع الجوارح: -- (ق)

٩٠ كما قال على رضي الله عنه: كما قال أمير المؤمنين على كرم الله وجهه (ق)

٩١ الجماع: وقت الجماع (ب)

٩٢ فاحفظه ... منه ان: فاحفظ نفسك ومن يعلم بتدبير الجماع وشروط فلا يضر بل ينفعه لأنه (ق) / أن: أنه (ب)

٩٣ الصفراوية والبلغمية: البلغمية والصفراوية (غ)

٩٤ يحصب: + من (ق)

٩٥ العلماء: الحكماء (غ/ب)

٩٦ أن الجماع: من أن الجماع مضر ردى (ب)

وزينته الظاهرة بوجود خمسة أشياء، **وهي** الحواسّ الخمسة الظاهرة كالسمع والبصر والشمّ والذوق واللمس. فأمّا الذوق الذي هو أحد الخمسة عبارة غالبة[٩٧] عن ذوق الجماع ولذّته (٥ظ) ونتيجة لذّة الجماع لحصول وجود[٩٨] الحيوانات وبه التوالد والتناسل في العالم الإنساني أيضًا فالقول بعدم جواز الجماع قولًا باطلًا.[٩٩]

والظاهر أنّ هذا القول ليس قولًا مطلقًا بل بالنسبة إلى الذين يجامعون مع جهلهم بأوقات المجامعة[١٠٠] وأحوال مباشرتها وعدم علمهم بشروطها وتدابيرها فبسبب ذلك الجماع يبتلون بتلك الأمراض المذكورة ويهلكون أنفسهم بخلاف من يعلم تدابير[١٠١] الجماع وشروطه[١٠٢] فلا يضرّه الجماع بل ينفعه نفعًا بليغًا[١٠٣] كما ذكرناه مع أنّه ما تمّ شيء في لذّات النفسانية الذّ من لذّة الجماع لأنّها جبلية ومختلطة في تراكيب[١٠٤] الإنسان وباقي الحيوانات ومنصبه في خلقهم ولهذا لم ير حيوان لم تركن تلك[١٠٥] اللذّة في نفسه ولم تحصل في دماغه إلا أن يكون (٦و) معلول المزاج مرخى الأعضاء ميت الشهوة.

فصل

اعلم أنّ البشرة لا تضعف ولا تبلى بمرض وألم إلّا إذا حصل للأعضاء الرئيسة

---

٩٧ غالبة: غالبا (ب)

٩٨ لحصول وجود: حصول وجود جميع (ب)

٩٩ قولا باطلا: قول باطل (ب)

١٠٠ المجامعة: الجماع (غ)

١٠١ تدابير: تدبير (غ)

١٠٢ الجماع وشرطه: المجامعة وشروطها (ب)

١٠٣ بليغا: عظيما (ب)

١٠٤ تراكيب: تركيب (ب)

١٠٥ لم تركن تلك: ترك هذه (ب)

ألم وما دام[١٠٦] الأعضاء[١٠٧] الرئيسة تقوية بالأدوية والمعالجات والاحتماء عن المخالفات والاحتراز عن المضرّات لها تكون الجوارح سالمة امنة من العلل والأسقام فلا يصيبها شيء من الآلام بإذن الله تعالى إلى وقت أجله فإن الأجل لا يمنعه شيء لا راد لقضائه ولا مانع لحكمه.[١٠٨]

واعلم أنّ الأعضاء الرئيسة هو الدماغ والقلب والكبد والخصى مع اعضائه وبعض الحكماء جعل الرئة من الأعضاء الرئيسة وبعضهم عدّ الكلى أيضًا [١٠٩] فينبغي للإنسان ان يقوّي هذه الأعضاء ويقوّي المعدة بالأدوية والمعاجين والأشربة[١١٠] والتمريخات كما سيأتي (٦ظ) شرحهم[١١١] وصفات أعمالهم وتدابيرهم إن شاء الله تعالى. كما ألقوا ذلك الحكماء المتقدّمون والأطبّاء المتأخّرون بتجاربهم واستعمالاتهم وبيّنوا ذلك في كتبهم كأفلاطون وأرطاطالوس[١١٢] وبقراط وبلطيوس[١١٣] وأرسطو أو أمثالهم.[١١٤]

---

١٠٦ دام: + الأعضاء الرئيسة سالمة من الآلام لم يحصل البشرة ضعف خصوصا إذا حصل (ب)

١٠٧ الأعضاء: للأعضاء (ب)

١٠٨ كما ذكره...حكمه: -- (ق)

١٠٩ وبعض الحكماء ... أيضًا: -- (ق)

١١٠ الأشربة: + والشيافات (ب/أ)

١١١ اشرحهم: بيانهم وشرحهم (أ)

١١٢ أرطاطالوس: أرسطاليس (ب/أ)

١١٣ بلطيوس: بطلميوس (ب/أ)

١١٤ يقوي هذه الأعضاء ... أو امثالهم: يقوي هذه الأعضاء بالأدوية والمعاجين والأشربة والتمريخات والاحتراز عن المضرات لتكون الجوارح سالمة من العلل والاسقام (ق)

فصل[115]

في بيان فائدة الجماع وضرره بحسب الفصول الأربع التي هي[116] الربيع والصيف والخريف والشتاء.[117]

واعلم أنّ أولى الفصول وأحسنها[118] وأنفعها للجماع هو فصل الربيع لأنّه[119] أعدل الفصول وهواه[120] أعدل الأهوية[121] و[122]فيها يصفوا[123] الدم ويعدل[124] ويزداد في عروق[125] الروح ويقوّي[126] الحرارة الغريزية ويزداد النشاط والذوق ويزول ضعف الذكر ويشتدّ فإذا كان الأمر كذلك[127] فلا يضرّه الجماع في هذا الفصل ولا يشقل البدن ولا يجلب السقم ولا آلام[128] سواء جامع بالأدوية والمعاجين (٧و) أو بغير المعاجين.[129] وأمّا الجماع في غير فصل الربيع فمضرّ[130] إذا كان بالأدوية فلا يضرّ لأنّ الذي ينصرف من الشهوة حصل عنده

---

١١٥ ساقط الفصل من (أ)

١١٦ هي: -- (غ)

١١٧ الصيف والخريف والشتا: الربيع والخريف والشتا والصيف (ق)

١١٨ أولى الفصول وأحسنها: أحسن الفصول (ق)

١١٩ لأنه: + هو (ب)

١٢٠ لأنه اعدل الفصول وهواه: لان هواه (ق)

١٢١ الأهوية: الهوائية (ب)

١٢٢ و: -- (ب)

١٢٣ يصفوا: يصف (ق)

١٢٤ ويعدل: -- (ق)

١٢٥ عروق: العروق (ب)

١٢٦ يقوي: تقوي (ب)

١٢٧ فإذا كان الامر كذلك: -- (ق)

١٢٨ ولا آلام: والآلام (ب)

١٢٩ لا يشقل ... المعاجين: -- (ق)

١٣٠ فمضرّ: + إلّا (غ)

بسبب قوى[١٣١] الأدوية[١٣٢] فذلك بالحقيقة ينصرف بالأدوية لا منك فحينئذ يحتاج من مجامع في فصل الصيف والخريف والشتاء إلى العلاج بالأدوية والمعاجين حتّى يفيد ولا يضرّ.[١٣٣]

الباب الأوّل

في تدبير ما يقتضيه مزاج كلّ إنسان وبيان العلامات التي يستدلّ بها على مزاج كلّ واحد.[١٣٤]

اعلم أنّ كلّ من كان أسمر اللون وحنطي اللون و[١٣٥]كان لحمه قويًا وليس بمرخي[١٣٦] واسع العروق وأسود الشعر ويكون معتدلًا نظيفًا أشهل العينين ويكون شعر حاجبيه كثيرًا[١٣٧] وخصيتيه قويًا[١٣٨] كان[١٣٩] مزاجه حارًّا يابسًا فهذه الطائفة تكون حمسًا[١٤٠] على (٧ظ) الجماع لا يبالون من الجماع.[١٤١]

وأمّا من يكون أصفرا اللون وأحمر الوجه وأبيض الجسم[١٤٢] كبير البطن

---

١٣١ قوى: قوة (ب)
١٣٢ فلا يضر ... الأدوية: -- (غ)
١٣٣ إذا كان ... ولا يضر: إلّا إذا كان بالأدوية فلا يضر ان شاء الله تعالي (ق)
١٣٤ على مزاج كلّ واحد: على المزاج (ق) / واحد: أحد (ب)
١٣٥ وحنطي اللون و: -- (ب)
١٣٦ وحنطى... بمرخى: ولحمه قوي (ق)
١٣٧ ويكون ... كثيرًا: يكون معتدلا لا اشهل العينين كثير شعر الحاجبين (ق)
١٣٨ قويًا: قويه (ق)
١٣٩ كان: -- (ب)
١٤٠ حمسا: حريصة (ب)
١٤١ فهذه ... الجماع: فلا يضره الجماع (ق) / من الجماع: -- (ب)
١٤٢ وأحمر الوجه وأبيض الجسم: أحمر الوجه أبيض الجسم (ق)

يكون مزاجه بارد رطب[١٤٣] مرطوب المزاج حريص على الجماع وليكن[١٤٤] لا يقوّي عليه وإذا زاد في الجماع ضعف بسببه.[١٤٥]

وأمّا من كان أسود اللون ونظيف الجلد والبدن هزيلًا مغيرًا[١٤٦] صغير العينين ويكون[١٤٧] لحم أسنانه شديد الحمرة يدلّ على أنّه حارّ المزاج وهذا[١٤٨] يكون حريصًا على الجماع.

وأمّا من كان أبيض اللون فهذا يكون على نوعين أحدهما من يكون لونه صافيًا وعينيه ملاحًا، والثاني هو الذي يكون بياضه مستويًا[١٤٩] بالصفرة ويكون شعره أصفر فهو يكون[١٥٠] حريصًا على الجماع.[١٥١]

ومن كان أبيض[١٥٢] وبلغمي المزاج يكون مرخي الأعضاء لا يكون له[١٥٣] قوة على الجماع وإن أفرط في[١٥٤] الجماع (٨و) هلك.[١٥٥] فينبغي لهذا أن يحترز من الجماع.

---

١٤٣ يكون... رطب: تكون أمزجتهم باردة رطبة (ب)

١٤٤ ليكن: لاكن (ب)

١٤٥ رطب ... بسببه: رطبا فيضره كثرية الجماع (ق)

١٤٦ مغيرا: -- (ب)

١٤٧ الجلد والبدن هزيلا صغيرا: البدن (ق)

١٤٨ وهذا: فهذا (ق)

١٤٩ مستويا: مشوبا (ب)

١٥٠ فهو يكون: فهؤلاء صفراويون المزاج ويكونون (ب)

١٥١ الجماع: + ويقوي عليه (ب/أ)

١٥٢ كان أبيض: كان منهم أبيضا (ب/أ)

١٥٣ يكون له: تكون لهم (ب)

١٥٤ في: على (ب)

١٥٥ هلك: هلكوا (ب)

فصل[١٥٦]

اعلم أنّ ضعف الجوارح ورخاوة الأعضاء تحصل من ضعف الدماغ وهذا يسمّى ضعيف الدماغ وعلامة ذلك دخان الرأس وتغوير العينين وضعف البصر[١٥٧] وضعف القوى وتغيّر[١٥٨] اللون وغلبة الحياء عند رخاوة الذكر والجماع[١٥٩] من غير نشا.[١٦٠] وإذا جامع لم تبق[١٦١] له قدرة على إعادة الجماع مرّة أخرى من غير توهمه[١٦٢] ورخاوة أعضائه.[١٦٣] فينبغي لمثله[١٦٤] أن يدفع هذه العلل بتقوية الدماغ،[١٦٥] فعلاج تقوية الدماغ بشراب السكّر لأنّ هذه العلل لا تحصل إلّا من زيادة الرطوبات و[١٦٦]تحلّ[١٦٧] الفضلات ويقوّي المنى ويكثر ويقوّي الجماع وله منافع شتى بطول شرحها.[١٦٨]

---

١٥٦ أمّا من كان... فصل: -- (ق)

١٥٧ ضعف الجوارح ... البصر: ضعف الجوارح الأعضاءء تحصل من ضعف الجماع وعلامته دوخان الراسن وضعف البصر والقواير العينين (ق)

١٥٨ تغير: تغيير (ب/أ)

١٥٩ رخاوت الذكر والجماع: الجماع ورخاوة الذكر (غ/أ)

١٦٠ نشا: نشاط (ب)

١٦١ تبق: يبق (غ)

١٦٢ غير توهمه: غاية توهمهم (ب/أ)

١٦٣ أعضائه: أعضائهم (ب/أ)

١٦٤ عند رخاوة ... لمثله: وقت الجماع ورخاوة الذكر وان جامع مره لم يقدر على الاعاده ولم يكن لنشاة لرخاوة اعضائه فهذا ينبغي له (ق) / لمثله: لمثل هذه الطائفة (ب)

١٦٥ الدماغ: + القول (أ)

١٦٦ و: + هذا الشراب (غ)

١٦٧ تحل: يحل (غ) / الرطوبات ... تحل: الرطوبات وشراب السكر يدفع الرطوبات وتحلل (ب)

١٦٨ شرحها: الكلام يذكرها تظهر استعمالها (أ)

صفة عمل تركيب السكّر[١٦٩]

قال[١٧٠] يؤخذ زنجبيل وقرفة (٨ظ) لفّ[١٧١] من الاثنين خمس دراهم بالسوية[١٧٢] وقاقلّة درهمين وقرنفل درهمين.[١٧٣] تدقّ[١٧٤] هذه الأدوية كلّ واحد وحده، ثم تجمعهم بالدقّ وتجعلهم في قدرة وتجعل[١٧٥] عليهم قدرهم[١٧٦] سبع مرّات ماء عذب ويغلى بنار ليّنة إلى أن تخرج قوة الأدوية فيه وينهرى[١٧٧] فيه الحوائج. ثمّ يصفّى الماء ويرمى التفل[١٧٨]، ثم يؤخذ قوامه بوزنه أربع مرّات سكّر يعنى بوزن[١٧٩] الحوائج أربع مرّات سكّر فيكون وزن السكّر اثنين وثلاثون درهم.[١٨٠] ثمّ يغلى إلى أن يمتزج ولا يعقد.[١٨١] ثم إذا أراد أن ينزلها يضع فيها نصف درهم زعفران وينزله ويستعمله في[١٨٢] كلّ يوم على الريق مقدار ملعقة ويصبر عن الأكل إلى الضحوة مفيد وشفاء إن شاء الله تعالى.

---

١٦٩ سكر: + شراب السكر (ب) / عمل تركيب السكر: تركيبة (أ)

١٧٠ فعلاج... قال: فعلاجه شراب السكّر فإنه يحل الفضلات ويقوي الجماع ويكثر المني وله منافع شيء (ق)

١٧١ لف: لب أي جيده (ب)

١٧٢ لفّ... بالسوية: لف خمسة دراهم منهما (ق) / قال.... بالسوية: زنجبيل وقرفة من كل واحد خمسة دراهم (أ)

١٧٣ درهمين: درهم وفي نسخة درهمين (ب) / درهم (أ)

١٧٤ تدق: يدق (أ)

١٧٥ تجعل: + يجعل (ب/أ)

١٧٦ عليهم قدرهم: عليه قدر الحوائج (أ)

١٧٧ ينهرى: تنهري (غ) / تهرا (ب) / يتهرا (أ)

١٧٨ التفل: تفله (ب)

١٧٩ بوزن: لوزن (ب) / بقدر وزن (أ)

١٨٠ ثلاثون درهم: ثلاثين (ب)

١٨١ يعقد: ينعقد (غ)

١٨٢ وقاقلة ... في: وقرنفل وقاقلة درهمين من كلّ منها نرقهم وتصب عليهم ماء عذبا حتي يعمهم ويغلى ذلك على النار الي ان تخرج قوة الأدوية في الماء فيصفي ويرمي التفل ثم تطوح فيه اثنين وثلاثين درهمًا سكرًا ويغلي على النار الي أن يمتزج فيلقى عليه نصف درهم زعفران وينزل ويرفع ويستعمل منه (ق)

وأمّا السبب الثاني في[١٨٣] ضعف الجوارح ورخاوة الأعضاء التي تحصل بحدث[١٨٤] (٩و) منها ضعف الجماع فهو ضعف القلب فعلامة من يكون ضعيف القلب أنّه إذا تحرّك بحركة أو مشي قوى في طلوع عقبه أو غضب[١٨٥] على أحد أو إذا بشروه ببشارة[١٨٦] أو إذا رأى مطلوبه أو إذا أراد أن يقارن جماعة يحصل له في هذه الصور كلّها[١٨٧] خفقان القلب وتأخذه الرعشة في يديه وركبه[١٨٨] ويحصل له اللهفان وضيق النفس ويتغيّر لونه ويجامع بالضعف ويحصل له بعد الجماع خفقان القلب فينبغي {لمثله أن يدفع هذه العلل بتقوية الجوارح ورخاوة الأعضاء بشراب التفاح لا يزيل هذه العلل} ويزيد[١٨٩] فضلات المعدة ويسخّن المني ويزيده[١٩٠] وله منافع كثيرة غير هذا لو ذكرناها لطال علينا كتابتها وفيه كفاية.

وأمّا صفة[١٩١] **تركيب شراب التفّاح، قال** يؤخذ التفّاح يقشّر وينقّى من[١٩٢] نواه

---

١٨٣ مفيد... في: فانه في شفاء بإذن الله وأمّا (ق)

١٨٤ تحصل بحدث: يحدث (غ) / (ب) / التي تحصل بحدث: الذي يحدث (أ)

١٨٥ غضب: في حال الغضب (أ)

١٨٦ إذا ... ببشارة: أو بشارة أو (أ)

١٨٧ تحصل ... كلها: تحدث عند الجماع نهي من ضعف القلب وعلامة انه إذا تحرك بحركة ومشي أو غضب يحصل له (ق)

١٨٨ ركبه: ركبتيه (ب)

١٨٩ فينبغي لمثله ... يزيد: وضربات العروق فإذا سكنت العروق يحصل لها الضعف والرخاوة ومتى أفرط هذه الأمراض في الجماع يهلك بلا شبه فينبغي ان يعالج في وقع هذه العلل بشراب التفاح فأنها يدفع هذه العلل ويقوي القلب ويزيل (غ) / وضربات العروق فإذا أسكن العروق يحصل لها الضعف ومتى أفرط صاحب هذه الأمراض في الجماع يهلك بلا شبهة فينبغي أن يعالج في دفع هذه العلل بشراب التفاح فإنه يدفع هذه العلل ويقوي القلب ويزيل (ب) / (أ)

١٩٠ يزيده: + كثرة (ب)

١٩١ صفة: + عمل (غ) / أما: -- (أ)

١٩٢ ويحصل... وينقي من: ويتغير لونه فهذا يضره الجماع فينبغي ان يعالج بشراب التفاح فانه يدفع هذه العلل ويقوي القلب ويزيل فضلات المعدة ويسخن المني ويزيده وله منافع شتي وصفة يؤخذ من التفاح جزء يقشر ويرمي (ق)

ويدقّ ويعصّر ماؤه من خرقة رفيعة أو[١٩٣] منخل رفيع، ثم (٩ظ) يؤخذ وزن ماء التفّاح ماء ورد، ثمّ يخلطهما. ثمّ يؤخذ[١٩٤] وزن الجميع عسل نحل مصفّى منزوع الرغوة ويأخذ قليلاً من ماء التفّاح وماء الورد المخلوطان يجعل في قدره وحده ويجعل عليه نصف درهم[١٩٥] زعفران ونضف درهم فلفل[١٩٦] ودرهم زنجبيل وقرنفل درهمين وتغليه حتّى تخرج قوة الأدوية فيه. ثمّ يصفّى ويرفع إلى وقت الحاجة، ثمّ يأخذ[١٩٧] وزن هذا الماء مرّتين من ماء المطر وتجعل الجميع مع الماء[١٩٨] الذي غليته بالبزور أن[١٩٩] في قدرة على نار ليّنة وأنت تحرّكه إلى أن ينعقد وترمى عليه قبل أن ينعقد قيراط مسك خالص، ثمّ تنزله وتبرده[٢٠٠] وتستعمل[٢٠١] منه كلّ يوم على الريق قدر ملعقة ونصف. نافع.[٢٠٢]

وأمّا[٢٠٣] **السبب الثالث** في رخاوة الأعضاء (١٠و) وضعف الجوارح والجماع، **قال** وأمّا[٢٠٤] ضعف الكبد فعلامته صفار الوجه مثل علّة اليرقان

---

١٩٣ او: له (غ)

١٩٤ يؤخذ: يأخذ (ب/غ)

١٩٥ يجعل عليه نصف درهم: تجعل عليهم وزن (غ) / من ... درهم: قدر نصف درهم (ب)

١٩٦ فلفل: دارفلفل (ب/غ) / قاقلة (ق)

١٩٧ من خرقة ... ثم يأخذ: ويصفي ثم يخلط بوزنه ماء ورد وكذا وزنهما عسل نحل منزوع الرغوة ويغلي على النار ويلقي عليه نصف زعفران ونصف درهم قاقلة ودرهم زنجبيل ودرهمان قرنفل ثم يصفي ثم تأخذ (ق)

١٩٨ الماء: -- (غ)

١٩٩ ثم ... أن: ونوع أخر تأخذ ماء التفاح وماء الورد على السوية إلخ ثم يؤخذ وزنها مرتين من ماء المطر وما ذكر من الأجزاء قبله وتغلى الجميع (ب)

٢٠٠ تبرده: + وترفعه (غ/ب)

٢٠١ وتجعل ... وتستعمل: ويغلي الجميع على النار ثم الق عليه قيراط مسك ثم نزل وارفع ويستعمل (ق)

٢٠٢ نافع: + إن شاء الله تعالى (أ)

٢٠٣ وأما: قال (أ)

٢٠٤ قال وأما: هو (ب) / -- (أ)

وينشف لسانه وشفتيه وتغور عينيه ويكون هزيلًا قليل الاشتهاء للطعام.[٢٠٥] وإذا أكل لا ينهضم وإذا وقف يرتعد ساقيه[٢٠٦] ولا يقدر على القيام إلّا بالتكلف ويكون مرخيًا لا يقدر على الجماع ، وإن قدر عليه لا يكون له حلاوة ولا لذّة ويكون منيه بارد[٢٠٧] ويكون يديه ورجليه باردتان[٢٠٨] ومثل هذا الرجل إذا أفرط في الجماع يبتلى بأحد هذه الأمراض الثلاثة إمّا أن يكون مفلوجًا أو مرخيًا[٢٠٩] وإمّا أن تنقطع[٢١٠] حرارته الغريزية فيحدث من ذللك موت المفاجأة،[٢١١] نعوذ بالله من ذلك.[٢١٢] فينبغي أن يدفع هذه العلّه[٢١٣] بشراب السنبل يسخّن معدته ويقوّي[٢١٤] كبده[٢١٥] ويقوّي[٢١٦] (١٠ظ) الحرارة الغريزية ويقوّي[٢١٧] الجماع وله ستّة وعشرون منفعة إن[٢١٨] ذكرناها يطول الكتاب.

---

٢٠٥ وأمّا السبب ...للطعام: لما ذكر وأمّا علامة ضعف الكبد تصفير الوجه وتنشف اللسان والشفتين ويكون هزيلا قليل الشهوة الأكل (ق)

٢٠٦ ساقيه: + وإذا وقع (أ)

٢٠٧ بارد: باردا (غ)

٢٠٨ باردتان: باردة (ب/أ)

٢٠٩ أن يكون مرخيا: فالوجا أو رخاوة (أ)

٢١٠ تنقط: تنطفي (ب) / انطفاء (أ)

٢١١ لا ينهضم ... المفاجأة: لا يهضم وليس له قدرة على الجماع وان جامع لم يجد له لذة ولا شهوة ومنيه بارد وكذا اعضائه باردة فهذا أيضًا يفره الجماع ويخشي عليه مرض الفالج لانقطاع الحرارة الغريزية عنه (ق)

٢١٢ من ذلك: -- (أ)

٢١٣ هذه العلة: + عنه (ق)

٢١٤ يقوي: تقوي (ب)

٢١٥ معدته ويقوي كبده: ويقوي الكبد (ق)
ويقوّى كبده: -- (غ)

٢١٦ يقوي: تقوي (ب)

٢١٧ يقوي: تقوي على (ب)

٢١٨ ان: إذا (ب)

وأمّا **صفة** شراب السنبل **قال** يؤخذ[219] قرفة[220] وقاقلّة وعود هندي[221] من كلّ واحد درهم وقرنفل نصف درهم تدقّ هذه الأدوية وتجعل[222] عليها قدر الحوائج[223] خمس مرّات ماء ويغلى حتّى ينهرى[224] الحوائج ويبقى[225] نصف الماء. ثمّ يصفّى ويجعل[226] قدر الماء عسل منزوع الرغوة ويغلى ساعة حتّى يمتزج، ثم يجعل[227] عليه نصف درهم زعفران يذاب[228] بماء الورد ويخلط، ويستعمل. نافع مفيد لما ذكرناه.[229]

السبب الرابع لضعف الجماع وضعف الذكر والخصيتين ورخاوتهما وهذا النوع يكون[230] على ثلاثة انواع.

أوّلها[231] أن تكون[232] هذه[233] التي ذكرناها من رخاوة الذكر والخصيتين

---

٢١٩ ويقوي ... يؤخذ: يزيد في الجماع وله منافع آخر يطول شرحها وصفته (ق)

٢٢٠ قرفة: سنبل وقرفة (ب) / يؤخذ قرفة: تأخذ سنبل وقرفة (أ)

٢٢١ عود هندي: + وجوز هندي (ق/ب)

٢٢٢ تجعل: يجعل (غ) / قرنفل ... تجعل: نسخة درهمين وقرنفل نصف درهم تدق هذه الأدوية ويجعل (ب)

٢٢٣ تجعل عليها قدر الحوائج: يجعل عليها بقدرها (ق)

٢٢٤ ينهرى: يتهري (غ/ب)

٢٢٥ ينهري الحوائج ويبقى: على النارحتي يبقي (ق)

٢٢٦ يجعل: + في (ب)

٢٢٧ ويجعل ... ثم يجعل: ويخلط بقدره عسلا منزوع الرغوة ويغلي حتي يمتزج ثم يلقي (ق)

٢٢٨ يذاب: مذاب (ب) / ينزله يذاب (أ)

٢٢٩ لما ذكرناه السبب: إن شاء الله تعالى (أ)

٢٣٠ يذاب... النوع يكون: مذوب بماء ورد ويرفع ويستعمل منه وقت الحاجة فانه نافع لما ذكر وأمّا رخاوة الذكر وضعفه فهو على ثلاثة انواع (ق)

٢٣١ أوّلها: -- (غ) / أحدها (ب) / أنواع أولها: وجوه أحدها (أ)

٢٣٢ تكون: يكون (ب)

٢٣٣ هذه: + العلل (غ/ب)

جبليًا له[٢٣٤] صحبه[٢٣٥] من بطن أمّه.

وثانيها (١١و) يكون[٢٣٦] من كثرة الجماع من[٢٣٧] صغره.

وثالثها كثرة الجماع من فوق الأربعين وبعد الأربعين[٢٣٨] وعلامة الأوّل يعنى الذي يكون رخاوته من بطن امه[٢٣٩] لا يقوم ذكره ويكون مع ذلك[٢٤٠] حريصًا على الجماع من غير اشتهاء له ويكون[٢٤١] مرخيًا. وعلاج هذا النوع معتدلًا على[٢٤٢] طول الزمان وعلامتها الذي حصل منها ذلك لكثرة الجماع في زمن[٢٤٣] صغره فعلامته[٢٤٤] قيام ذكره في أوائل الليل وأواخره ووقت الصبح أو في فصل الربيع. فعلاج هذا النوع هين يصلح سريعًا سنذكره إن شاء الله في موضعه. وما[٢٤٥] حصل له من كثرة الجماع في كبره من فوق الأربعين فعلامته قيام ذكره[٢٤٦] في الجملة في الأوقات القليلة وبعض الأيّام و[٢٤٧]جماعه[٢٤٨]

---

٢٣٤ له: -- (ب)

٢٣٥ هذه التي... صحبته: خلفته (ق)

٢٣٦ يكون: تكون (ق)

٢٣٧ من: في (ق)

٢٣٨ فوق الأربعين وبعد الأربعين: فوق الأربعين من عمره (ق)

٢٣٩ من بطن امه: من بطن من بطن امه (ق) / امه: + كذلك (غ)

٢٤٠ مع ذلك: -- (ق)

٢٤١ (الجماع) من.... يكون: وعلامة ال ي يكون من بطن أمه ولد فذلك لا يقوم ذكره أبدا ويكون حريصا على الجماع غير شهوة (أ)

٢٤٢ معتدلا: معقد والا (غ)

٢٤٣ منها... زمن: منه كثرة الجماع في حال (ب)

٢٤٤ اشتهاء... فعلامته: شهوة فلا علاج له وعلامته الثانية (ق) / زمن ...فعلامته: حال صغره (أ)

٢٤٥ وما: وأما الذي (ب/أ)

٢٤٦ ذكره: ذكرهم (ب)

٢٤٧ في اوايل... الأيّام و: آخر الليل فعلاجه بالأدوية والمعاجين الاتية وعلامته الثالثة (ق)

٢٤٨ جماعه: جماعهم (ب)

بلا نشاط ينزل منيه بارد[٢٤٩] أو تارة (١١ظ) منيه[٢٥٠] بالحرقان ومثل هذا لا يكون له[٢٥١] أولاد ولا بنين وسبب هذا النوع من البرودة في ظهره ووسطه[٢٥٢] فإن البرودة تكون غالبة عليه.[٢٥٣] فينبغي أن يعالج في مثل هذه[٢٥٤] بمعجون المسك فإنه يزيل البرودة والرطوبة[٢٥٥] التي في الظهر وفي[٢٥٦] الوسط ينقّى المثانة ويجري المنى ويجري[٢٥٧] الدم في العروق ويفتح السدد.

فينبغي أن يحتمى من الماء كلّ المتخالفات[٢٥٨] حتّى يتخلّص سريعًا ولا يبتلي بزيادة المرض وسنذكر احتمائه وما يفيد[٢٥٩] من الاغذية إن شاء الله تعالى. ولهذا المعجون ثلاثة وثلاثون فائدة غير ما ذكرناه.[٢٦٠]

---

٢٤٩ بارد: باردا (غ)
٢٥٠ ينزل ... منيه: وينزل منيهم بارد وتارة منيهم (ب) / أو تارة منيه: ينزل مني بعهم (أ)
٢٥١ له: لهم (ب)
٢٥٢ ظهره ووسطه: ظهورهم وأوساطهم (ب)
٢٥٣ ينزل منيه ... لبة عليه: ومنيه بارد ينزل بحرقان بلا شهوة وسببه بروده في ظهره (ق) / عليه: عليهم (أ)
٢٥٤ في مثل هذه: -- (ق) / + العلل (ب)
٢٥٥ والرطوبه: -- (ق) / والرطوبات (ب)
٢٥٦ في: -- (ب/أ)
٢٥٧ يجرى: -- (ق)
٢٥٨ المتخالفات: المخالفات (ب) / مخالفة (أ)
٢٥٩ يفيد: يصلح (ب)
٢٦٠ المتخالفات... تعالى: الرديه الحامضة ليتخلص من هذا المرض ولهذا المعجون ثلاث وثلاثون فائدة (ق)

وصفة تركيب[٢٦١] معجون المسك

قال[٢٦٢] يؤخذ[٢٦٣] مسك قيراط وسليخة وسنبل وساذج هند[٢٦٤] مليح[٢٦٥] وجنطيانة رومي، من كلّ واحد درهمين وزعفران[٢٦٦] وكمّون وبزر جزر ومصطكى، من كلّ واحد ثلاث (١٢و) دراهم[٢٦٧] وعود وقرنفل[٢٦٨] ومرّ تركي، من كلّ واحد نصف درهم، يدقّ هذه الأدوية وينخل[٢٦٩] ويؤخذ قوامهم[٢٧٠] بقدر الأدوية ثلاث مرّات عسل نحل ويجعله[٢٧١] معجونًا ويستعمل منه كلّ يوم مثقال. نافع إن شاء الله تعالى.[٢٧٢]

علاج آخر

يؤخذ ديوك صغار قبل أن يصيحوا ويذبحهم[٢٧٣] ويجمع[٢٧٤] مرارتهم مقدار[٢٧٥] عشرة دراهم. ثمّ يؤخذ مرداسنك مقدار[٢٧٦] ما يعجن به المرائر المجموعة ويعجنه

---

٢٦١ تركيب: -- (ق)
٢٦٢ قال: ان (ق)
٢٦٣ يؤخذ: تأخذ (أ)
٢٦٤ هند: هندي (ق/ب)
٢٦٥ مليح: -- (ب)
٢٦٦ وزعفران: زعفران (ق)
٢٦٧ ثلاث دراهم: درهم (ق)
٢٦٨ وقرنفل: -- (ق)
٢٦٩ ينخل: تنخل (ب)
٢٧٠ قوامهم: قوامه (ب)
٢٧١ يدقّ ... يجعله: وعسل نحل قدر الجميع ثلاث مرات ويغلي على النار ويجعل (ق)
٢٧٢ تعالى: لما ذكر (ق)
٢٧٣ يذبحهم: يذبحو (ق)
٢٧٤ يجمع: يؤخذ (ق)
٢٧٥ مقدار: بقدر (ق)
٢٧٦ مقدار: بقدر (ق)

بها عجنًا رقيقًا[٢٧٧] ، ثمّ يضعه في الشمس حتّى يمتزج ويخلط[٢٧٨] بعضه في بعض وإيّاك أن لا يجفّ ولا يغلظ.[٢٧٩] ثمّ يدخل الحمام[٢٨٠] وكلّما خرج من الحمام[٢٨١] يطلى به ذكر وتحت إبطيه ومقعده وليكن ذلك على الريق. ثمّ يستعمل من ذلك المعجون أيّ معجون المسك الذي تقدّم.[٢٨٢] ثم يطبخ الأدياك[٢٨٣] المذبوحة التي[٢٨٤] جمعت مرائرهم بقدرة مع بصل[٢٨٥] (١٢ظ) ويرشّ عليه بزر[٢٨٦] فجل وبزر رشاد أجزاء سواء ويأكله. نافع مفيد إن شاء الله تعالى.[٢٨٧]

فينبغي أن يجعل غداؤه ما يناسبه ويصلح له[٢٨٨] مثل الهريسة بلحم الفراريج أو بلحم الغنم الشيشاع[٢٨٩] والخبز الفطير المخدوم بالعجن القوي من دقيق الجراية[٢٩٠] وماء الحمّص كعادة الحكماء وذلك أن يأخذ الحمّص الأبيض وينقع[٢٩١] ويقشر ويطبخ في قدرة إلى أن ينهري[٢٩٢] وتخرج قوته إلى الماء.[٢٩٣]

---

٢٧٧ المجموعه ... رقيقا: -- (ق)

٢٧٨ يخلط: يختلط (ب)

٢٧٩ ويخلط ... ولا يغلظ: -- (ق)

٢٨٠ الحمام: + مرارا (ب)

٢٨١ وكلّما خرج من الحمّام: صباحا و(ق)

٢٨٢ وتحت... تقدم: ومقعدته وتحت ابطيه ثم يأكل من معجون المسك بعد خروجه من الحمام (ق)

٢٨٣ الادياك: الديوك (ق)

٢٨٤ التي: الذي (ب)

٢٨٥ بقدرة مع بصل: ببصل (ب)

٢٨٦ ويرشّ عليه بزر: ترش الفجل (أ)

٢٨٧ التي جمعت ... تعالى: بقدرها بصلا ويرشّ عليه بزنجبيل وبزر رشاد اجزاء سواء ثم يأكلها فانه نافع المذكور (ق)

٢٨٨ يناسبه ويصلح له: يناسب (ق)

٢٨٩ الشيشاع: -- (ب)

٢٩٠ الجراية: صافي (ب)

٢٩١ الشيشاع ... وينقع: وصفه أمّا ماء الحمّص وهوان يؤخذ منه جزء ونقطع (ق)

٢٩٢ ينهرى: يتهري (غ/ب)

٢٩٣ الماء: الماء المطبوخ فيه (ق)

ثمّ يصفّى الماء ويرمى التفل، ثم يجمع[٢٩٤] العصافير الدورية[٢٩٥] وتذبح[٢٩٦] وينقوا من أوساخهم ويقطعوا كلّ قطعة قدر الحمّصة تجعلهم في القدرة[٢٩٧] في ماء الحمّص وتطبخهم به[٢٩٨] وتسدّ فم القدرة حتّى لا يخرج البخار وتقد عليه بنار لينّه حتّى لا يحترق وينهري[٢٩٩] وعلامة ذلك أن تطلع[٣٠٠] (١٣و) رائحته مثل اللحم المشوي. ثمّ ينزل عن النار ويجعل فيه هذه الحوائج، وهي[٣٠١] زنجبيل خمسة دراهم ودار فلفل درهمين ونصف وستجات جوزة[٣٠٢] وعشرة دراهم قرفة. يدقّ الجميع ويرفعوا[٣٠٣] وترش على ما ذكرناه ويستعمل وكلّما أكل مثل هذا الطعام يرشّ عليه من هذه الأبازير ويأكل وإن لم يلتقي[٣٠٤] العصافير يأخذ[٣٠٥] عوضهم فراخ الحمام فان ذلك يقوم مقام العصافير. وكذلك يأكل تقلية الجزر بلحم الشيشك أو الفراريج[٣٠٦] والديوك قبل أوان صياحها ولا يطبخ الجزر إلّا بعد غلسه وتنظيفه من قشره. ثمّ يقطع صغارًا ويطبخ مع ما تيسر من اللحوم التي[٣٠٧]

---

٢٩٤ بجمع: يجعل (ب)

٢٩٥ يجمع العصافير الدورية: تجمع العصافير (ق)

٢٩٦ تذبح: يذبح (غ)

٢٩٧ القدرة: القدر (ب)

٢٩٨ اوساخهم ... به: الاوساخ وتقطع كلّ قطعه مقدار الحمّص وتطبخ في ماء الحمّص (ق)

٢٩٩ ينهرى: تتهري (غ) / يتهري (ب)

٣٠٠ تطلع: يطلع (ب)

٣٠١ وتقد ... هى: فإذا ظهرت رائحته ينزل عن النار ويغلي عليه (ق)

٣٠٢ ستجات طيب: ست حبات جوزة الطيب (ب)

٣٠٣ يرفعوا: يرفعها (غ)

٣٠٤ وستجات ...لم يلتقى: وست جوزات وقرفة عشرة دراهم وتمزجهم ثم ترفعهم فإذا اكلت طعامًا نفيسا فرشها عليه منه ويستعمل فانه نافع لما ذكرناه وان لم يجد (ق)

٣٠٥ بأخذ: يؤخذ (ب)

٣٠٦ فينبغي (أن يجعل) ... الفراريج: -- (أ)

٣٠٧ تيسر... التي: قليل من اللحم الذي (أ)

ذكرناها. ثمّ يرشّ عليه من الأبازير المذكورة يؤكل[٣٠٨] ويشرب عليه[٣٠٩] من الألبان الحليب البقري مطبوخًا[٣١٠] (١٣ظ) بالتمر مقدار أن تحليه ويأكل أيضًا السمك المشوي[٣١١] بالبصل الأبيض وإذا أكل التسليق ياكله[٣١٢] بالثوم. نافع.

صفة عمل التسليق[٣١٣] الثوم

قال هو أن[٣١٤] يأخذ الثوم الشامي الجديد ويقشر[٣١٥] فصوصًا، ثمّ[٣١٦] يؤخذ[٣١٧] دهن البقر[٣١٨] يسلى،[٣١٩] ثمّ يصفّى. ثمّ يؤخذ من سلاه قليلًا ويدقّ ويخلط مع الدهن ويطبخ حتّى ينهرى،[٣٢٠] ثمّ يوضع في سكّروجة[٣٢١] ثمّ[٣٢٢] يعجن باليد عجنًا قويًا حتّى ينماع ويكون رائق،[٣٢٣] ثمّ يجعله على النار الليّنة إلى أن يشتدّ قليلًا.[٣٢٤] ثمّ يجعل عليه الثوم المقشّر[٣٢٥] ويخلط ويضرب حتّى يتّحدا، ثمّ ينزله عن النار ويرمى

---

٣٠٨ يؤكل: يأكل (أ)

٣٠٩ عليه: -- (أ)

٣١٠ مطبوخا: مطبوخ (أ)

٣١١ مطبوخا ... المشوي: المستوي (غ)

٣١٢ التسليق يأكله: التصليق فاكله (ب) / التسليق: التصليق (أ)

٣١٣ التسليق: التصليق (ب) / نافع ... هو أن: الشامي. عمل الثوم الشامي (أ)

٣١٤ فان ذلك... هوان: فانها تقوم بمقامها وكذا طبيخ الجزر باللحم أو الفراريج يرشّ عليه وصفة التسليق (ق)

٣١٥ يقشر: تقشر (ب)

٣١٦ ويقشر فصوصا ثم: يقشر و(ق) / يقشر: تقشر (أ)

٣١٧ يؤخذ: تأخذ (أ)

٣١٨ البقر: + وفي أخرى سمن البقر(ب)

٣١٩ يسلى: ويسلي (ق) / تسليه (أ)

٣٢٠ ينهرى: يهتري (غ/ب)

٣٢١ سكّروجة: سكّرجة (غ/ب)

٣٢٢ ثم: -- (أ)

٣٢٣ رائق: رائقا (ب/أ)

٣٢٤ قليلا: حتّى يتحد (غ)

٣٢٥ المقشر: المقشور (ب/أ)

عليه[٣٢٦] من الأبازير والحرارات المذكورة وقدر ما يعمل مزاجه[٣٢٧] مع نصف درهم زعفران[٣٢٨] في وعاء قزاز[٣٢٩] ويرفع ويستعمل منه في كلّ يوم ثلاث مثاقيل[٣٣٠] وهذا (١٤و) هو تسليق[٣٣١] الثوم الذي ذكرناه يدفع البرودة من الظهر والوسط وينقّي المعدة من البلاغم وينقّى الصدر من البلغم والفضلات ويخرج جميع العلل من البدن بإذن الله تعالى. **ويستعمل** أيضًا الورد المربّى بالعسل النحل الصافي.

وصفنته[٣٣٢] هو أن تأخذ الورد وتجعله في الشمس في وعاء قزاز وتجعل عليه العسل وتبسه معه وكلّما جفّ العسل عنه[٣٣٣] تزيده عسلًا إلى أن يأخذ قوامه ويتربّى ويأكل أيضًا الخبز الفطير المبسوس بالسمن البقري الطري ويستعمل التفّاح الحلو البالغ الاحتماء[٣٣٤] الذي ذكرناه، فينبغي أن يحتمى من أكل الحوامض جميعها ومن الألبان ومن قديد البقري والطري منه[٣٣٥] ويحترز من لحم الماعز ومن الزبيب الأسود ويتناول من الأشربة الحلو منها ويحترز من حامضها ومرّها (١٤ظ) نقل الخواجا[٣٣٦] الطوسي أنّه سمع روايات عن الحكيم[٣٣٧] بقراط وعن أرطاطاليس[٣٣٨] وغيرهم أنّه من عالج نفسه بما تقدّم

---

٣٢٦ يؤخذ ... عليه: ويلقي عليه الثوم المقشر ثم يطبخ على النار اللينة ويرمي عليها (ق)
٣٢٧ وقدر ما يعمل مزاجه: -- (ق) / ما يعمل مزاجه: ما كيل مزاجه (غ)
٣٢٨ زعفران: + يجعل في (ب)
٣٢٩ في وعاء قزاز: -- (ق)
٣٣٠ كل.... مثاقيل: في كلّ يوم ثلاث مثاقيل فانه نافع بإذن الله (ق)
٣٣١ تسليق: تصليق (ب)
٣٣٢ صفته: -- (أ)
٣٣٣ عنه: منه (ب)
٣٣٤ الاحتماء: وأما الاحتماء (ب/أ)
٣٣٥ الطري منه: الطير (أ)
٣٣٦ الخواجا: + حكيم (أ)
٣٣٧ الحكيم: حكيم (ب)
٣٣٨ ارطاطاليس: ارسطاطاليس (ب/أ)

من الأغذية والأشربة الحامضة[٣٣٩] يأمن من جميع ما ذكرناه من المضرّات ومن جميع الآلام[٣٤٠] والأسقام ويزول عنه الرخاوة وتقوّي جميع أفعاله خصوصًا على الجماع ولو جامع ما شاء لا يضعف ولا يتغيّر وجهه من الجماع ولا يملّ أبدًا ويجمل حاله وينصلح أمره والسلام.[٣٤١]

الباب الثاني

في بيان الأغذية المفردة النافعة المقوّية المصلحة لبدن الإنسان وطبيعته[٣٤٢]

فمن ذلك **الحلاوة** العجمية التي يكون دقيقها من دقيق جراية[٣٤٣] معتدل الملح والنضج.

قال الحكيم خواجا الطوسي رحمه الله تعالى رواية[٣٤٤] عن الحكماء المتقدّمين أنّه من كلّ من أوّل عمره على (١٥و) الدوام خبزًا ناشفًا ولا يأكل معه شيئًا آخر لا يبتلى في عمره بمرض[٣٤٥] إلى أجله لأنّ الابتلاء بالمرض لا يكون إلّا من زيادة الأخلاط،[٣٤٦] وزيادة الأخلاط لا تكون إلّا من[٣٤٧] اختلاف

---

٣٣٩ الحامضة: غير الحامضة (ب)

٣٤٠ أيضا: + وأما (أ)

٣٤١ وهو تسليق ... والسلام: -- (ق) / ويجمل ... السلام: -- (أ)

٣٤٢ المصلحة ...وطبيعته: لبدن الإنسان والله اعلم (ق)

٣٤٣ دقيق جراية: الدقيق الصافي في دقيق الجارية (ب)

٣٤٤ رواية: روايات (ب)

٣٤٥ لا يبلى ... بمرض: فلا يبتلى جسمه بمرض مدة عمره (ب)

٣٤٦ زيادت الأخلاط: الأخلاط وزيادة (غ)

٣٤٧ وهو تسليق ... والسلام: -- (ق) الحامضة ... السلام: واحتمي عن المواكيل المخالفات والمشاريب الحامضة كما ذكرنا يأمن ان شاء الله تعالى من من جميع الأمراض والأسقام ويزول عنه الرخاوة وتقوي جميع أفعاله خصوصا على الجماع ولو جامع ما شاء لا يضعف ولا يتغير وجهه من الجماع أبدا (أ)

الأطعمة وأيضًا[٣٤٨] من الأغذية النافعة مثل لحم الغنم المشوي المهري حتّى لا تشوش المعدة منه بسرعة هضمه. وما أتمّ أحسن غذاء الطبيعة الإنسان والطف من هذه الاثنين وبعد ذلك[٣٤٩] لحم الحمام وأفراخه وأفراخ[٣٥٠] الإوزّ والدجاج والفراريج والديوك قبل أوان صياحها[٣٥١] ولحم[٣٥٢] السمك الطري وبيض الدجاج والإوزّ والبرشت[٣٥٣] وبيض غيرها يضرّ ويؤكل بيض السمك[٣٥٤] ولحم العصافير الدورية[٣٥٥] وأدمغتهم وحليب البقر والغنم الطري والبصل الأبيض المستوى على النصف[٣٥٦] والجزر واللفت (١٥ظ) والحمّص والكرّاث والسكّر والعسل والسمن البقري[٣٥٧] واللوز والبندق والفستق والرطب والتين الأخضر والعنب والرمّان الحلو البلدي[٣٥٨] والتفّاح البلدي البالغ[٣٥٩] الحلو والسفرجل الحلو المستوى[٣٦٠] البالغ[٣٦١] حتّى لا يبْقى فيه أثر الحموضة وهذه الأشياء التي ذكرناها جميعها مقوّيات للجماع ملطّفات تقوّي الدماغ والأعضاء وإن كانت الأدوية كثيرة لكنّ المختار منها

---

٣٤٨ زيادة الأخلاط: الأخلاط وزيادة (غ)

٣٤٩ التي يكون دقيقها ... بعد ذلك: وهي مأخوذة من الدقيق الجارية والسمن البقري والعسل النهل وكذا أكل الخبز الناشف و(ق)

٣٥٠ افراخه وافراخ: لحم (ق) / افراخ: فرخ (غ/ب) / من هذه ... فراخ: بعد هذا الأفراخ الحمام والحمام أيضا وفرخ (أ)

٣٥١ قبل اوان صياحها: -- (ق)

٣٥٢ لحم: -- (ق)

٣٥٣ البرشت: النمرشت (ب)

٣٥٤ برشت... والسمك: -- (ق)

٣٥٥ الدروية: -- (ق)

٣٥٦ على النصف: -- (ق)

٣٥٧ والسمن البقري: -- (ق) / البقري: + دهن (أ)

٣٥٨ الحلوى البلدي: -- (ق) / البلدي: المليسي (ب)

٣٥٩ البالغ: -- (ق)

٣٦٠ المستوى: -- (ق)

٣٦١ الحلو ... البالغ: -- (أ)

هذا المذكور. والسلام.[٣٦٢]

(فائدة ومما يقوي الباه، يؤخذ بزر الكرافس ويدقّ ويحله مع مثليه سكّر ويؤكل منه على الريق فإنّه مجرّب وفي رجوع الشيخ إلى صباه بزر كرفس درهمين ومثله سكّر يخلط بالسمن ويستعمل ثلاث أيّام وجامع مع شئت منه.)[٣٦٣]

الباب الثالث

في بيان الأدوية المفردة التي هي خلاصة الأدوية النافعة لجميع الأمراض التي يعالج بها[٣٦٤] خصوصًا[٣٦٥] لتقوية الأفعال في الجماع[٣٦٦] وزيادة المنى وقوة الباه.

قال أوّلها[٣٦٧] المسك والعنبر والزعفران والشقاقل وقنطريون وكبابة وفلفل وزنجبيل وقرنفل (١٦و) وأبو زيدان ولكّ وقرفة وعود هندي ولسان العصافير[٣٦٨] وقشر أترنج وأنيسون وفستق وخيار[٣٦٩] ودار فلفل وقسط وخطمية[٣٧٠] الثعلب والبض[٣٧١] الأحمر والأبيض[٣٧٢] والخولنجان وعاقرقرح[٣٧٣] وشحم الأسد ولحية

---

٣٦٢ حتّى لا يبقى ... والسلام: فهذه كلها نافعه تقوي الدماغ والأعضاء (ق)

٣٦٣ في (ب) فقط (في الهامش)

٣٦٤ بها: + الانسان (أ)

٣٦٥ خصوصا: -- (ب)

٣٦٦ الأفعال في الجماع: أفعال الجماع (غ) / (ب)

٣٦٧ قال أولها: فأولها (أ)

٣٦٨ العصافير: + قشر نارنج (ب)

٣٦٩ خيار: جلنار(ب)

٣٧٠ خطمية: خصية (ب/أ)

٣٧١ البض: البهمن (ب/أ)

٣٧٢ البض الأحمر والأبيض: الهنا الأبيض والأحمر (غ)

٣٧٣ عاقرقرح: عاقرقرحا (غ/ب) / عود القرح (أ)

التيس وزفت رومي وخشخاش وبزر الجزر وبزر اللفت وبزر الرشاد وجوزة[٣٧٤] وبسباسة وسنبل ومصطكى وقاقلّة وبورق أرضي[٣٧٥] أرمني ولؤلؤ غير مثقوب وزرنباد وساذج هندي وهليلج وبليلج وأملج وحرير[٣٧٦] والحبّة السوداء وجوز الهندي وسعد[٣٧٧] وجميع هذه الأدوية المذكورة لتقوية الجماع والباه وزيادة المنى ودفع الأمراض وهؤلاء[٣٧٨] خاصّة[٣٧٩] الأدوية المستعملة المفيدة ولأجل هذا ذكرناها فانتبه[٣٨٠] لها إذا ذكرت كلّ (١٦ظ) واحد منها في مقامه كما سيأتي ذلك عند الاحتياج إلى ذكرها.[٣٨١]

الباب الرابع[٣٨٢]

في بيان الأدوية والأغذية المركبّة[٣٨٣] والحلويات[٣٨٤] التي تصلح مزاج[٣٨٥] الإنسان وتزيل علّة[٣٨٦] الفالج ورخاوة الأعضاء وتقوّي أفعال الجماع والباه.

---

٣٧٤ جوزة: جوزة الطيب (ب)

٣٧٥ أرضى: -- (غ/ب/أ)

٣٧٦ حرير: + خام (ب)

٣٧٧ سعد: السعد (غ) / جوز الهندي وسعد: جوز الهند والسعد (ب) /الهندي: هندي (أ)

٣٧٨ هؤلاء: -- (ب)

٣٧٩ خاصة: خلاصة (أ)

٣٨٠ فانتبه: فتنبه (ب)

٣٨١ مقامه ... ذكرها: موضعه فيما يأتي بيانه (أ)

٣٨٢ في بان الأدوية المفردة... الباب الرابع: -- (ق)

٣٨٣ المركبّة: -- (ق)

٣٨٤ الحلويات: الحلاوات (ب)

٣٨٥ مزاج: -- (ق)

٣٨٦ علة: -- (ق)

قال[٣٨٧] يؤخذ من[٣٨٨] البصل الأبيض و[٣٨٩]يقشر ويقطع ويطبخ[٣٩٠] بقليل زيت وماء حتّى ينهري،[٣٩١] ثمّ يطبخ أفراخ الحمام بالملح الأندراني[٣٩٢] فإذا استوى وتهرى[٣٩٣] يصبّ عليه البصل الذي طُبخته بالزيت وتقليه معه حتّى يختلطا[٣٩٤] جيدًا. ثمّ يؤخذ[٣٩٥] وزن درهم قرفة ودرهم خولنجان ودرهم عود صليب تسحق هذه الأدوية وترشّ[٣٩٦] على البصل[٣٩٧] المطبوخ ويؤكل بالخبز الفطير ويشرب مرقته. نافع مفيد[٣٩٨] يصلح المزاج الفاسد وينوّر الوجه ويصفّى اللون والدم ويقوّي (١٧و) الجماع وله سبعة عشر فائدة غير ما ذكرناه ولو عددناها لطال الكلام وتظهر تلك الفوائد عند استعمالها إن شاء الله تعالى.[٣٩٩]

غيره: قال[٤٠٠] يؤخذ لحم الخروف يكون لا سمينًا ولا هزيلًا معتدلًا بين

---

٣٨٧ قال: فمن ذلك (ق)
٣٨٨ من: -- (ق) / قال يؤخذ من: خذ أولا من (أ)
٣٨٩ و: -- (ق)
٣٩٠ يطبخ: يطبخه (أ)
٣٩١ ينهري: يتهري (غ/ب/أ)
٣٩٢ بالملح الانذراني: -- (ق)
٣٩٣ وتهرى: -- (ق)
٣٩٤ تقليه ... يختلطا: يقليه معه حتى يخلط (أ)
٣٩٥ يؤخذ: يأخذ (أ)
٣٩٦ تسحق ... ترش: يسحق هذه الحوائج ويرشهم (أ)
٣٩٧ الذي طبخته... البصل: ويغلي حتي تختلط به ثم يؤخذ قرفة وخولنجان وعود صليب من كلّ واحد درهم يدقّ ويرشّ على ذلك المطبوخ (ق)
٣٩٨ يشرب مرقته نافع مفيد: يشرب عليه المسرفه فانه نافع (ق)
٣٩٩ ولو... تعالى: ولكن تظهر فائدته لأكله (أ)
٤٠٠ وله سبعة .... قال: نوع آخر (ق) / غيره قال: صفة أخرى (أ)

الشيئين وتدقّ[٤٠١] كبيبات ويطبخ بقدره[٤٠٢] بصل أبيض حتّى ينهرى.[٤٠٣] ثمّ يؤخذ قليل[٤٠٤] من دهن الجوز ويجعل عليه قاقّلا[٤٠٥] ودرهم قرفة ونصف درهم قرنفل[٤٠٦] وقيراط مسك ويسحق هذه الأدوية[٤٠٧] وتخلط[٤٠٨] بدهن الجوز وتصبّ[٤٠٩] على اللحم[٤١٠] في القدر وتحرّك[٤١١] حتّى تختطا[٤١٢] جميعًا ويغلى شويه[٤١٣] فينزل وهو مسدود[٤١٤] الغطاء[٤١٥] حتّى لا يخرج بخاره ويترك ساعة حتّى يبرد ويعتدل يؤكل[٤١٦] منه وقت الغداء فإنّه يصلح المزاج الفاسد ويزيل الرخاوة ويشدّ الباه[٤١٧] ويزيد المنى ويقوّي الجماع كما ينبغي[٤١٨] وله منافع كثيره هذا تظهر (١٧ظ) عند استعمالها والسلام.[٤١٩]

---

٤٠١ معتدلا ... تدق: قويا ولا هزيلا قويا ويدق (ب) / سمينا ... تدق: سمينا جدا ولاهزيلا جدا ويدقه (أ)

٤٠٢ الخروف... بقدره: الضاءن الصغير ويدقّ ويعمل الكباب ويطبخ ويرمي عليه (ق) / يطبخ: يطبخه (أ)

٤٠٣ ينهرى: يتهرى (غ/ب)

٤٠٤ ثم يؤخذ قليل: ويؤخذ (ق)

٤٠٥ قاقلا: درهم قاقلا (ب) / قاقلة (أ)

٤٠٦ ويجعل ... قرنفل: جزء وقاقلة وقرفة وقرنفل من كلّ واحد درهم (ق)

٤٠٧ ويسحق هذه الأدوية: -- (ق) / يسحق: تسحق (أ)

٤٠٨ تخلط: يخلط (ق/أ)

٤٠٩ تصب: يصب (ق/أ)

٤١٠ لحم: + الخاروف (أ)

٤١١ القدر وتحرك: القدرة ويحرك (ب/أ)

٤١٢ تخلطا: يخلط (أ)

٤١٣ شويه: قليلا (ب)

٤١٤ مسدود: مشدود (ب)

٤١٥ الغطا: الفم (غ)

٤١٦ يؤكل: فيؤكل (ب) / يبرد ... ويؤكل: يبرد شويه ويعتدل ثم يأكله (أ)

٤١٧ ويشد الباه: -- (أ)

٤١٨ كما ينبغي: -- (أ)

٤١٩ والسلام: -- (أ)

غيره: قال[٤٢٠] يؤخذ الفراريج و[٤٢١] تذبح وتنشف[٤٢٢] وتغسل، ثمّ تشرح شرحات وترشّ على ناحية منها[٤٢٣] ملح اندراني وتشوى[٤٢٤] على جمر وتقلب[٤٢٥] ظهرًا وبطنًا حتّى تستوي معتدلًا، فيؤخذ قدر[٤٢٦] خمسة دراهم حبّة السوداء وثلاثة دراهم[٤٢٧] من لحية التيس وأربعة دراهم لسان عصفور ونصف درهم جوز الهند[٤٢٨] الجميع ويرشّ منهم على اللحم. ثمّ يتعشّى به من حين فإنّه يقوّي الأعضاء الرئيسة ويزيد في الحرارة الغريزية ويزيل البرودات من الظهر والوسط ويخرج الرطوبات والفضلات من البدن ويحمر الوجه ويصفّي الدم ويقوّي الجماع، ولو جامع ثلاثة أيّام متوالية[٤٢٩] لا يبالى ولا يضعف ومع ذلك يرضى كلّ ليلة عشرة من الجواري ومن النساء (١٨و) الأحرار[٤٣٠] من غير تشويش[٤٣١] وانزعاج كذا ذكروه[٤٣٢] الحكماء والأطبّاء المتقدّمون وقالوا إن هذه الأسرار لا ينبغي {لأحد} كشفها إلّا على أهلها وإذا استعملها الإنسان ودوام عليها يظهر له فوائد ومنافع في أسرع وقت، والسلام.

---

٤٢٠ تحرك حتّى ... قال: يحرك حتي يمنزج بها وينزل ويشرب فانه نافع لما ذكر ان شاء الله وغيره (ق) / قال: -- (أ)

٤٢١ و: -- (ب)

٤٢٢ تنشف: تنتف (ب)

٤٢٣ منها: منهم (غ/ب) / الواحد (أ)

٤٢٤ تشوى: يشوي (أ)

٤٢٥ تقلب: يقليه (أ)

٤٢٦ قدر: -- (ب) / تستوي ... قدر: يستوي معتدلا ثم وزن (أ)

٤٢٧ دراهم: -- (غ)

٤٢٨ الهند: الهندي + يسحق (غ) / الهندي (ب) / هندي + يسحق (أ)

٤٢٩ متوالية: -- (ب)

٤٣٠ الأحرار: -- (ب) / من النساء الأحرار: -- (أ)

٤٣١ تشويش: تشوش (ب)

٤٣٢ كذا ذكروه: وتغيير مزاج كذا ذكره (ب/أ)

فصل في بيان الحلاوات إذا استعملها الإنسان يصلح[٤٣٣] مزاجه[٤٣٤] وتصلح المفلوج وتزيل الرخاوة وتقوّي[٤٣٥] الأعضاء الرئيسة وتزيد الحرارة الغريزية وتقوّي[٤٣٦] الجماع وتزيد المنى وذلك أن يأخذ وزن[٤٣٧] مائة درهم عسل نحل الأبيض منزوع الرغوة مع وزنه بصل أبيض يقشّر ويقطّع صغارًا، ويطبخ مع العسل ويجعل عليه قليل ماء[٤٣٨] حتّى ينهرى[٤٣٩] البصل. ثمّ يجعل عليه قليل زيت وينقل[٤٤٠] ويجعل في قدرة ويوقد[٤٤١] على نار ليّنة[٤٤٢] إلى أن ينعقد نصف انعقاد. ثمّ يصفّى (١٨ظ) ويصبر قليلًا حتّى يبرد، ثمّ يرشّ على[٤٤٣] هذا المسحوق وهو من القرفة خمسة دراهم ومن قشر الأترنج[٤٤٤] خمسة دراهم وعود هندي درهمين ونصف درهم[٤٤٥] زعفران يدقّوا ناعمًا[٤٤٦] وينخلوا من خرقة[٤٤٧] حرير ويضافوا إلى العسل والبصل ويضربوا بالملعقة وترفعهم في إناء قزاز وتستعمل

---

٤٣٣ يصلح: تصلح (غ)

٤٣٤ مزاجه: + الفاسد (ب) / المزاج الفاسد (أ)

٤٣٥ تصلح... تزيل ... تقوي: يصلح... يزيل ... يقوي (أ)

٤٣٦ وتزيد ... تقوي: يقوي (أ)

٤٣٧ وتذبح وتنشف.... وزن: وتطبخ ويرمي عليها خمسة دراهم لسان عصفور ودرهم جوز هندي ودرهم قرفة وقرنفل ويحرره حتي يمتزج بها وينزل ويتعشا به فانه غاية لما ذكر وأمّا الحلويات في أصلح المزاج وتقوي الأعضاء الرئيسة وتزيل الرخاوة وتزيد الحرارة الغريزية ومنها يؤخذ (ق)

٤٣٨ ماء: الماء (غ)

٤٣٩ ينهرى: تتهري (غ) / حتى ينهرى: إلى أن يتهرأ (ب/أ)

٤٤٠ ينقل: يقلى (أ)

٤٤١ يوقد: يغلي (غ/ب) / في قدرة ويوقد: -- (أ)

٤٤٢ وتزيد ... تقوي: يقوي (أ)

٤٤٣ على: عليه (غ)

٤٤٤ ثم يجعل ... الأترنج: ويأخذ العسل في الانعقاد فيرشّ عليه وقرفة وقشر الأترنج من كلّ (ق)

٤٤٥ خمسة ... درهم: -- (أ)

٤٤٦ ناعمًا: + ويسحقوا (غ/ب)

٤٤٧ خرقة: -- (ب/أ)

منه كلّ ليلة عند النوم ترى[٤٤٨] العجب.

نوع آخر

قال[٤٤٩] يؤخذ حمّص أصفر ينقع في الماء ثمّ يقشّر و[٤٥٠] يغلى في سمن بقري إلى أن يحمر وإيّاك أن[٤٥١] يسود ويحترق. ثمّ يدقّ ناعمًا ويجعل عليه وزنه لبّ صنوبر[٤٥٢] شامي مدقوق ويخلط في عسل نحل أبيض منزوع الرغوة، ويرشّ عليه هذه الأدوية مسحوقة، وهي نصف درهم زعفران وخمسة دراهم قشر اترنج ودرهم[٤٥٣] قرفة[٤٥٤] لفّ ونصف درهم عود هندي وعشرة (١٩و) دراهم دار صيني يسحقوا ناعمًا، وترشّ[٤٥٥] على الأدوية ويحرّكوا. ثمّ ترفعوا ويستعملوا[٤٥٦] عند النوم كلّ يوم ترى العجب ولو كان لك عشر جوار ترضيهن في ليلة[٤٥٧] من غير انزعاج ولا تغيير مزاج.[٤٥٨] مجرّب، والسلام.[٤٥٩]

---

٤٤٨ نار لينة: النار اللينة (أ)

٤٤٩ قال: -- (أ)

٤٥٠ أصفر... و: مقشر بعد نقعه في ماء ثم (ق)

٤٥١ أن: + لا (أ)

٤٥٢ واياك ... صنوبر: ثم يدقّ ناعمًا ويضاف وزنه لب شونيز (ق)
صنوبر: شونيز (غ)

٤٥٣ درهم: درهمين (ب)

٤٥٤ قرفة: قرنفل (أ)

٤٥٥ ترش: يرش (أ)

٤٥٦ ترفعوا: يرفعوا (غ) / يرفعوا ويستعملوا: يرفع ويستعمل (ب/أ)

٤٥٧ في ليلة: -- (ب)

٤٥٨ ولا تغيير المزاج: -- (أ)

٤٥٩ مدقوق ويخلط... والسلام: ويصب عليه بقدره عسل نحل منزوع الرغوة حتي يمتزج به ثم يرشّ عليه قشر اترنج خمس دراهم وزعفران نصف درهم ويحرك وينزل ويستعمل منه كلّ يوم عند النوم مثقال تر العجب العجيب لما ذكر (ق)

الباب الخامس

في بيان الأشربة التي تصلح المزاج الفاسد وتصفّى الدم وتقوّي[٤٦٠] جميع الأفعال للجماع والباه.

اعلم أنّ الشراب إذا كان حلوًا وأحمر اللون يقال له الشراب العلى فهو مفيد. وأمّا الشراب الذي يميل إلى الصفرة يقال له الشراب اليزدي[٤٦١] ويكون حلوًا[٤٦٢] أبيض[٤٦٣] مفيد. وأمّا الشراب الذي يعتصر من العنب الأبيض المستوى البالغ يقال له الشراب الريحاني وهو أيضًا مفيد. ولكن أحسنهم[٤٦٤] أن يكون ممزوجًا مطبوخًا لأنّ الشراب[٤٦٥] يضرّ، بل ينبغي أن يكون مثلثًا (١٩ ظ) كعادة الحكماء مطبوخًا بالأدوية حتّى يناسب الطبيعة ويحصل[٤٦٦] الفوائد كما علموا ذلك بالتجارب.

صفة الشراب المثلّث[٤٦٧]

قال هو على عادة الحكماء هو يؤخذ[٤٦٨] من أيّ نوع أردت من الأشربة المذكورة وتجعل[٤٦٩] عليه قدره ثلاث مرّات ماء عذب صافي ويغلى حتّى يذهب ثلثي الماء

---

٤٦٠ تصفى ... تقوي: يصفى ...ويقوي (أ)

٤٦١ اليزدي: الزمردي (ب)

٤٦٢ حلوا: + فهو (غ/ب)

٤٦٣ أبيض: أيضا (ب) / وهو أيضا (أ)

٤٦٤ أحسنهم: الأحسن (ب)

٤٦٥ الشراب: + الصرف (غ/ب)

٤٦٦ يحصل: تحصل (غ) / يجعل (أ)

٤٦٧ على هامش النص في (ب): وفي نزهة الشيخ داود ما نصه ومن أخذ مثقلا من العود الهندي قيراط من المسك وثلاثة من الزعفران ونصف رطل من العسل وستة أرطال من الشراب وإثني عشر رطلا من الماء العذب وطبخ الكل حتى يذهب النصف كفا قليلة سكرا وتفريحا ونفعا ولم يحتج إلى إصلاح.

٤٦٨ هو... يؤخذ: إن تأخذ (ب) / قال... يؤخذ: يأخذ (أ)

٤٦٩ تجعل: يجعل (أ)

ويبقى الثلث، فيؤخذ[470] من هذا المطبوخ وزن ثلاثمائة درهم ووزن خمسين درهم من عسل النحل الأبيض[471] أو سكّر أبيض ويغلى الى أن يؤخذ رغوته. ثمّ يؤخذ[472] زنجبيل ودار صيني من كلّ واحد درهمين وعود هندي وعنبر وسنبل من كلّ واحد درهم.[473] يدقّ الجميع ناعمًا كالغبار وينخلوا من خرقة حرير. ثمّ يضعهم[474] على الشراب، ثمّ يغلى ثانيًا بنار ليّنة ساعة لطيفة حتّى يمتزج بعضها[475] (٢٠و) ببعض.[476] ثمّ ينزل وتصبر عليه[477] حتّى يبرد. ثمّ يرفع في إناء زجاج وإذا أراد الاستعمال منه يأخذ[478] منه وزن أربعين درهمًا وتمزج بوزنهم ماء وتشربهم[479] نافع إن شاء الله تعالى. يقوّي المعدة ويسخّن الكبد وينوّر الوجه ويصفّى الدم ويقوّي الحرارة الغريزية والجماع ولو جامع عشر جوار لأرضاهن[480] من غير تعب ولا ضعف ولا إزعاج بل يزداد نشاطًا ولكن يصبر بعد[481] ساعتين، ثمّ يجامع ولا يأكل شيئًا إلّا بعد الجماع يرى عجبًا إن

---

٤٧٠ فيؤخذ: ثم يؤخذ (أ)

٤٧١ جميع الأفعال... الأبيض: الجماع ويسمي بالشراب المثلث يؤخذ من ماء العنب جزء ويجعل عليه ماء عذب قدره بثلاث مرات ويغلي حتي يبقي الثلث فيؤخذ منه وزن ثلاث مائة درهم ومن العسل النحل خمسين درهما (ق)

٤٧٢ إلى ان ... يؤخذ: ثم يضاف له (ق)

٤٧٣ درهم: + مسك درهم (أ)

٤٧٤ يضعهم: تضعهم (غ) / وينخلوا ... يضعهم: منخولا من المنخل الخرير الرفيع ويصبهم (أ)

٤٧٥ يمتزج بعضها: تمتزج بعضهم (غ)

٤٧٦ بضعها ببعض: بعضهم بالبعض (ب/أ)

٤٧٧ عليه: ساعة (ب)

٤٧٨ يأخذ: يؤخذ (ب)

٤٧٩ تشربهم: يشربه (ب) / تمزج ... تشربهم: يمزجه بوزنه ماء ويشرب فإنه (أ)

٤٨٠ لارضاهن: لارضى الجميع (ب)

٤٨١ بعد: + شربه (غ/ب) / لارضاهن ... عجبا: ارضا بنشط وانبساط ولكن يصير بعد شربه ساعتين (أ)

شاء الله تعالى.[482]

(وشراب اللوز أيضًا نافع مفيد، وكيفية تأخذ اللوز وتسلقه بالماء الحارّ حتّى يذهب جميع قشره وتدقّه في هوان رخام أو عود وتنقعه في ما يكفيه من الماء العذب وتعصره بعد أن يخرج نفعه كلّه وتضيف له شيئًا من المصطكى وما يكفيه من السكّر الأبيض ويطبخ على نار ليّنة حتّى يعقد قليلاً، ويرفع.)[483]

الباب السادس

في بيان المعاجين والجوارشات[484] المفرحة الدافعة للملال[485] التي تقوّي المعدة وتدفع[486] البلغم والسوداء وتدفع[487] سدد الدماغ والأعضاء[488] وتصفّى الدم وتحلل الرياح الفاسدة وتقوّي (٢٠ظ) الأعضاء الرئيسة وتزيل[489] الصداع ووجع الرأس والنزلات و[490]الحرارة الغريزية[491] وتقوّي[492] الجماع قوة عظيمة حتّى لو جامع عشرين إمرأة لم يحصل له كلل ولا ملل ولا ارتخاء عضو بسبب هذا المعجون وفوائده لا تعدّ ولا تحصى خصوصًا فائدته عند

---

٤٨٢ يدقّ الجميع... تعالى: حتي يمتزج وينزل ثم يرفع في اناء زجاج فإذا اراد استعمال يؤخذ منه وزن أربعين درهما ويمزج بوزنه ماء عذب ويشرب فانه نافع لما ذكر ان شاء الله (ق)

٤٨٣ زيادة في (ب) في الهامش.

٤٨٤ والجوارشات: -- (ق)

٤٨٥ الدافعة للملال: -- (ق)

٤٨٦ وتدفع: + الصفراء (غ)/ + الصفر و(ب) / تقوي ... تدفع: يقوي...يدفع (أ)

٤٨٧ تدفع: تفتح (ب) / يفتح (أ)

٤٨٨ البلغم ... الأعضاء: الصفراء والبلغم والسوداء وتفتح السدد في المعدة (ق)

٤٨٩ تزيل: يزيل (أ)

٤٩٠ و: + تقوي (غ) / (ب)

٤٩١ ووجع... الغريزية: (ق)

٤٩٢ تقوي: يقوي (أ)

الجماع والاستعمال.[٤٩٣]

صفة جوارش القاقلّة

قال مؤلّفه عفا الله عنه[٤٩٤] يؤخذ حصا لبان[٤٩٥] وقاقلّة وبسباسة من كلّ واحد أربعة دراهم ودار فلفل وزنجبيل[٤٩٦] من كلّ واحد ثمانية دراهم وعنبر وعود هندي من كلّ واحد درهم ومن الزعفران عشرة دراهم[٤٩٧] تدقّ[٤٩٨] الأدوية وتنخل[٤٩٩] ناعمًا كالكحل، ويؤخذ قوامه[٥٠٠]عسل نحل منزوع الرغوة ويكون على نصف قوامه. ثمّ يضاف إليه الأدوية ويرفع ويستعمل عند الحاجة إليه ترى عجبًا، والسلام.[٥٠١]

(صفة ماء مفرج ومقوّي للباه مجرّب

يؤخذ وقه من الزيت الجيد ونصف أوقية من خمير الحنطة ورطل من الملح يغمر الجميع بقدر عبار ماء عذب ويختمر ليلة، ثمّ يلقى عليه ثلاثة أرطال شيبة

---

٤٩٣ خصوصا ... و: تشاهد فائدة عند (ب) / خصوصا ... الاستعمال: يحصى وعند الاستعمال تظهر فائدة (أ)

٤٩٤ حتّى لو... الله عنه: صفة جوارش القاقلة (ق)

٤٩٥ حصا لبان: + ذكر (ق)

٤٩٦ فزنجبيل: وزنجبيل (ق) / (غ)

٤٩٧ وعنبر ... عشرة دراهم: وعوده درهم وعنبر درهم وزعفران ثلث دراهم (ق)

٤٩٨ تدق: يدقّ (غ)

٤٩٩ تنخل: ينخل (ب/أ)

٥٠٠ وتنخل... قوامه: وترمي في (ق)/ يؤخذ قوامه: يأخذ له قوام (أ)

٥٠١ ويكون... والسلام حتي ينعقد ويرفع ويستعمل منه وزن مثقال بعد العشاء تر العجب (ق) / عسل... السلام: العسل ويجعلهم في إناء زجاج ويستعمل منه عند الحاجة فإذا أراد الجماع يشرب على المعجون قدحين ثلاثة من الشراب المثلثي الذي تقدم وصفة ترى العجب (أ)

وقفة نعناع ويقطر ويرفع فإنّه جيد.)[502]

(٢١و) صفة معجون السنبل[503]

قال يؤخذ سنبل وبسباسه وجوز[504] وقرنفل وحبّة السوداء[505] وقاقلّة ودار صيني من كلّ واحد نصف[506] درهم وسمسم أبيض[507] مقشّر ستين درهمًا تدقّ الأدوية وحدهم والسمسم وحده ناعمًا كالغبار. ثمّ يخلطا[508] ويعجن[509] بعسل منزوع الرغوة[510] على نصف قوامه ويستعمل منه عند الحاجة إليه وزن ثلاث دراهم ترى عجبًا خصوصًا عند الجماع.

صفة معجون ذوي[511] الحسك[512]

قال يؤخذ[513] شوك الحسك ما أردت يقطع صغار[514] ويوضع في قدرة[515] ويغلى عليه بالماء حتّى يخرج قوة الحسك[516] في الماء، ثمّ يصفّى الماء المنتخب

---

٥٠٢ زيادة في (ب) في الهامش.

٥٠٣ الوصفة ساقطة من (أ)

٥٠٤ جوز: جوز بوا (ب)

٥٠٥ السوداء: سوداء (ق)

٥٠٦ نصف: -- (ق)

٥٠٧ أبيض: -- (ق)

٥٠٨ تدقّ... ويخلطا: -- (ق)

٥٠٩ يخلطا ويعجن: يخلطان ويعجنوا (ب)

٥١٠ الرغوة: -- (ب)

٥١١ ذوي: -- (ب)

٥١٢ هذه الوصفة ساقطة من (أ)

٥١٣ يعجن ... يؤخذ: بعد الدقّ بالعسل النحل حتي ينعقد ويستعمل منه عند الحاجة ثلاث دراهم تر العجب معجون الحسك يؤخذ من (ق)

٥١٤ يقطع صغار: تقطع صغارا (ب)

٥١٥ قدرة: قدر (ب)

٥١٦ ما أردت... الحسك: جزء يقطع ويغمر بالماء ويغلي على النار حتي تخرج قوته (ق)

في[٥١٧] الحسك الذي يبقى قشره، ويؤخذ قشره وورقه ويسقى الماء الذي صفيته في الشمس الحارّة أيّام الصيف وكلّما جفّ ونشف تسقيه[٥١٨] وحرّكه (٢١ظ) إلى أن يشرب الماء الذي صفيته ويبقى لينًا مستويًا.[٥١٩] فيؤخذ منه درهم وعاقرقرح[٥٢٠] درهم وزنجبيل نصف درهم وعشرة دراهم من أدمغة العصافير الدورية، ثمّ تسحق[٥٢١] الأدوية سحقًا بليغًا وتخلط مع الأدمغة خلطًا جيّدًا ويضاف إليهم قوامهم من السكّر أو من عسل النحل المنزوع الرغوة ويعقد معجونًا[٥٢٢] ويجعل في إناء زجاج ويستعمل منه عند الحاجة إليه وإذا[٥٢٣] أراد الجماع يشرب عليه قدحين أو[٥٢٤] ثلاثة من الشراب المثلث الذي تقدّم وصفه يرى عجبًا حتّى لو جامع عشر[٥٢٥] من النساء في ليلة لا رضاهن، والسلام.[٥٢٦]

٥١٧ المنتخب في: المتخشب من (ب)

٥١٨ تسقيه: اسقيه (ب)

٥١٩ ثم يصفى... مستويا: فيصفي ويتبقي من قشره ومرقه ثم يوضع في الشمس الحارّة فكلّما نشف اسقه من ذلك الماء حتي يلين (ق)

٥٢٠ عاقرقرح: عاقرقرحا (غ/ب)

٥٢١ تسحق: يسحق (غ)

٥٢٢ درهم وزنجبيل ... معجونا: وزنجبيل من كلّ درهم وادمغة العصافير عشرة دراهم ويسحقهم سحقا جيدًا ثم يعقد بالعسل النحل (ق)

٥٢٣ وإذا: فإذا (ق/ب)

٥٢٤ أو: -- (ب)

٥٢٥ عشر: عشرة (غ/ب)

٥٢٦ يشرب ... والسلام: تشرب عليه قد حين الشراب المثلث المتقدم ذكره فانه غايه والله اعلم (ق)

صفة الإطْرِيفَل[٥٢٧]

وله منافع عظيمة وفوائد لا تعدّ ولا تحصى منها أنّه يزيد في العقل[٥٢٨] وينقّى[٥٢٩] الدماغ من جميع العلل والنزلاء[٥٣٠] ويحدّ البصر ويزيد (٢٢و) نوره ويفتح سدد الرأس والعين[٥٣١] ويقوّي سمع الأذن ويصفّي الدم ويسمّن ويقوّي الأعضاء الرئيسة والحرارة الغريزية ويقوّي الباه[٥٣٢] ويشدّ الأعصاب[٥٣٣] وعروق الذكر والخصيتين ويسخّن الكلى والمثانة والمنى ويقوّي الجماع تقوية عظيمة بحيث لو جامع ما شاء لا يملّ ولا يضعف ولا يرتخي ولا يضرّه.[٥٣٤]

وصفته: يؤخذ[٥٣٥] قشرة وهليلة[٥٣٦] صفراء وبليلج[٥٣٧] وأملج[٥٣٨] ودار فلفل من كلّ واحد ثلاثة دراهم، وبسباسة وزنجبيل من كلّ واحد أربعة دراهم، وشقاقل[٥٣٩] درهم، ولسان عصفور[٥٤٠] خمسة دراهم ودار صيني سبعة دراهم وسمسم أبيض مقشور عشرون[٥٤١] درهمًا، يدقّ هذه الأدوية ناعمًا وينخل من

---

٥٢٧ الإطريفال: +الصغير (ب)

٥٢٨ وله ... العقل: -- (ق) / وله... منها: الذي قدره عظيم ونفع جسيم وفرائده لا تعد ولا تحصى فمن بعض منافعه أنه (أ)

٥٢٩ ينقى: ينفع (ق)

٥٣٠ النزلاء: النزلات (غ/ب) / النزلات ويدفعها (أ)

٥٣١ نوره ويفتح سدد الرأس والعين: العقل (ق)

٥٣٢ ويقوي الباه: فالذكر (أ)

٥٣٣ الرئيسه ...الاعصاب: -- (غ)

٥٣٤ ما شاء... يضره: بها جامع (أ)

٥٣٥ يؤخذ: قال يؤخذ: قدر (ب)

٥٣٦ وهليله: أهليلج (ب)

٥٣٧ بليبج: بليله (أ)

٥٣٨ يقوي الباه... وأملج: يشد العصب والذكر ويسخن الكلا والمثانه ومني ويقوي الجماع قوة عطيمة وصفة اهليلج وأملج وبليلج (ق)

٥٣٩ وبسباسه ... وشقاقل: بسباسه وشقاقل (ق)

٥٤٠ عصفور: العصافير (ق/غ/ب)

٥٤١ عشرون: عشرين (ق/أ)

خرقة رفيعة[٥٤٢] ويضاف إليهم نصف قوامهم[٥٤٣] سكّر أبيض (٢٢ظ) أو[٥٤٤] عسل نحل منزوع الرغوة ويعجن الحوائج به ويرفع[٥٤٥] في إناء قزاز[٥٤٦] ويسدّ رأسه[٥٤٧] ويدفن[٥٤٨] في الشعير أربعين يومًا، ثمّ يستعمل منه عند الحاجة إليه ثلاث مثاقيل ويشرب بالماء. نافع إن شاء الله تعالى.[٥٤٩] مجرّب.[٥٥٠]

الباب السابع

في بيان الشيافات التي تدفع الرطوبات من الأعضاء ويزيل[٥٥١] البرودات من الظهر والوسط[٥٥٢] وتجذب البلغم والصفراء والسوداء ويقوّي[٥٥٣] الجماع بالغًا.

وصفته: قال[٥٥٤] يؤخذ سكّر أبيض خمسة[٥٥٥] دراهم و[٥٥٦] زنجبيل درهمين[٥٥٧]

---

٥٤٢ هذه الأدوية... رفيع: الأدوية وتنخل (ق)

٥٤٣ إليهم نصف قوامهم: إليها (ق) / قوامهم: قوام (أ)

٥٤٤ أبيض أو: و(أ)

٥٤٥ منزوع ...يرفع: أبيض ويعجنهم ثم يرفعه (أ)

٥٤٦ الرغوة... قزاز: ويرفع في اناء زجاج (ق)

٥٤٧ رأسه: رأس الإناء (ب)

٥٤٨ يدفن: يدفنه (أ)

٥٤٩ إن شاء الله تعالى: -- (ب)

٥٥٠ نافع ... مجرب: فانه نافع لما ذكر ان شاء الله (ق) / مجرب: -- (أ)

٥٥١ يزيل: تزيل (غ/أ)

٥٥٢ تدفع .... والوسط: -- (ق)

٥٥٣ يقوي: تقوي(ب)

٥٥٤ بالغا وصفته قال: جدًا ويهيج الشهوة يهيجا عظيما وصفة (ق)

٥٥٥ خمسة: خمس (ق)

٥٥٦ قال...و: خمسة دراهم سكر (أ)

٥٥٧ درهمين: درهمان (ق)

وعاقر قرح[٥٥٨] قيراط يسحق الجميع ناعمًا كالكحل[٥٥٩] ويعجن[٥٦٠] بعسل نحل منزوع الرغوة مأخوذ القوام ويجعلوا أشيافًا ويشتفّ منه[٥٦١] عند النوم نافع إن شاء الله تعالى.

نوع آخر

قال[٥٦٢] المفيد[٥٦٣] يؤخذ أدمغة[٥٦٤] ثلاث عصافير وقيراط عاقر قرح[٥٦٥] أجزاء (٢٣و) سواء يدقّوا ناعمًا وينخلوا ويعجنوا بعسل النحل ويجعلوا أشيافًا ويشتفّ منها عند النوم يحصل المقصود. نافع.[٥٦٦]

نوع آخر

قال يؤخذ[٥٦٧] لبّ القطن وسورنجان من كلّ واحد ثلاث[٥٦٨] دراهم يدقّ ناعمًا

---

٥٥٨ عاقر قرح: عاقرقرحا (غ)

٥٥٩ يسحق الجميع ناعمًا كالكحل: ويدق (ق)

٥٦٠ يعجن: يعجنوا (ب)

٥٦١ مأخوذ القوام ويجعلوا أشيافا ويشتف: ويستعمل (ق) / يشتف: يشيف (غ) / يشتف: ينشف (ب) / يشتف: يتتشيف به (أ)

٥٦٢ ان شاء الله تعالى نوع آخر قال المفيد: لما ذكر نوع آخر (ق)

٥٦٣ المفيد: -- (غ)

٥٦٤ قال ... أدمغة: دماغ (أ)

٥٦٥ عاقر قرح: عاقرقرحا (غ/ب) / عرق القرح (أ)

٥٦٦ اجزا... المقصود: يدقّ ناعمًا وينخل من خرقة رفيعة ويخلط مع الأدوية ويوضعهم فوامهم عسل نحل ويجعل شيافا ويستعمل عند النوم ويكون بعد الاحتماء والتنقية من المغلظات نافع (غ) / (ب) / يدقّ ناعمًا وينخل من خرقة فيه ويخلط معه الأدوية ويؤخذهم فوام عسل نحل ويجعلهم شيافا ويستعمل عند النوم ويكون بعد الاحتماء والشتية من المغلظات (أ)

٥٦٧ اجزا... يؤخذ: وقرفة وقرنفل وزنجبيل من كلّ درهم ويجق ويخلط مع العسل ويستعمل عند النوم نافع لم ذكر جدًا ونوع يؤخذ لب القطن وعاقرقرحا وزنجبيل يدقّ ويعجن بالعسل ويستعمل عند النوم يحصل المقصود نوع آخر (ق)

٥٦٨ ثلاث: ثلاثة (ق)

ويعجن بشحم الأسد ويجعلا[569] أشيافًا[570] ويتشفّ[571] به[572] عند النوم بالقطن يري عجبًا خصوصًا في قوة الجماع يحصل المقصود. نافع إن شاء الله تعالى.[573]

الباب الثامن[574]

في بيان الحقن التي تمنع وجع المفاصل وذات[575] عرق النساء ووجع الظهر والوسط ويدفع الأرياح الفاسدة والقولنج ويشدّ الظهر ويقوّي أفعال الجماع.

قال يؤخذ خصي[576] الخرفان[577] يدقّ دقًّا جريشًا، ويؤخذ قدره[578] قمح أحمر[579] وقبضة بزر لفت ويجعل في قدر برام[580] ويصبّ فوقه غمره[581] ماء[582]

---

٥٦٩ يعجن ... يجعلا: يعجنوا بدهن شخم الأسد ويجعل (ب)

٥٧٠ والسورنجان ... أشيافًا: وعاقرقرحا اجزاء سواء ويدقّوا ناعمًا وينخلوا ويعجنوه بالعسل النحل ويجعلوا أشيافا (غ)

٥٧١ يشنف: ينشف (ب)

٥٧٢ به: بها (غ)

٥٧٣ ناعمًا... تعالى: ويعجن بشحم الاسد مع السل ويستعمل عند النوم يري العجب معجب (ق) قال... تعالى: لب بزر القطن وسورنجان من كل ثلاثة دراهم يدقا ناعما ويعجنان بدهن شحم الأسد ويجعلهم شايافا ويتشيف يهم عند النوم لابقطن ترى العجب (أ)

٥٧٤ ساقط الأبواب الثامن والتاسع والعاشر من (أ)

٥٧٥ ذات: + الجنب و(ب)

٥٧٦ التي تمنع... خصي: لوجع المفاصل وعرق النساء والقولنج وتدفع الأرياح الفاسدة وتقوي الجمع ونتفع وجع الظهر وصفة يؤخذ خصا (ق)

٥٧٧ الخرفان: + في نسخة لحم خصى الضأن و(ب)

٥٧٨ قدره قدر الجميع (ب)

٥٧٩ دقًّا جريشًا ويؤخذ قدره قمح أحمر: وقدره قمح (ق)

٥٨٠ ويجعل في قدر برام: ويوضع في قدر (ق)

٥٨١ غمره: غمرهم (ب)

٥٨٢ غمره ماء: ماء حتي يغمره (ق)

(٢٣ظ) ويسدّ رأس القدر بغطاء ويوضع[٥٨٣] في الفرن ليلة حتّى يتهرى، فإذا أصبح يخرجه ويأخذ[٥٨٤] من مائة وزن ثلاثين درهمًا يوضع عليه وزن درهمين من دهن الجوز الهندي[٥٨٥] ويحتقن به وقت الصبح[٥٨٦] بعد الاحتماء ويكون خالي البطن[٥٨٧] وبجعل تحت وسطه مخدّة لا عالية حتّى رأسه إلى أسفل ورجليه إلى فوق[٥٨٨] بحيث يصل الماء إلى بطنه وتجري في مصارينه يرى[٥٨٩] عجبًا ولو احتقن به في كلّ سنة مرّتين مرّة في فصل الربيع ومرّة في فصل الخريف يأمن من جميع الأمراض والأسقام بإذن[٥٩٠] الله تعالى.

نوع آخر

قال[٥٩١] يؤخذ بزر الجزر وبزر القرع وشبت[٥٩٢] وبزر بصل وكرّاث وقرفة وزنجبيل وفلفل[٥٩٣] ودار فلفل من كلّ واحد ثلاثة دراهم وكبشة حمّص مقشّر وكبشة قمح مدقوق (٢٤و) وقطعة ليّنة[٥٩٤] وقليل من دهن[٥٩٥] الخروف الضأن

---

٥٨٣ رأس ...فرن: رأسها ويرفع (ق)

٥٨٤ يأخذ: يؤخذ (ب)

٥٨٥ الجوز الهندي: جوز الهند (غ) / + فإن لم يوجد فدهن الجوز (ب)

٥٨٦ يتهرى ... الصبح: يتهرا فيؤمنماية صباحا وزن ثلاثين درهما ويوضع عليه درهمان من دهن جوز الهند ومحتقون به صباحا (ق)

٥٨٧ ويكون خالى البطن: -- (ق)

٥٨٨ فوق: + ويحقن (غ)

٥٨٩ يرى: ترى (غ)

٥٩٠ بإذن: إن (ب)

٥٩١ لا عالية ... قال: بحيث يصل الدواء الي بطنه ويجري في مصارينه فانه نافع لجميع الأمراض فيفعل في فصل الريع مرة وفي فصل الصيف وعجبًا نوع آخر (ق)

٥٩٢ وشبت: -- (ق)

٥٩٣ وكراث وقرفة وزنجبيل وفلفل: بزر كراث وبزر شبت وقرفة وقرنفل وزنجبيل (ق) / فلفل: قرنفل (غ) / فلفل: -- (ب)

٥٩٤ لينة: ليلة (ب)

٥٩٥ دهن: + مخُ (ب)

وخصى الخروف ويجعل هذا المجموع[596] في قدره ويسدّ رأسها بغطاء، وتوضع في تنور حامي أو فرن حامي ليلة حتّى يتهري. ثمّ يؤخذ ويحتقن به وهي {التي} يسمّونها[597] الحقنة المليّنة ولها سبعة وعشرون فائدة إذا[598] احتفن بها في فصل الربيع مرّة، يأمن في سنة إلى الربيع الآخر من[599] جميع الأمراض والأسقام بإذن الله تعالى.

الباب التاسع

في بيان الشدود والثياب التي تناسب طبيعة الإنسان إذا اشتدّ بها في وسطه في كلّ فصل من الفصول الأربعة.[600]

فإنّ الشدود إذا خالف طبيعة الإنسان بحسب الفصول ربما يبتلى بمرض من الأمراض.

فينبغي أن يكون الشدود والثياب منسابًا للأوقات التي (٢٤ظ) ينبغي فيها لبس ذلك حتّى تشدّ أعضاؤه وتقوّيها ولا يفسد مزاجه فطهرات المناسب من الشدود ومن ذلك اللباس والملابس في فصل الربيع الذي هو أعدل الفصول الذي يستوي فيه الحرّ والبرد أن يكون من القطن لأنّه معتدل الحرارة والبرود لا يخرج الأعضاء من الاعتدال ولا يفسد المزاج.

وأمّا الفصل الثاني الذي هو فصل الصيف الذي يقوّي فيه الحرّ فينبغي أن تكون الدكك والشدود في هذا الفصل كلّها ملمعه منسوجة من الحرير والكتّان أو الكتّان

---

٥٩٦ المجموع: الجميع (غ)

٥٩٧ وقطعة لينة ... يسمونها: وقليل دهن ضأن وقطعه لينه خروف ويوضع في قدر ويغمر بالماء ويسدّ رأسها ويوضع في الفرن ليله حتى يتهري ويحتقن به وتسمي بالملينة (ق)

٥٩٨ إذا: فإذا (ق)

٥٩٩ إلى الربيع الاخر من: – (ق)

٦٠٠ يحتوي هذا الباب في (ب) على فصل قي استخراج البيان الذي في الباب الحادي عشر في المخطوطات الأخرى

وحده، ولا تكون من الحرير وحده. وأمّا فصل الخريف، فينبغي أن تكون الشدود والملابس في هذا الفصل من الصوف والمنسوج من التنكيك.[٦٠١]

وأمّا الفراء فينبغي أن تكون من (٢٥و) السمّور والقاقم والسنجاب أو فراء الخرفان الأبيض منه والأسود منه، ويكون شدّه من صوف الجمال ومن جلد السمّور الذي يصفونه على هيئية شدّ يقال له بالتركي كمر قشاق. فإذا دبّر على هذا التدبير مشي على هذا المنوال يحصل له الأمن من ارتخاء[٦٠٢] الأعضاء الرئيسة ضعفًا ويأمن من أوجاع المفاصل والضربان والقولنج ومن الأمراض المختلفة[٦٠٣] بمشيئة الله تعالى.[٦٠٤]

الباب العاشر

في بيان شروط الجماع وكيف ينبغي أن يجمع حتّى لا يصل إليه ضعف ولا ضرر[٦٠٥] ولا سرعة الشيب والشيخوخة.

قال اعلم أنّ الجماع[٦٠٦] قائمًا يضرّ الإنسان غاية الضرر[٦٠٧] ويورث له[٦٠٨]

---

٦٠١ من التنكيك: والتفكيك (غ)

٦٠٢ الارتخاء: + وضعف الجراح والمنى بسبب اختلاف الأدوية ولا يكون (غ)

٦٠٣ فان الشدود...القولنج ومن: وكذا لبس الثياب المناسب للأوقات لاشتداد الأعضاء وتقويتها فمما يناسب في فصل الربيع لبس القطن فانه لايخرج الأعضاء من الاعتدال ولا يفسد المزاج ومما يناسب لبسه في فصل الصيف لبس الكتّان وحده وفي فصل الخريف لبس الصوف المنسوج وأمّا لبس الفر فالسمون والقاقم والسنجاب والغنم الأبيض والأسود فينفع من ارتخاء الأعضاء ومنعوا المزاج و(ق)

٦٠٤ فإنّ الشدود... تعالى: -- (ب)

٦٠٥ وكيف ... إليه: وكيفيته حتي لا يحصل منه (ب)

٦٠٦ وكيف... اعلم ان: وكيفيته فالجماع (ق) / قال: -- (ب)

٦٠٧ غاية الضرر: -- (ق) / الضرر: -- (ب)

٦٠٨ يورث له: يتولد منه (ب)

الخفقان وذات الجنب وعرق النساء وذات[٦٠٩] الرئة والنقرس والصداع، نعوذ بالله ذلك كلّه. فإنّها أمراض مهلكة (٢٥ظ) صعبة المداواة[٦١٠] يحدث غالبها من الجماع واقفًا وبعض الناس لا يعتمد على هذا الكلام، ويقول أنا جامعت هكذا ولا حصل لى من هذا الأمراض شيء.[٦١١] فنقول إن هذه الأمراض التي تحصل من الجماع قائمًا تارة تحدث[٦١٢] على الفور، وتارة[٦١٣] على التراخي إلى[٦١٤] آخر عمره[٦١٥] عند ضعف الحرارة الغريزية بحسب قوة المزاج وضعفه. من أين علم هذا القائل بأنّه سلم من لحوق شيء من هذه الأمراض ربّما يعرض له ذلك على التراخي على إنا قلنا هذا القول إذا أكثر من الجماع قائمًا.

أمّا إذا لم يكثر بل فعله مرّة أو مرّتين في عمره فلا لأن الذي يفعل هذا الشيء ما يفعله الأمر كثرة الشغف والمحبّة في حال الشبوبية فربّما دافع الم ذلك (٢٦و) وضرره كثرة حرارته الغريزية وقوة أعضائه الرئيسة وبعض هذه الأبدان يؤثر فيه ضرر ذلك لأنّه لم يميّز حاله لجهله بأحوال نفسه وقواه. هذا القدر يكفي للعاقل والسلام.

وأمّا الجماع وهو قائم على ضلعه فهو مضرّ غاية الضرر[٦١٦] يحدث منه[٦١٧] وجع الفؤاد {والقلب} والكبد ويبتلى عرض[٦١٨] القولنج وسلس البول نعوذ بالله ذلك كلّه، خصوصًا إذا اجامع على شقّه الأيمن فإنه أضرّ وأنحس من اليسر

٦٠٩ ذات: -- (ق)

٦١٠ المداواة: المعالجة (ب)

٦١١ يحدث ... شيء: كلها تحدث من النكاح قائما وقد يقول قائل أنا نكحت قائما ولم يصيبني شيء من ذلك (ب)

٦١٢ تحدث: تحصل (ب)

٦١٣ تارة: + تحصل (ب)

٦١٤ إلى: في (ب)

٦١٥ عمره: العمر (ب)

٦١٦ نعوذ بالله...الضرر: نائما (ق)

٦١٧ منه: -- (ق)

٦١٨ يبتلى عرض: -- (ق)

وكذلك الجماع قائمًا على قفاه والمرأة من فوقه[٦١٩] يورث وجع المثانة وانعقاد البول والتنقيط واحتراق البول ويبتلى بوجع المرء وهو سيلان الدم والقيح مع البول إذا بال أو وحده بلا بول نعوذ بالله من ذلك.

فينبغي (٢٦ظ) للعاقل أن يحترّز من الجماع على الهيئات المذكورة المضرّة حينئذ حتّى لا يبتلى بما ذكرناه من الأمراض.

أمّا علاج هذه الأمراض هو أن يؤخذ[٦٢٠] من عنب الذئب المستوى البالغ ويعصره. ثمّ يأخذ الأردج البالغ المستوى ويستخِرج ماؤه بالطبخ. ثمّ يجعل عليه من سكّر القند قوامه. ثمّ يخلط المائين ماء عنب الذئب وماء الأردج، ويأخذ قوامها على النار الليّنة. ثمّ يستعمل منه قدر ملعقة على الريق وملعقة عند النوم. نافع إن شاء الله تعالى.[٦٢١]

فصل[٦٢٢]

واعلم أنّ أحسن الهيئات وأولى الأشكال من الجماع أن تستلقي المرأة على

---

٦١٩ نعوذ بالله ... فوق: والجماع على الأيمن اضرّ من الأيسر وقائم على القفاء وهو على المرأة عليه (ق)

٦٢٠ يؤخذ: يأخذ (غ)

٦٢١ بحسب قوة ... تعالى: وضعف المزاج وهذه الآلام تصيب الذي يجامع قائما بحسب مداومته عليه. وأما إذا كان نادرا فلا بأس، وأما جماع الإنسان وهو نائم على شقه فهو أيضا مضر غاية الضرر، فيحدث منه وجع الكبد والفؤاد والفلج وسلس البول وخصوصا إذا جامع على شقه الأيمن، فإنه أضر من الشق الأيسر. وأما جماع الإنسان زوجته وهو نائم وهي مستعلية عليه، فإنه يحصل منه وجع المثانة وانعقاد البول والنقطة واحتراق البول ومرض البرودة وهي سيلان الدم والقيح مع البول أو من غير بول، يعوذ بالله من ذلك. فينبغي للعاقل أن يتحرى عن هذه الأمور التي تكون له سببا في هذه الأمراض. (ب)

٦٢٢ اعلم أن أحسن الهيئات وأولها أن يأتي الرجل وزجته وهي مستلقية على قفاها مستوية وتجعل تحت وسطها مخدة رقيقة وترفع فخذيها بنفسها فإذا وقع الإنزال من الرجل يضع ركبتيه على الأرض ويلقى نفسه على المرأة وهي تعانقه بيديها ورجليها وتضمه

قفاها استلقاء مستويًا وتضع تحت وسطها مخدّة رقيقة وترفع المرأة فخذيها بنفسها ولا يرفعها الرجل فإنّ ذلك مشقّة على (٢٧و) الرجل عند المجامعة تضرّه وأن يقوم الرجل على يديه وأصابع رجليه إلى أن يقرب إنزال المنى. فإذا اخذ في الانزال يضع الرجل ركبتيه على الأرض ويلقى نفسه على المرأة تعانقه بيديها ورجليها وتلمّ الرجل على صدرها لمًّا قويًا إلى أن يتمّ إنزال المنى وينقطع إنزاله في الرحم مستقيمًا مستويًا، ولا ينتصب منحرفًا ولا يضيع المنى فيحصل من إضاعته عدم حصول التولّد والتناسل، ويحصل الضرر للرجل. وإذا وقع الجماع على الوجه والشروط الذي ذكرناه يحصل له الفوائد التي ذكرناه ويأمن العلل التي قدّمناها.

الباب الحادي عشر

في بيان الأدوية التي إذا طلا[٦٢٣] بها على الذكر تغلظه وتشدّه وتجعله[٦٢٤] قائمًا من غير رخاوة خصوصًا إذا كان الرجل (٢٧ظ) لا يقدر على أكل الأدوية الحارّة يعالج بالأدوية التي تطلى[٦٢٥] على الذكر.[٦٢٦] وذلك[٦٢٧] أن تأخذ بصل

عل صدرها حتى تفرغ الأنزال في الرحم ولا يميل وقت الإنزال عن صدرها. فإن المني لا ينزل في الرحم كما هو المطلوب منه وإن لم ينزل المنى في الرحم لا تحمل المرأة منه وينقطع التناسل وإن وقع الجماع بشروط يحصل منه النفع ويمنع العلل التي شرحناها. (ب)

٦٢٣ طلا: يطلى (ب)

٦٢٤ تشدها وتجعله: يشده ويجعله (أ)

٦٢٥ تطلى: يطلى به (ب)

٦٢٦ تغلظه ... للذكر: فتغلطه وتشد رخاوته حتى يصير متينا جدا. (ب)

٦٢٧ ذلك: هو (أ)

النرجس[٦٢٨] وعاقر قرح[٦٢٩] وزبيب أحمر منزوع النوى أجزاء سواء وتدقّ[٦٣٠] الأدوية مع ربعها جوز الهند[٦٣١] وتسحق[٦٣٢] الجميع ناعمًا. ثمّ تغسل ذكره[٦٣٣] قبل الجماع بساعة بالماء الحارّ ويدلكه دلكًا قويًا حالة الغسل. ثمّ يطلى ذكره بالأدوية مقابل حرارة النار يحصل له ما ذكرناه من الغلظ والقوة وأحكامه[٦٣٤] كما ينبغي.

نوع آخر[٦٣٥]

قال يؤخذ[٦٣٦] لبّ بزر القطن نصف درهم وسعد درهمين ونصف ولبّ نوى[٦٣٧] الخروب الشامي نصف درهم وقيراط جوز الهند يدقّ الجميع ناعمًا[٦٣٨] ويجعل

---

٦٢٨ انعقاد البول ... النرجس: احتراق البول والنقطة وسيلان الدم فينبغي للعاقل ان يحترز من الجماع على الهيأت المذكورة فينبغي هذا ان تستلقي المرأة على قفاه وتضع تحتها وسطها يجده وترفع مخدتها ويقوم الرجل على أصابع رجليه إلى ان يقرب إنزال المني يلقي نفسه على المرأة وتعانقه بيديها الي الن يتم انزال المني فيحصل له الفائدة ويامن العلل المتقدمة إن شاء الله تعالي الباب الحادي عشر في بيان الأدوية لتقويته وتغليظه يؤخذ بصل نرجس (ق)

٦٢٩ عاقر قرح: عاقرقرحا (غ/ب) / عرق القرح (أ)

٦٣٠ تدق: يدق (أ)

٦٣١ تدقّ الأدوية مع ربعها جوز الهند: يدقّ مع ربعه جوز الهندي (ق) / الجوز الهندي (ب)

٦٣٢ النوى ... تسحق: العجم وقدر ربع هذه الأجزاء من الجوز الهندي يسحق (ب) / تسحق: يسحق (أ)

٦٣٣ تغسل ذكره: يغسل ذكر (أ)

٦٣٤ ثم .... أحكامه: حتى يمتزجوا ويوضع في انية فإذا أردت أن تجامع فاغسل كرك قبل الجماع بساعة بماء حار دلكا قويا حلا الغسل ثم دهنه بالدواء ودلكه به وهو مقابل النار فإنه يغلظ وينبغي. (ب) / الغلظ والقوة.: غلظة الذكر وقوته (أ)

٦٣٥ هذه الوصفة ساقطة من (أ)

٦٣٦ قال يؤخذ: نوع أخر وهو أن تأخذ (ب)

٦٣٧ نوى: بزر (ب)

٦٣٨ ناعمًا: -- (غ)

عليه ماء العنب أو الزبيب الرازقى[٦٣٩] ويغلى على النار الليّنة إلى أن يمتزجا ويشدّ[٦٤٠] الماء. ثمّ ينزل ويرفع ويطلى به (٢٨و) الذكر عند الحاجة إليه.[٦٤١]

نوع آخر[٦٤٢]

قال[٦٤٣] هذا العمل لمن به رخاوة في أعضائه وذكره وليس له قوة[٦٤٤] على الجماع وهذا لا يخلو إمّا أن يعرض له بعد أو من عدم استعماله الجماع وعلى أيّ تقدير كان، فعلاجه ان[٦٤٥] يؤخذ مرارة تيس[٦٤٦] وعاقرقرح[٦٤٧] عشرة دراهم يسحق ناعمًا.[٦٤٨] ثمّ يخلط مع دهن[٦٤٩] السعد الريحاني وتوضع[٦٥٠] في الشمس ثلاثة أيّام حتّى يمتزجوا في بعضهم بعضًا.[٦٥١] ثمّ تأخذ من جوز الهند[٦٥٢] درهم ونصف يدقّ ويخلط معهم خلطًا جيدًا ويرفع فإذا أراد الجماع يطلى به ذكره[٦٥٣]

---

٦٣٩ الرازقي: -- (ب)

٦٤٠ يشد: ينعصر (ب)

٦٤١ إليه: -- (غ) / ينزل ... أليه: احفظه في زجاجة واطلى به ذكرك وقت الحاجة والسلام. (ب)

٦٤٢ ساقط "نوع آخر" و"فصل" من (ب)

٦٤٣ قال: -- (أ)

٦٤٤ قوة: قدرة (أ)

٦٤٥ وتسحق ...فعلاجه ان: يدقّ ناعمًا ويرمي في ماء العنب والزيت ويغلي على النار الي ان ينزل ويطلى به الذكرنوع آخر (ق)

٦٤٦ تيس: التيس (ق)

٦٤٧ عاقرقرح: عاقرقرحا (غ) / عرق القرح (أ)

٦٤٨ ناعما: + غاية (أ)

٦٤٩ ثم يخلط مع دهن: ويخلط بدهن (ق)

٦٥٠ السعد الريحاني: سعد (ق) الريحاني وتوضع: ودهن الريحان وتضعه (أ)

٦٥١ بعضا: في بعض (أ)

٦٥٢ توضع... الهند: يوضع في الشمس ثلاث أيام ثم يوضع عليه جوز هندي (ق) / جوز الهندي (أ)

٦٥٣ يدق ... ذكره: ويخلط ويطلى الذكر (ق)

قبل الجماع بثلاثة أيّام كلّ يوم مرارًا فإنّه ينصلح أمره ويقوّي رخاوته وذكر جالينوس أنّه من عالج نفسه بهذا العلاج[٦٥٤] يصلح حاله ويشتدّ رخاوته عضوه ويلقى قوة الشباب في حالة الشيخوخة فكيف (٢٨ظ) إذا كان شابًا لا ينبغي فيه رخاوة أبدًا ولو كان من عشرين سنه لزالت وانصلح أمره.[٦٥٥]

فصل[٦٥٦]
في بيان عمل دهن الريحان وهو دهن السعد وسائر الأدهان

قال إذا أردت[٦٥٧] عمل دهن من الأدهان فحذ من أيهما شيئت مثلاً فيؤخذ من الريحان فيقطع أو من السعد فيدقّ فيوضع[٦٥٨] في قنّينة ويوضع عليه قدره مرّتين زيت طيّب[٦٥٩] ويسدّد رأسها سدًّا محكمًا[٦٦٠] بالشمع حتّى لا يداخل هو أو يعلّق[٦٦١] في الشمس الحارّة في أيّام الصيف أربعين يومًا في موضع لا تنقطع الشمس عنه من طلوعها إلى غروبها، فإذا تمّ الأربعين يوما تمّ الدهن. ثمّ يصفي من منخل رفيع أو خرقة رفيعة ويرفع.

واعلم أنّ هذا دهن الريحان والسعد والبنفسج يخرج على هذا المنوال وعلى هذه الطريقة.[٦٦٢] وأمّا دهن القلوب مثل (٢٩و) دهن[٦٦٣] الفستق ودهن اللوز والبندق وقلب حبّ القطن وقلب الجوز وسائر القلوب ودهن جلنّار وامثاله

---

٦٥٤ العلاج: + عشرة أيّام (غ)

٦٥٥ ويشتد ... أمره: إن شاء لله (أ)

٦٥٦ ساقط الفصل من (أ)

٦٥٧ بثلاثة أيام ... إذا أردت: ثلثة أيام ير العجب فصل في الأدهان فأردت (ق)

٦٥٨ من الأدهان... فيوضع: السعد فيؤخذ جزء من السعد ويوضع (ق)

٦٥٩ قدره مرتين زيت طيب: زيت طيب قدره مرتين (ق)

٦٦٠ سدا محكما: -- (ق)

٦٦١ حتى لا يداخل هو أو يعلق: ويعلق (ق)

٦٦٢ في أيّام الصيف ... الطريقة: في الصيف أربعين يوما ثم يصفي من منخل رفيع ويرفع (ق)

٦٦٣ مثل دهن: كدهن (ق)

على غير هذه الطريقة، بل يخرج على هذا الوجه[٦٦٤] هو أن تأخذ ما شيئت من القلوب فيدقّ دقًّا ناعمًا حتّى يبقى مثل الكسب الناعم. ثمّ تأخذ[٦٦٥] صينية نحاس مبيضه وتجعل على النار[٦٦٦] رماد سخن وتبل يدقّ بالماء الفاتر وتعرك القلب المدقوق على الصينية وتلفه وتدحرجه على الصينية تفعل به ذلك حتّى يخرج جميع دهنه وكذا تفعل بسائر القلوب والسلام.[٦٦٧]

الباب الثاني عشر[٦٦٨]

في بيان الأدوية التي تطلى على الذكر فتطوله تقويه كما تريد وتشهى.

واعلم أنّ الذكر كلّه[٦٦٩] مركّب من جميع العروق وهو[٦٧٠] يطول بالجماع وبالدلك، ولكنّ لا يكون ذلك مثل الطلى. فإن الطلى يكون (٢٩ظ) أقوى بسبب الأدوية كما ذكره أفلاطون وأرطاطاليس[٦٧١] وبقراط وجالينوس الحكيم وقالوا بوقوعه وممّا عملوا به وجرّبوه.[٦٧٢] وروي محمّد الدامغاني[٦٧٣] والإمام الرازي رحمة الله تعالى[٦٧٤] عن أفلاطون هذا العمل تطويل الذكر.[٦٧٥]

---

٦٦٤ وقلب حب القطن ... الوجه: القطن والجوز والجلنار (ق)

٦٦٥ يدقّ دقًّا ... تأخذ: تدقّ ناعم حتي يبقي كالكحل ثم تضع في (ق)

٦٦٦ مبيضه وتجعل على النار: -- (ق)

٦٦٧ تعرك ... السلام: تعجن القلب المذكور حتى تخرج دهنه وكذا تفعل سائر القلوب (ق) / والسلام: -- (غ)

٦٦٨ ساقط الباب كله من (أ)

٦٦٩ فتطوله... كله: لتنعيظه وتقويته وتطويله اعلم ان الذكر (ق)

٦٧٠ هو: قد (ق)

٦٧١ أرطاطاليس: أرسطاطاليس (ب)

٦٧٢ وقالوا .... جربوه: -- (ب)

٦٧٣ الدامغاني: الدمغاني (ب)

٦٧٤ رحمه الله تعالى: -- (غ) / رحمة الله علينا وعليهم (ب)

٦٧٥ روي ... الذكر: صفة تطويل الذكر قال محمد الدمفاني والإمام الرازي رحمهما الله

قال[٦٧٦] يؤخذ أصل الحسك الذي نبت أكثر من سنة وتغسله نظيفًا وتجفّفه وتسحقه ناعمًا وتنخله[٦٧٧] من منخل[٦٧٨] رفيع. وتدخل[٦٧٩] الحمّام وتدلك به ذكرك بالماء السخن[٦٨٠] وتغسله[٦٨١] حتّى يحمر وتدرّ[٦٨٢] عليه من أصل الحسك المسحوق بعد دلكه. ثمّ يدهن بدهن السعد المسحوق معه وزن نصف درهم جوز الهند، وإن كنت عملت هذه النسخة عندك ودهنت به منها في الحمّام ثلاث مرّات إلى أن يخرج من الحمّام. فإنّه يطول إلى أن تتعجب منه، لكنّ حكمه من ذلك (٣٠و) اليوم إلى عشرة أيّام فقط ويريد أن تجدّده،[٦٨٣] والسلام.[٦٨٤]

نوع غريب[٦٨٥] وهو من أسرار الحكماء يطول الذكر ويجعله قدر نفسه مرّتين.[٦٨٦] قال[٦٨٧] يؤخذ بعر الغنم الطري المرق والعنبر اليابس مقدار ما تطلى

عن افلاطون هذا العمل لتطول (أ)

٦٧٦ بالد لك ... قال: الدلك (ق)

٦٧٧ تنخله: ينخله (ب)

٦٧٨ تغسله... منخل: يغسيله نظيفا ويجففه غاية ويسحقه ناعما وينخله (ب/أ)

٦٧٩ تدخل: يدخل (ب/أ)

٦٨٠ السخن: الحار (ب)

٦٨١ تدلك ... تغسله: يدلك ذكره دلكا قويا (أ)

٦٨٢ تدر: يدر (ب/أ)

٦٨٣ تجدده: يجدده (ب)

٦٨٤ وإن كنت ... سلام: وتكون سحقها واحضرتها عندك في الحمام تطلي به ذكرك ثلاثة مرات إلى إن تخرج من الحمام فإنه غاية ونهاية لكن حكمه إلى عشرة أيام فقط (أ)

٦٨٥ نوع غريب: نوع آخر تركيب غريب (أ)

٦٨٦ وسلام ... مرتين: -- (ب)

٦٨٧ قال: نوع آخر (ب)

به الذكر[٦٨٨] وقيراط مسك يسحق ويؤخذ من جوز الهند[٦٨٩] درهمين ويدقّ ناعمًا[٦٩٠] في غاية النعومة ويخلط الجميع في بعضهم بعضًا خلطا قويًا. ثمّ تدخل الحمّام وتدلك ذكرك[٦٩١] بدهن السعد دلكا قويًا إلى أن[٦٩٢] يحمر. ثمّ يطلا[٦٩٣] بالحوائج الذي خلطت بالبعر مثل ما تطلى الخاتم. ثمّ يلفّ بخرقة من الصبح إلى المغرب. ثمّ تحلّه وتغسله. ترى عجبًا لأنّه يطول الذكر قدر ما كان مرّتين، ولكنّ حكمه إلى عشرين يومًا. ثمّ تجدّد العمل، والسلام.[٦٩٤]

الباب الثالث عشر

في بيان الأدوية التي يطلى بها بين أصابع اليدين (٣٠ظ) والرجلين[٦٩٥] فيقوّي الجماع ويشدّ الذكر[٦٩٦] ومهما جامع لم يضعف ولم يملّ ولم يرتخي أبدًا.

---

٦٨٨ الذي نبت أكثر ...الذكر: فيغسل ويجفف ويسحق وينخل ويدلك به الذكر في الحمام بعد غسل بالماء الساخن ثم يدهن بدهن السعد مع نصف درهم بفعل ذلك ثلاث مرات أو أكثر فإنه غاية في تطويله نوع يؤخذ عنبر يابس جزء (ق) / المرق ... الذكر: الرقيق وعود العنبر (ب)

٦٨٩ الهند: هندي (ب)

٦٩٠ يسحق ... ناعما: تسحقه وتأخذ جوز الهند أربع دراهم وقدقه في غاية (أ)

٦٩١ ويسحق ... ذكرك: وبعر غنم طري جزء ودرهمان جوز هند يدقّ ناعمًا الي ان يختلطوا فيدخل الحمام ويدلك الذكر (ق) / ناعما ... ذكرك: ويخلط ثم يدخل الحمام ويدلك الذكر (ب)

٦٩٢ إلى أن: حتى (ب)

٦٩٣ يطلى ... العمل: ثم يدهن بهذا الدواء ويلف عليه خرقة من الصباح إلى المساء وعند الجماع ينزع الخرقة ويغسل الذكر بالماء الحار فإنه يتعجب من طوله (ب)

٦٩٤ ثم يطلا ... الخام: فيطلي بالأدويه ثم يلف بخرقه من الصبح الي الغروب ثم يغسله ير العجب من تطويله ولكن حكمه الي عشرين يوما لم يجدد العمل والله أعلم (ق) / ثم... السلام: -- (أ)

٦٩٥ اليدين والرجلين: الرجلين واليدين (غ) / اليد والرجل (أ)

٦٩٦ بين أصابع اليدين والرجلين فيقوى الجماع ويشد الذكر: على أصابع الرجلين واليدين لتقوية الجما وشد الذكر (ق)

قال[٦٩٧] يؤخذ فراخ العصافير[٦٩٨] الدورية قبل أن ينبت عليهم الريش وتربط بخيط وتعلّق[٦٩٩] على باب بيت النحل. ثمّ يهوّش على[٧٠٠] النحل حتّى تلدغ الفراخ. فإذا ألدغوها مرارًا، تؤخذ بالعجلة وتذبح ولا يدع دماهم يقطر أبدًا[٧٠١] بل في وعاء. وتضعهم في قدره وتغمرهم[٧٠٢] من دهن الريحان المذكور، وتسدّ فم القدر[٧٠٣] وترفع على النار إلى أن ينهري[٧٠٤] الأفراخ. ثمّ يخرجوا ويصفّوا من خرقة حتّى تخرج[٧٠٥] قوتهم في الدهن. ثمّ يسحق قيراط أفربيون[٧٠٦] ناعمًا مثل الكحل ويخلط مع الدهن خلطًا جيدًا. ثمّ يجعل الدهن في قنّينة ويسدّ فمها وتوضع[٧٠٧] في الشمس الحارّة ثلاثة أيّام. فإذا كان وقت الحاجة يؤخذ منه بقطنة ويدهن (٣١و) بها بين أصابع اليدين والرجلين[٧٠٨] يرى عجبًا ولو جامع[٧٠٩] ما شاء لا يضعف ولا يرتخى ولا يملّ أبدًا[٧١٠] ولا ينام ذكره ولا يزال منتصبًا حتّى يغسله بالماء البارد مرارًا كثيرة، والسلام.

---

٦٩٧ قال: -- (أ)
٦٩٨ العصافير: عصافير (أ)
٦٩٩ تربط ... تعلق: يربط ... يعلق (أ)
٧٠٠ يهوش على: يشوش (أ)
٧٠١ يقطر أبدا: ولا يدثم مائهم ينقط برا بلا وعاء (ب)
٧٠٢ تؤخذ... تغمرهم: يؤخذو بالعجلة ويذبح ولا ينقط دماهم برا بل يأخذ دماهم في قدر صغير ويجعل عليهم غمرهم (أ)
٧٠٣ تسد فم القدر: يشد فم القدرة (ب) / تسد: يسد (أ)
٧٠٤ ينهرى: تتهري (غ) / (ب) / ترفع ... ينهري: يغليه علي نار لينة إلى أن تنهري (أ)
٧٠٥ يخرجوا ،،، تخرج: يخرجهم ويصفيهم (أ)
٧٠٦ أفربيون: فربيون (ب/أ)
٧٠٧ توضع: يعلقها (أ)
٧٠٨ اليدين والرجلين: أيديه ورجليه (ب/أ)
٧٠٩ يرى... حامع: ترى العجب ويجامع (أ)
٧١٠ لا يضعف... أبدا: لا يمل (أ)

نوع آخر

قال[٧١١] يؤخذ مائة نملة من النمل الأسود الكبار والصغار يجعلوا[٧١٢] في قنّينة ويسكب[٧١٣] عليهم خمسة[٧١٤] دراهم من دهن السوس الازرق ويسدّ فم القنّينة[٧١٥] وتعلق[٧١٦] في الشمس الحارّة عشرين يومًا، و[٧١٧]بعد ذلك يسحق الجميع سحقًا قويًا حتّى يتخمر.[٧١٨] فإذا كان وقت الحاجة يؤخذ[٧١٩] قيراط عود هندي يدقّ[٧٢٠] ناعمًا ويجعل في ماء حارّ وزن عشرة دراهم. ثمّ يغسل ذكره من هذا الماء ويغسل يديه ورجليه وتحت أبطئه. ثمّ يأخذ من ذلك الدهن[٧٢١] الذي في القنّينة دهن النمل[٧٢٢] نقطه (٣١ظ) أو شيء قليل صرفًا[٧٢٣] بلا ماء ويدهن به أصابع يديه ورجليه وأبطئه ومرافقه. ثمّ يلبث ساعة، ثمّ يجامع فلو جامع عشرة من النساء[٧٢٤] في ليلة لم يعجز ولم يرتخى.[٧٢٥]

---

٧١١ ومهما جامع ... قال: -- (ق) / قال: نوع آخر قال (ب) / قال: -- (أ)

٧١٢ يجعلوا: تجعلها (ق)/ ويجعلوا (ب)/ يجعلهم (أ)

٧١٣ يسكب: تسكب (ب)

٧١٤ خمسة: وزن خمسة (ب)

٧١٥ يسكب ... القنينه: يسكب عليها من دهن السوسن الازرق وشد فمها (ق)

٧١٦ تعلق: يعلقها (أ)

٧١٧ و: ثم (أ)

٧١٨ يتخمر: يتخذوا (ب) / يخلط في بعضهم بعضا (أ)

٧١٩ يؤخذ: يأخذ (أ)

٧٢٠ بعد ذلك ... يدق: ثم يسحقها قويًا ثم قيراط عود هند يسحق (ق) / يدق: +ويسحق (ب/أ)

٧٢١ ذلك الدهن: -- (أ)

٧٢٢ دهن النمل: -- (أ)

٧٢٣ (ذلك) الدهن ... صرفا: القنينة نقطة وينقط على الماء الذي فيه العود ثم يدهن به بين أصابع يديه ورجليه وتحت ابطيه. ثم يأخذ من ذلك الماء الذي في القنينة نقطة أو شيئا قليلا صرفا (ب/أ)

٧٢٤ ثم ... النساء: ويشتغل بالجماع ترى العجب ولو جامع جوار (أ)

٧٢٥ وزن عشرة ...يرتخى: ويغسل ذكر بهذا الماء وكذا يديه ورجليه وابطيه ثم يدلك الدهن أصابع اليدين والرجلين والابطين والمرفقين ير العجب (ق)

الباب الرابع عشر

في بيان الحبوب التي إذا أمسكها الإنسان تلذّذ الرجل بالجماع لذّة عظيمة. قال يؤخذ[٧٢٦] درهم مصطكى[٧٢٧] وقيراط ونصف مسك، ونصف درهم قرنفل، وخمس دراهم سكّر، ونصف درهم جوزة هند[٧٢٨]، ويسحق الجميع ناعمًا كالكحل. ثمّ تضعهم[٧٢٩] في قنّينة وتغمرهم بدهن[٧٣٠] وتعلّق[٧٣١] في الشمس ثلاثة أيّام حتّى تمزج بالدهن. ثمّ يؤخذ له قوامه[٧٣٢] عسل نحل أبيض منزوع الرغوة ويعقد الحوائج ويحبّب[٧٣٣] كلّ حبّة وزن درهم وقت الحاجة (٣٢و) للجماع[٧٣٤] يجعل في فمه حبّة يرى عجبًا والسلام.[٧٣٥]

نوع آخر

قال[٧٣٦] يؤخذ فستق بقشر[٧٣٧] ويؤخذ قلبه ويشوى على النار ويحترز من

---

٧٢٦ إذا امسكها ... قال: تمسك في الفم تلذذ الجماع جدًا (ق) / التي... يؤخذ: الذي إذا أمسكها في فمه يلذذ الرجل وهذه في الجماع لذة عظيمة. يأخذ (أ)

٧٢٧ مصطكى: مستكى (ب)

٧٢٨ جوزة هند: جوز هندي (أ)

٧٢٩ تضعهم.: يجعلهم (أ)

٧٣٠ بدهن: + السعد (ب)

٧٣١ قنينة... تعلق: دهن سعد في قنينة ويعلقها (أ)

٧٣٢ يؤخذ له قوامه: يأخذ له قوام (أ)

٧٣٣ يحبب: يحببوا حبيبات (ب) / يجعلهم حبيبات (أ)

٧٣٤ وقت... للجماع: ووقت الجماع (ب)

٧٣٥ ونصف مسك... السلام: مسك وقرنفل نصف درهم وسكّر خمسة دراهيم وجوز هند درهم يسحق ناعمًا ويوضع في قنينه ويغمر بدهن زنبق وتعلقها في الشمس ثلاث أيّام ثم يؤخذ عسل نحل ويعقد بها ويحبب كلّ حبه وزن درهم ويجعل في فمه حبه وزن درهم ويجعل في بمه حبه وقت الجماع ير العجب (ق) / وقت ... السلام: ويجعلهم في فمه على الحاجة ترى الععجب (أ)

٧٣٦ قال: -- (ق/أ)

٧٣٧ بقشر: بقشره (ب) / ويقشر (أ)

حرقه.[٧٣٨] فإذا انقلى وجفّ، يسحق منه قدر[٧٣٩] درهم ويضاف إليه وزن درهم قرنفل وقيراط مسك[٧٤٠] ودرهم عنبر، ويسحق ناعمًا كالكحل ويدرّوا على دهن الفستق الذي قلاه حتّى يبقى كالعجين. ثمّ يوضع[٧٤١] في الشمس ثلاثة أيّام، ثمّ يحبّب بالسكّر أو بالعسل النحل[٧٤٢] المنزوع الرغوة ويعقد كالعادة كلّ حبّة وزن درهم ويرفع. فإذا أردت ذلك ضع[٧٤٣] في فمك[٧٤٤] حبّة وجامع[٧٤٥] ترى عجبًا.[٧٤٦]

الباب الخامس عشر

في بيان حالة الجماع التي يحصل منها لذّة عظيمة للرجل[٧٤٧] والمرأة مثل ما ذكره الحكماء المتقدّمون والأطبّاء المتأخّرون (٣٢ظ) وعلموا اذلك بتجاربهم.

---

٧٣٨ حرقه: الحرق (أ)

٧٣٩ قدر: وزن (غ)

٧٤٠ مسك: المسك (أ)

٧٤١ يوضع: يضعهم (أ)

٧٤٢ النحل: + الأبيض (ب/أ)

٧٤٣ ضع: يضع (غ/ب)

٧٤٤ فمك: فمه (ب)

٧٤٥ جامع: يجامع + فانه (غ)

٧٤٦ فستق ... عجبًا: قلب فستق ويحط في طاسيه على النار ويسحق منه درهم حتي يظهر دهنه فيؤخذ قرنفل درهم ودرهم عنبر وقيراط مسك ويدرهن الفستق ويمزج ويجعل في الشمس ثلاث أيّام ثم يحلب بالسكر والعسل ويحبب كلّ حبه درهم ويؤخذ في الفم حبه وقت الجماع فانه ير العجب (ق) / عجبًا: + والسلام (غ) / ترى عجبا: فإنه يرى عجبا والسلام (ب) / يرفع ... عجبا: يرفعهم فإذا احتاج إليهم يمسك في فمه واحده ويشتغل بالجماع لإن الفائدة واللذة التي تخصل لا تحصى (أ)

٧٤٧ التي ... الرجل: من ألذة التي تحصل للفاعل والمفعول يعني الرجل (أ)

قال[٧٤٨] يؤخذ وزن درهم قرفة لفّ ونصف درهم عاقرقرح[٧٤٩] وقيراط قاقلّة. يسحق الجميع كالغبار، ثمّ يخلطوا[٧٥٠] بماء عنب رازقي[٧٥١] ويطلى به على جميع ذكره ويصبر[٧٥٢] ساعة. ثمّ يغسله بماء سخن، ثمّ يأخذ في فمه نصف درهم دارصيني ويمضغه. ثمّ يأخذ ريقه ويطلى به ذكره ويجامع[٧٥٣] يرى الرجل والمرأة عجبًا من اللذّة ولا يتشوش منهما واحد، والسلام.[٧٥٤]

نوع آخر

قال[٧٥٥] يؤخذ كبابة وعاقرقرح[٧٥٦] ودار صيني وزنجبيل[٧٥٧] وجوز هندي، من كلّ واحد قيراط، ويسحق الجميع ويعجنوا[٧٥٨] بالعسل النحل المعقود. ثمّ يأخذ منه في فمه ويطلى من ريقه على ذكره ويجامع.[٧٥٩] يرى عجبًا من اللذّة للرجل والمرأة ما لم يوصف، والسلام.[٧٦٠]

---

٧٤٨ تجاربهم قال: تجاريب استعمالاتهم وذلك أن (أ)

٧٤٩ عاقرقرح: عاقرقرحا (غ/ب) / عرق القرح (أ)

٧٥٠ حالة الجماع... يخلط: ما يحصل للرجل والمرأة من لذة النكاح يؤخذ قرفة درهم وعاقر قرحا نصف درهم وقاقلة قيراط يخلط (ق) / كالغبار ثم يخلطوا: ناعما كالغبار ثم يخلط (أ)

٧٥١ رازقي: الرازق (أ)

٧٥٢ على جميع ذكره ويصبر: الذكر (ق) / ذكره ويصبر: ذكر ويتوقف (أ)

٧٥٣ يجامع: يشتغل بالجماع (أ)

٧٥٤ يمصغه ... السلام: ويطلي الذكر بريقه ويجامع فانهما يجد ان لذة عظيمة (ق) / ولا ... والسلام: ما لا يوصف (أ)

٧٥٥ قال: -- (ق)

٧٥٦ عاقرقرح: عاقرقرحا (غ/ب/أ)

٧٥٧ كبابه ... وزنجبيل: كبا ودار صيني وزنجبيل وعاقر قرحا (ق)

٧٥٨ الجميع ويعجنوا: الجميع كالغبار ويعجنه (أ)

٧٥٩ يجامع: يشتغل بالجماع (أ)

٧٦٠ الجميع ... السلام: ويعقد بعسل ثم يأخذ منه في فمه ويطلي ذكره بريقه ويجامع يري من اللذة شيء عجيب (ق) / يرى ... السلام: ترى العجب من لذة الرجل والمرأة ما لا يوصف (أ)

الباب السادس عشر

في بيان الأدوية التي إذا تحمّلت[٧٦١] بها المرأة تصير في ضيق رحمها وحرارتها ولذّتها. وذلك (٣٣و) أن تأخذ [٧٦٢] عاقرقرح[٧٦٣] وزن[٧٦٤] درهمين ولحية تيس خمسة دراهم، وشراب صرف[٧٦٥] ستّة عشر درهمًا، وتمر مرسين. يدقّوا ناعمًا ويجعلوا في قدرة ويغمروا بالماء. ثمّ[٧٦٦] يغلوا على النار إلى أن ينقص ثلاث[٧٦٧] الماء وبعض الشراب. فإذا بقيت القدرة على هذه الحالة[٧٦٨] تقف المرأة على بخارها[٧٦٩] سبع مرّات. ثمّ تنزل القدرة وترفع،[٧٧٠] فإذا احتاجت المرأة إليها[٧٧١] تبلّ صوفه وتتحمّل بها فإنّها تصير أقوى من البكر في الضيق والحرارة.[٧٧٢]

نوع آخر

يؤخذ من ثمرة[٧٧٣] المرسين وقشر رمّان وعاقرقرحا[٧٧٤] أجزاء سواء ويدقّوا[٧٧٥]

---

٧٦١ تحملت: احتملت (أ)

٧٦٢ إذا تحملت ...تأخذ: تضيق الرحم وتسخنه يؤخذ (ق)

٧٦٣ عاقرقرح: عاقرقرحا (غ/ب/أ)

٧٦٤ عاقرقرح وزن: عاقرقرحا (ق)

٧٦٥ صرف: حرف (ب)

٧٦٦ ويغمره... ثم: ويجعل على القدرة ماء و(أ)

٧٦٧ ثلاث: -- (أ)

٧٦٨ فإذا... الحالة: وإذا نزلت الشراب (أ)

٧٦٩ يدقّ و... بخارها: يدقّ ناعمًا ويغمر في قدر بالماء ويغلي الان ينقص الثلث من المء فتتلقى المرأة بخاره (ق)

٧٧٠ تنزل... ترفع: ينزل ويرفع (أ)

٧٧١ تنزل ... إليها: ثم ترفع القدره عندها فإذا احتجاجت (ق) / إليها: بها (غ)

٧٧٢ الحرارة: + والسلام (غ/ب) / تصير... الحرارة: تبقا أقوى من البكر في الضيق (أ)

٧٧٣ ثمرة: تمر (ق/أ) / تمرة (ب)

٧٧٤ عاقرقرحا: + وقرنفل (ب)

٧٧٥ يدقوا: يدق (ب)

ناعمًا ويغلوا[٧٧٦] شراب عتيق صرف. ثمّ تبلّ صوفه وتتحمّل بها[٧٧٧] ساعة فإنها تصير كالبكر في الضيق والحرارة.[٧٧٨]

نوع آخر

يؤخذ بلّوط وبزر عصفر[٧٧٩] وسعد وكليل[٧٨٠] وحيّ عالم أجزاء سواء. يخلطوا في[٧٨١] بعضهم (٣٣ظ) بعضًا بالدقّ الجريش ويغلوا ويصفوا، ويصفّى عليهم[٧٨٢] وزن خمسة دراهم عاقرقرحا، ثمّ[٧٨٣] يغلى على النار غليًا[٧٨٤] قويًا. ثمّ ينزل فإذا احتاجت المرأة إليه تستنجى منه مرّتين أو ثلاثة فإنّها تصير كالبنت البكر في الضيق والحرارة والسلام.[٧٨٥]

الباب السابع عشر

في بيان الأدوية التي إذا تحمّلت بها المرأة ما تحبل ما دامت[٧٨٦] تستعملها وتصير كالبنات ضيقًا وحرارة.

---

٧٧٦ ويدقّوا ناعمًا ويغلوا: تدق ناعمًا وتغلي (ق)

٧٧٧ بها: + المرأة (غ)

٧٧٨ ثم تبل ... الحرارة: -- (ق) / الضيق والحرارة: ضيقها وحرارتها وحلاوتها (أ)

٧٧٩ وبزر عصفر: ونور عصفور (ق)

٧٨٠ كليل: اكليل (ق/ب)

٧٨١ يخلطوا في: ويخلط (أ)

٧٨٢ يغلوا... عليهم: يغلى ويصفى ثم يضع عليه (ب) / يغلى ويصفى ثم يجعل عليه (أ)

٧٨٣ يخلطو ... ثم: تدق وتغلي وتصفي ثم يضاف إليها عاقرقرحا خمسة دراهم و(ق)

٧٨٤ ثم ... غليا: مدقوق ثم يغلى غليانا (ب/أ)

٧٨٥ ثم ينزل... السلام: وينزل وتستجي به الماء مرتين أو ثلاث فانه تصير كالبنت في الضيق والحرارة واللذة والله اعلم (ق) / والسلام: -- (ب) / منه مرتين ... السلام: منه المرأة مرتين أو ثلاثة تصير كالبكر في ضيقها وحرارتها (أ)

٧٨٦ ما دامت: أبدا لم (أ)

قال يؤخذ مرارة دبّ تخلط مع ماء العنب الرازقي[787] خلطًا قويًا. ثمّ تتحمّل منها المرأة بقليل دقيق لم تحبل وتبقى[788] كالبكر.

نوع آخر

قال يؤخذ من[789] مرارة البقر وزن مثقال ومثله[790] من مرارة الذئب يجعلا بقدر ما يغمرها شيرج.[791] ثمّ تتحمّل منه المرأة[792] بقطنة أو صوفة، فإنّها تصير كالبكر[793] ولا تحبل أبدًا.[794]

نوع آخر

قال من أخذ[795] قطران زجاجي[796] وطلى به وقت (٣٤و) الجماع ذكره تلذّذ به غاية اللذّة ولا تعود المرأة تحبل أبدًا إلّا إذا كان بالعلاج.[797]

---

٧٨٧ الرازقي: رازق (أ)

٧٨٨ الأدوية التي... تبقى: ما يمنع الحمل ويسخن الحم يؤخذ مرارة دب تخلط في ماء العنب الراز في بكف دقيق وتعمل صوفه وتتحمل بها لم تحبل مده وتسخن الرحم وتضيقه (ق)

٧٨٩ قال يؤخذ من من: يؤخذ (أ)

٧٩٠ مثله: مثلها (أ)

٧٩١ يجعلا ... شيرج: يسحقان بقدر مائها بشيرج (ب) يسحقان بقدر ما يجتماع شيرج (أ)

٧٩٢ منه المرأة: المرأة كالعادة (أ)

٧٩٣ فإنها... كالبكر: ترى العجب تصير بكرا (أ)

٧٩٤ قال يؤخذ ... ابدا: يؤخذ مرارة بقر مثقال وكذا مرارة ذئب ويغمر بشريج وتحمل المرأة بصوفه منه فإنها تصير ولم محبل (ق)

ابدا: + والسلام (غ)

٧٩٥ قال من اخذ: يؤخذ (ق)

٧٩٦ زجاجي: + نصف درهم (أ)

٧٩٧ طلى به ...بالعلاج: يطلي به الذكر وقت الجماع يمنع الحبل منه ويلذ نوع آخر أقاقيا وجنت البلوط من كلّ واحد عشرة دراهيم وعفص وباذنجان يابس من كلّ واحد خمسة عشرة درهما تدقّ ناعمًا وتنخل ثم تسحق في هاون سحقا بليغا وتتحمل

الباب الثامن عشر

في بيان الأدوية التي إذا تحمّلت بها المرأة تحبل[798] بإذن الله تعالى.

قال[799] يؤخذ عود هندي[800] وورق مرسين أخضر، من كلّ واحد نصف درهم، ومن[801] المسك[802] قيراط. يدقّ الجميع[803] ناعمًا ويصرّوا[804] في[805] خرقة رفيعة ويجعل[806] في قدرة، ويصبّ عليه[807] قليل شراب عتيق، ويغلى على نار[808] ليّنة حتّى تخرج قوة الأدوية فيه. ثمّ يصفّى بالماء ويجعل[809] في قنّينة، فإذا احتاجت المرأة إليه تتحمّل منه بصوفة تكون كالبكر وتحبل بإذن[810] الله تعالى.

المرأة منها بقطعه مبلولة بالماء في ثلاث أيام فإنها تر العجب في الضيق والحرارة (ق)/ بالعلاج: + والسلام (ب) / تلذذ ... الجماع: يلذذ به غاية اللذة ولا تعود تحبل أبدا بالعلاج (أ)

٧٩٨ تحملت بها: إذا استعملتها المرأة تحمل (ب) / في بيان... تحبل: في ذكر الأدوية التي إذا استعملتها المرأة التي لم تحبل تحبل (أ)

٧٩٩ إذا تحملت ...قال: تحبل بها المرأة (ق) / قال: ذاكر (أ)

٨٠٠ هندي: هند (ق)

٨٠١ من: -- (ق)

٨٠٢ .مرسين أخضر.. المسك: مرسين أخضر وبلح أخضر من كل والواد نصف درهم مسك (أ)

٨٠٣ الجميع: -- (ق)

٨٠٤ يصروا: تصر (ق) / يصر (ب) / ناعمًا ويصروا: دقا ناعما ويصير (غ)

٨٠٥ في: -- (غ)

٨٠٦ رفيعة ويجعل: من شاش وتوضع (ق)

٨٠٧ عليه: عليها (أ)

٨٠٨ على نار: بنار (ق)

٨٠٩ ثم... يجعل: يصفى الماء ويجعله (أ)

٨١٠ حتّى تخرج ...بإذن: وصفي الماء ويحبل في قنينه وتحبل منها بصوفه قبل الجماع فانها تحبل ان شاء (ق)

نوع آخر

قال يؤخذ[٨١١] عفص أخضر وادخر مكّي من كلّ واحد[٨١٢] درهمين، وبلح أخضر درهم يسحقوا[٨١٣] ناعمًا[٨١٤] حتّى تخرج قوة الأدوية في الشراب. ثمّ يرفعوا[٨١٥] عند الحاجة تتحمّل منه المرأة[٨١٦] بصوفة[٨١٧] تحبل بإذن الله تعالى.[٨١٨]

(٣٤ظ) نوع آخر

قال يؤخذ[٨١٩] قشر كافور خام[٨٢٠] أربعة دراهم وشبّ أحمر درهمين، و[٨٢١] سعد درهم، وعفص أخضر مدقوق[٨٢٢] أربعة دراهم ونصف، وتراب مكّة نصف قيراط. يسحق الجميع غير العفص فإنّه يدقّ جريشًا لا ناعمًا. ويغلى بشراب[٨٢٣] كالعادة ويصفّى ويؤخذ[٨٢٤] ماؤه ويرفع وعند الحاجة إليه تبلّ المرأة

---

٨١١ قال يؤخذ: -- (ق/أ)

٨١٢ من كل واحد: -- (أ)

٨١٣ يسحقوا: يسحق (غ)

٨١٤ ناعما: + ويغلوا شراب (ب) / + فيغلي و في شراب (أ)

٨١٥ ناعمًا حتّى تخرج قوة الأدوية في الشراب ثم: بقليل شراب ويرفع (ق) / يرفعوا: يرفع (ب/أ)

٨١٦ منه المرأة: المرأة منه (ق) / المرأة منها (أ)

٨١٧ بصوفه: + قبل الجماع (ق) / بصوفه: بصوف (غ)

٨١٨ تعالى: والسلام (أ)

٨١٩ يؤخذ: -- (ق) / قال يؤخذ: -- (أ)

٨٢٠ خام: + مدقوق (غ/ب) / مدقوقا (أ)

٨٢١ و: -- (ق)

٨٢٢ مدقوق: + جريش (غ)

٨٢٣ بشراب: بالشراب (أ)

٨٢٤ يؤخذ: يأخذ (أ)

منه بصوفة[٨٢٥] وتتحمّل بها[٨٢٦] وهي مستلقية على قفاها قبل الجماع بساعة[٨٢٧] فإنّها تصير كالبكر وتحبل بإذن الله تعالى.

نوع آخر

قال[٨٢٨] يؤخذ لحية التيس تدقّ وتسحق[٨٢٩] ويستخرج ماؤها. ثمّ يؤخذ عفص أخضر وقشر[٨٣٠] رمّان وعود هندي[٨٣١] وقشر أترنج، من كلّ واحد نصف درهم وشبّ أحمر أربعة دراهم وسعد درهم. يسحق[٨٣٢] الجميع ويغلى[٨٣٣] بشراب عتيق حتّى تخرج[٨٣٤] قوة الأدوية في الشراب. ثمّ (٣٥و) تتحمّل منها المرأة فإنّها[٨٣٥] تصير كالبكر[٨٣٦] وتحبل بإذن الله تعالى.

نوع آخر

قال[٨٣٧] يؤخذ قاقلّة نصف درهم وصمغ عربي وحبّة سوداء، من كلّ واحد

---

٨٢٥ بصوفة: صوفه (غ) / منه بصوفة: منها صوفة (أ)
٨٢٦ وتتحمل بها: -- (أ)
٨٢٧ أربعة دراهم ... بساعة: يغلي بالشراب ويصفي ماءه ويرفع وتتحمل منه المرأة بصوفي وهي مستلقيه قبل الجماع (ق)
٨٢٨ قال: -- (ق/أ)
٨٢٩ تدق وتسحق: يدقّ (ق/أ) / تدقّ وتسحق: يدق ويسحق (غ/ب)
٨٣٠ قشر: قشور (ق) / يؤخذ عفص أخضر: يأخذ العفس الأخضر (أ)
٨٣١ هندي: هند (ق)
٨٣٢ يسحق: تسحق (ق)
٨٣٣ يغلى: تغلي (ق)
٨٣٤ تخرج: يخرج (ب/أ)
٨٣٥ فإنها: بصوفة مبلولة عند الحاجة (أ)
٨٣٦ حتّى تخرج ... كالبكر: وتتحمل المرأة منه بصوفه (ق)
٨٣٧ قال: -- (ق) / قال يؤخذ: -- (أ)

قيراط، وكحل اصبهاني[٨٣٨] نضف دراهم، وقشر أترنج[٨٣٩] نصف درهم. يسحق الجميع ويغلى بشراب عتيق حتّى تخرج[٨٤٠] قوة الأدوية في الشراب. ثمّ تتحمّل منه المرأة بصوفة عند الحاجة فإنّها[٨٤١] تصير كالبكر الذي[٨٤٢] لم يصبها رجل وتحبل[٨٤٣] بإذن الله تعالى.[٨٤٤]

تمّ ذلك بحمد الله وعونه وحسن توفيقه والحمد لله على كلّ حال[٨٤٥] وصلّى الله على سيّدنا محمّد وعلى آله وصحبه وسلّم تسليمًا كثيرًا إلى يوم الدين يا ربّ العالمين.[٨٤٦] [سنة ١٢٠٨]

---

٨٣٨ اصبهاني: اصفهاني (أ)

٨٣٩ أترنج: نارنج (ب/ق/غ)

٨٤٠ بشراب ... تخرج: بالشراب العتيق حتى يخرج (أ)

٨٤١ فإنها: كالعادة (أ)

٨٤٢ الذي: التي (أ)

٨٤٣ يصبها ... تهبل: يصيبها الرجل وتحمل (ب)

٨٤٤ تعالى: + وقدرته وهو على كل شيء قدير. (ب)

٨٤٥ ثم ذلك... حال: -- (غ)

٨٤٦ أترنج ... الرحيم: نارنج درهم تسحق وتغلي بشراب عتيق وتتحمل منه بصوفه قبل الجماع فإنها تصير بكر وتحبل بحول الله تم الكتاب بعون الملك الوهاب ثمانية عشر أيام من شهر ربيع الأول ليلة الربوع ١٣٣٩ (ق) / تسليمًا ... العالمين: ولا حول ولا قوة إلا بالله العلى العظيم تم وكمل لحمد الله وعون وحسن بالله (غ) / تم ... الحريم: تم الكتاب بعون الملك الوهاب وهذه اللطيفة هي التركيبات العجيبة النافعة المفيدة هي من أسرار الأطباء ومن اختصاراتهم المفيدة لأنها جعلت لخزانة سلطان من السلاطين المسلمين لنفع. انتهى على يد كاتبه العبد الفقير الراجي رحمة ربه القدير الغازي في بحر ذنوبه محمد علي بن حسين بن حسن الجزائري غفر الله له والجميع المسلمين والمسلمات الأحياء منه والا موات. (ب) / تم... العالمين: وقدرته انه على كل شيء قدير وهذا التركيب الذي ذكرناه في هذا الكتاب من أسرار الأطباء ولهذا ذكرنها والله سبحانه (أ)

فهرس الأعلام

فهرس المصطلحات

ث

ج

ح

خ

د

ذ

ر

ز